An Insider's Guide to the Medical Specialties

An Insider's Guide to the Medical Specialties

Edited by

Ian Reckless,

Specialist Registrar in General Medicine, Oxford;
Honorary Fellow, Nuffield Department of Medicine,
University of Oxford, Oxford, UK.

John Reynolds,

Consultant Physician and Clinical Pharmacologist,
John Radcliffe Hospital, Oxford, UK.

with

Raghib Ali,

Clinical Lecturer in General Medicine and
Clinical Pharmacology, University of Oxford,
Oxford, UK.

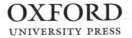

OXFORD
UNIVERSITY PRESS

OXFORD
UNIVERSITY PRESS

Great Clarendon Street, Oxford OX2 6DP

Oxford University Press is a department of the University of Oxford.
It furthers the University's objective of excellence in research, scholarship,
and education by publishing worldwide in

Oxford New York

Athens Auckland Bangkok Bogotá Buenos Aires Cape Town
Chennai Dar es Salaam Delhi Florence Hong Kong Istanbul Karachi
Kolkata Kuala Lumpur Madrid Melbourne Mexico City Mumbai Nairobi
Paris São Paulo Shanghai Singapore Taipei Tokyo Toronto Warsaw

with associated companies in Berlin Ibadan

Oxford is a registered trade mark of Oxford University Press
in the UK and in certain other countries

Published in the United States
by Oxford University Press Inc., New York

British Library Cataloguing in Publication Data

Data available

Library of Congress Cataloging-in-Publication Data

An insider's guide to the medical specialties / edited by Ian Reckless, John Reynolds, Raghib Ali.
p. ; cm.
1. Clinical medicine. 2. Medicine--Specialties and specialists. I. Reckless, Ian. II. Reynolds,
John, Dr. III. Ali, Raghib.
[DNLM: 1. Specialties, Medical. W 90 I81 2006]
RC48.I47 2006
616--dc22

2006031691

ISBN 13: 978-0-19-856970-1 (pbk. : alk. paper)
ISBN 10: 0-19-856970-x (pbk. : alk. paper)

10 9 8 7 6 5 4 3 2 1

Typeset in Minion
by CEPHA Imaging Pvt Ltd, India.
Printed in Great Britain on acid-free paper by
Biddles Ltd., King's Lynn

Contents

Foreword *vii*

Preface *ix*

1. Cardiology *1*
   Ian Reckless & Jeremy Dwight

2. High-Dependency Medicine *41*
   Razeen Mahroof & Jonathan Salmon

3. Poisoning *55*
   Jamie Coleman & Robin Ferner

4. Endocrinology & Lipids *67*
   Paul Newey & John Reckless

5. Diabetes & Obesity *93*
   Aparna Pal & David Matthews

6. Hypertension & Nephrology *115*
   Peter Hill & Chris O'Callaghan

7. Neurology *151*
   Christopher Kipps & Martin Lee

8. Stroke Medicine *185*
   Matthew Giles & Andrew Coull

9. Infectious Diseases *193*
   John Frater & Nicola Jones

10. Hepatology *217*
    William Gelson & Graeme Alexander

11. Gastroenterology *239*
    William Gelson & Anthony Ellis

12. Respiratory Medicine *273*
    Fiona McCann & Lorraine Hart

13. Oncology *309*
    Kate Scatchard, David Church & Ed Gilby

14. Haematology *329*
    Katherine Lowndes & David Perry

15. Palliative Care Medicine *347*
   Chi Chi Cheung & Bee Wee

16. Geriatric Medicine *359*
   Matthew Giles & Andrew Coull

17. Rheumatology *373*
   Wendy Holden & Joseph Joseph

18. Immunology *387*
   Catherine Sargent, Aamir Aslam & Richard Steele

19. Dermatology *401*
   Ashley Cooper & Barbara Leppard

20. Obstetric Medicine *413*
   Deborah Harrington & Christopher Redman

21. Liaison Psychiatry *427*
   Michael Browning & Christopher Bass

Foreword

It is inconsiderate of patients to have more than one disease. The patient with a single disease who manages to reach a specialist or super-specialist stands a good chance of getting high quality care. Unfortunately, not all patients have only one disease. Indeed, there are many patients, for whom it is impossible to ascertain precisely the cause of signs or symptoms, who are very difficult to triage to a particular specialty.

These patients pose a major challenge to the health service, and a major intellectual challenge to the physician faced with someone who is severely ill with a number of existing diagnoses, none of which readily explains their current predicament. It is essential for some clinicians to maintain the ability to manage these most complex problems that often present acutely and may occur in patients who are unable to give an accurate and succinct account of the origin and evolution of their problems when first assessed.

While specialization has improved the care of people who both have the relevant disease and manage to access the appropriate specialist (for not all people who are eligible for a service are engaged by it), the development of specialization has posed problems for patients for whom no diagnosis has been reached or who have multiple diagnoses.

Increasing specialization, along with an (appropriate) drive to reduce waiting times for outpatient opinions and certain investigations has led to some difficulties in staffing acute general medical services, particularly as the European Working Time Directive has begun to bite. In some hospitals, there may be few physicians interested in, or able to focus on, general medicine.

This phenomenon is perhaps felt even more keenly in teaching hospitals, where trainees may give priority to their specialties, often at the expense of general medicine. It first became apparent to me in Oxford in the early 1990s during my first month in the job as Regional Director of Public Health. Holding the contracts of hundreds of doctors-in-training and responsible for the delivery of healthcare to a population of a million, I found that a potential staffing crisis threatened general medicine in the teaching hospital. Fortunately, the then newly appointed Nuffield Professor of Medicine, John Bell, also recognised this problem and the need for the teaching hospital to have a solid platform of general medicine expertise.

General medicine is too valuable to wither on the vine of specialization. It is essential, and this book will contribute to its survival and indeed its recovery.

Long live general medicine, and if it does, long and well will live the patient who has more than one disease and who does not neatly fall into the scope of any single specialist.

Sir J A Muir Gray, CBE, DSc, MD, FRCPSGlas, FCLIP
Director of Clinical Knowledge, Process and Safety,
NHS Connecting for Health;
Programme Director, UK National Screening Committee

Preface

Medicine is complex – increasingly so. As the pool of knowledge grows deeper, the chances of drowning in it are ever greater. One response for the busy physician is to specialise and then sub-specialise in order to become absolutely familiar with just one lane of the knowledge pool. For many though, sub-specialising is not the answer and much of the appeal of medicine lies in its variety. Indeed, for the patient (and for the running of an acute healthcare service), we believe that the survival of the generalist is essential.

So how can a doctor for whom general medicine may make up just a fraction of the working week hope to remember snippets of information first encountered many years ago? How can a physician manage to keep on top of advances in medicine in the round? The answer, unfortunately, is *'with difficulty'*. There are of course many educational opportunities for doctors with the time, funds and inclination, at all stages of their careers: academic conferences; taught courses; clinical meetings; online learning resources and learned texts. Some of these opportunities can prove useful at the bedside; others are used at a distance. None is perfect.

An Insider's Guide to the Medical Specialties aims merely to provide an additional tool upon which the general physician may call. In it, pairs of authors – one an established consultant, the other a trainee – write about aspects of their specialty for a 'generalist' audience. They enable the reader to revise their existing knowledge of a specialty, to update themselves on key advances that have taken place, to share in the odd 'specialty secret', and to take a glimpse at the evolving context in which the specialty operates. *An Insider's Guide to the Medical Specialties* brings together epidemiology, evidence from trials and the day-to-day clinical experience of the authors. It is written in conversational prose and never shies away from controversy. Above all, it is intended to allow physicians of any grade to absorb knowledge with the minimum of effort, and a degree of pleasure.

In editing the contributions of over forty colleagues, we have tried to develop a cogent and coherent book. Each individual chapter has been externally peer-reviewed. However, that is not to say that the forensic reader will find neither repetition nor contradiction: boundaries between specialties are not fixed, and differences between the opinions of various specialists on the same issue are, for us, a source of interest and intrigue, rather than one of frustration. Any errors of fact, as opposed to opinion, are of course those of the editors, and the editors alone.

An Insider's Guide to the Medical Specialties is a new type of book, rather different from its companions in the bookstore. It is written to be read, not to be left nestling in the pocket of a white coat or gathering dust on a shelf.

We hope you enjoy it. We certainly have.

Ian Reckless
John Reynolds
Oxford
November 2006

Contributors

Graeme Alexander,
Consultant Physician and
Hepatologist, Cambridge, UK.

Aamir Aslam,
Specialist Registrar in Clinical
Immunology, Oxford, UK.

Michael Browning,
Specialist Registrar in Psychiatry,
Oxford, UK.

Christopher Bass,
Consultant in Liaison Psychiatry,
Oxford, UK.

Chi Chi Cheung,
Specialist Registrar in Palliative Care,
London, UK.

David Church,
Specialist Registrar in Medical
Oncology, Bristol, UK.

Jamie Coleman,
Specialist Registrar in Clinical
Pharmacology, Birmingham, UK.

Ashley Cooper,
Specialist Registrar in Dermatology,
Southampton, UK.

Andrew Coull,
Consultant Physician in
Geriatric and General Medicine,
Edinburgh, UK.

Jeremy Dwight,
Consultant Physician and
Cardiologist, Oxford, UK.

Anthony Ellis,
Consultant Gastroenterologist,
Oxford, UK.

Robin Ferner,
Consultant Physician and Clinical
Pharmacologist, Birmingham, UK.

John Frater,
Specialist Registrar in Infectious
Diseases and General Medicine,
Oxford, UK.

William Gelson,
Specialist Registrar in
Gastroenterology and Hepatology,
Cambridge, UK.

Ed Gilby,
Consultant Oncologist, Bath, UK.

Matthew Giles,
Specialist Registrar in Gerontology,
Oxford, UK.

Deborah Harrington,
Subspecialty Trainee in Maternal and
Foetal Medicine, Oxford, UK.

Lorraine Hart,
Consultant Chest Physician,
Ascot, UK.

Peter Hill,
Specialist Registrar in Nephrology,
Oxford, UK.

Wendy Holden,
Specialist Registrar in
Rheumatology, Oxford, UK.

Nicola Jones,
Consultant General and Infectious
Disease Physician, Oxford, UK.

Joseph Joseph,
Consultant Rheumatologist,
Nicosia, Cyprus.

Christopher Kipps,
Honorary Consultant Neurologist
and Wellcome Trust Research Fellow,
Cambridge, UK.

Martin Lee,
Consultant Neurologist,
Norwich, UK.

Barbara Leppard,
Consultant Dermatologist,
Southampton, UK.

Katherine Lowndes,
Specialist Registrar in Haematology,
Cambridge, UK.

Razeen Mahroof,
Specialist Registrar in Anaesthesia
and Critical Care Medicine,
Oxford, UK.

David Matthews,
Professor of Diabetes Medicine,
Oxford, UK.

Fiona McCann,
Specialist Registrar in Respiratory
Medicine, Oxford, UK.

Paul Newey,
Specialist Registrar in Diabetes and
Endocrinology, Oxford, UK.

Chris O'Callaghan,
Honorary Consultant Nephrologist,
Oxford, UK.

Aparna Pal,
Specialist Registrar in Diabetes and
Endocrinology, Oxford, UK.

David Perry,
Consultant Haematologist,
Cambridge, UK.

Ian Reckless,
Specialist Registrar in General
Medicine, Oxford, UK.

John Reckless,
Consultant Physician and
Endocrinologist, Bath, UK.

Christopher Redman,
Professor of Obstetric Medicine,
Oxford, UK.

Jonathan Salmon,
Consultant in General Medicine and
Intensive Care, Oxford, UK.

Catherine Sargent,
Specialist Registrar in Infectious
Diseases, Oxford, UK.

Kate Scatchard,
Specialist Registrar in Medical
Oncology, Bristol, UK.

Richard Steele,
Clinical Immunologist, Wellington,
New Zealand.

Bee Wee,
Consultant in Palliative Medicine;
Senior Clinical Lecturer in Palliative
Medicine, Oxford, UK.

Chapter 1

Ian Reckless and Jeremy Dwight

CARDIOLOGY

ISCHAEMIC HEART DISEASE

Moving the goal posts

The basic problem of the ischaemic heart has not changed in the last 50 years. Now, as then, the myocardium finds itself requiring more fuel than the arteries are able to deliver. The heart can react to this inadequacy of supply in one of two ways: it can grumble in a predictable manner (stable angina), or it can protest in a far more dramatic and abrupt fashion, infarcting and giving rise to potentially fatal dysrhythmias.

For the main part, the pathology behind these more acute presentations is well established. Rupture or erosion of an atheromatous plaque provides an irresistible substrate for thrombus formation. However, there is also a less well-defined group of patients presenting with clinically identical anginal chest pain who go on to have ostensibly normal coronaries at angiography. These individuals, who may respond well to conventional antianginals, are variably labelled as having microvascular angina, syndrome X or coronary spasm. It is of concern that the frequently held assumption of a good prognosis in such cases has been questioned.[1]

What has changed, however, is the nomenclature that we attach to the various troubles that may brew in the coronaries. No longer do we find ourselves meticulously mapping out the rise and fall of the traditional 'cardiac' enzymes over time. No longer do we necessarily relax in the absence of ST elevation. With the advent of the routine measurement of the cardiac troponins, a whole new range of ischaemic entities, previously defying classification, has been born. Indeed, the term myocardial infarction is no longer primarily defined

---

[1] Opherk *et al.* Circulation (1989) 80: 1610–1616.

in terms of the ECG alone, rather by an elevation in cardiac troponin in the presence of a compatible history.[2] It is now recognized that patients with acute myocardial infarction characterized traditionally in terms of ST segment elevation represent the minority of those with high-risk coronary disease presenting to the general take. Whereas our old friend stable angina is still a permitted term, the acute end of ischaemic heart disease has been rebranded.

Patients with ischaemic-sounding chest pain now attract the label of acute coronary syndrome. Their initial ECG then allocates them to one of two groups: those who are potentially eligible for immediate reperfusion therapy (usually thrombolysis) and those who are not. The ticket to thrombolysis looks very much as it used to – ST elevation or left bundle branch block that is not known to be old. The passage of time will confirm whether these patients are indeed experiencing myocardial infarction and whether or not they are destined to have Q waves appear on their ECG. It is worth remembering that when a patient is seen to have ST elevation on the ECG, even after the complete resolution of typical pain, they remain eligible for thrombolytic reperfusion therapy until 12 h have passed.[3] Those who do not qualify for thrombolysis are defined as having a non-ST elevation acute coronary syndrome. Elevation of cardiac markers or enzymes in these patients will identify those with a non-ST elevation MI (NSTEMI), whereas those without elevated cardiac markers have unstable angina. This is not semantics; these categories provide a framework for estimating prognosis and directing clinical management.

Although a major advance, the advent of troponin measurement is no diagnostic panacea. Three particular difficulties have arisen: whether to use troponin T or I, the imperfect specificity of the test, and the timing of the blood sample. Happily, for most physicians, the choice of troponin assay (and any associated anxiety) is academic, having been taken out of their hands by the clinical biochemist! The troponin T assay is universal and has behind it a wealth of data to guide its use in risk stratification in acute coronary syndrome. The main drawback, however, is its tendency to generate the odd false positive, particularly in cases of renal impairment. Troponin I assays are numerous, and this can lead to a degree of confusion for the itinerant hospital junior, moving from place to place. False positives are perhaps less of an issue.

As experience of troponin use in clinical practice has built up, there has been an increasing recognition that while a troponin rise is highly likely to signify

[2] Joint European Society of Cardiology & American College of Cardiology Committee, Eur Heart J (2000) 36: 959–969.

[3] LATE Study Group, Lancet (1993) 342: 759–766.

myocardial damage, this damage need not relate to partial or total coronary occlusion. Myocarditis, cardiac failure and even cardiac infiltration (with amyloid for example) may all be associated with a small elevation in troponin. Indeed, in patients who are critically ill for a variety of reasons, an increase in troponin may be seen, either consequent to a period of perioperative hypotension or perhaps hypotension secondary to sepsis. Whatever the cause, these troponin peaks are markers of poor prognosis. Some authors have suggested that a significant proportion of patients with pulmonary embolism (up to half in one study) have a modest troponin rise.[4]

With regard to timing, a negative troponin after as little as 6 h, in combination with a normal exercise tolerance test, provides a good level of reassurance and facilitates discharge for outpatient management. In the real world though, exercise facilities are rarely sufficiently dynamic, and the 12-h troponin (or 8 h, as a compromise) is used instead, with exercise testing often being deferred to a later date.

Returning now to ST elevation myocardial infarction (STEMI), it is encouraging that although the fundamental principles behind thrombolysis have not changed, timings have been squeezed. In hospitals throughout the UK, door-to-needle times have plummeted, often following wholesale reconfiguration of service delivery. Now that goals for thrombolysis door-to-needle times have largely been met, there is no resting on laurels. Attention has now shifted to improving call-to-needle times and, indeed, considering the role of primary angioplasty within everyday healthcare systems.

Needles and balloons

Before immersing oneself in the debate on thrombolysis versus primary angioplasty, it is perhaps worthwhile to be reminded of the background. It is estimated that around a quarter of a million people suffer acute STEMI in the UK each year.[5] Of these, half are dead in 30 days. Of these deaths, half never reach hospital, and, for them, the development of primary angioplasty services offers nothing. Many of the other deaths occur in the first few hours from symptom onset. The primary aim of any treatment for acute MI ought to be to reestablish good flow in the coronaries, with few complications and as rapidly as possible. Time is important, and the golden hour ought not

---

[4] Gunnewiek *et al.* Curr Opin Crit Care (2004) 10: 342–346.

[5] National Service Framework for Coronary Heart Disease, Department of Health (2000) (www.dh.gov.uk)

to be forgotten.[6] While door-to-needle times may have tumbled in recent years, call-to-needle (and indeed symptom-onset-to-needle) times have not. In the UK, the median time taken to get to hospital, having called the emergency services, remains close to 1 h.

The benefit of thrombolysis is clear in those presenting with left bundle branch block or anterior ST elevation, with a life being saved for every 20 or 25 treated patients, respectively. Although the benefit of thrombolysis in terms of relative risk reduction is similar for inferior infarcts, absolute risk reduction is markedly lower (especially where the right ventricle is not involved). Inferior infarction carries a far lower mortality than the other territories. Administering thrombolysis to patients without indication will result in the death of 1 or 2 per 1000.[7]

Thrombolysis has transformed the management of myocardial infarction. However, it has three major limitations. The first is the risk of stroke, the second a rather long list of contraindications to the use of thrombolytic agents and, finally (and perhaps most importantly), the failure to provide adequate reperfusion of the infarct-related territory in anything up to 65% of patients. The enthusiasm for primary angioplasty, which boasts a success rate of greater than 90% in opening occluded arteries, arises largely from dedicated interventionalists who provide this service to patients on a round-the-clock basis in well-equipped and well-staffed centres in Europe and the US. The key to the argument for this effective but labour- and resource-intensive strategy is the open-artery hypothesis. Based on an analysis of the GUSTO thrombolytic trial, normal flow in the infarct-related coronary artery following thrombolysis is a major predictor of good outcome.[6] There is no doubt that angioplasty is far more effective in achieving this objective than thrombolysis but do the logistic difficulties of taking the patient to the catheter lab in an interventional centre, with the delay that this inevitably entails, mitigate (or even outweigh) this important benefit? There have been large numbers of trials comparing primary angioplasty to traditional thrombolysis, and none of them is perfect in design. For example, many of the trials fail to record door-to-intervention times for all patients, and few attempt to analyse the impact of call-to-intervention. A meta-analysis of 22 trials involving almost 7000 patients did demonstrate significant benefits to those undergoing primary angioplasty in terms of death, reinfarction and stroke.[8] Where it could

6 GUSTO Investigators, NEJM (1993) 329: 1615–1622.
7 ISIS-2, Lancet (1988) 2: 349–361.

be assessed, there appeared to be a median delay to treatment of around 50 min for those having angioplasty. Clearly, outside the artificial trial environment, delays will tend to be longer. Average door-to-balloon times in a real life observational study in the US were approximately 2 h.[9] Where transfer is required, this is not free of risk. Subgroup analysis of several different trials clearly shows that much of the benefit of primary angioplasty over thrombolysis takes place in those patients who present more than 3 h after the onset of pain.

Given that in the first 3 h following symptom onset, there is little to be chosen between thrombolysis and angioplasty in terms of crude outcome, an alternative strategy is to consider the use of prehospital thrombolysis. The available data regarding symptom-to-call and call-to-door times remind us that this is an entirely valid approach. Happily, a small study shows that paramedics are skilled at assessing a patient's suitability for thrombolysis. When compared to the 'gold standard' of two consultant cardiologists, paramedics have been shown to diagnose STEMI with a sensitivity of 97% and, importantly, a specificity of 91%.[10] It may be that some hospitals would be satisfied if their doctors achieved these rates! Technology now allows 12 lead ECGs from the field to be transmitted direct to coronary care units for further advice. While the attractions of prehospital thrombolysis are more obvious in remote geographical areas, it should be remembered that median call-to-needle times in 'urban' populations living within 15 km of the hospital are around 80 min.[11]

So then, a debate is taking place, and one needs to take a position. Invest in primary angioplasty or in prehospital thrombolysis? Fence sitting has never been overly comfortable but the results of the CAPTIM study would appear to advocate it.[12] When the two techniques were compared, there was a mean in-hospital delay of 60 min to angioplasty, and there was no significant difference in mortality. A quarter of those patients receiving prehospital thrombolysis required a trip to the catheter suite later in their inpatient stay, and enthusiasts for primary angioplasty would perhaps assert that they should have gone there directly. The view that primary angioplasty for all patients with STEMI is

[8] Keeley et al. Lancet (2003) 361: 13–20.

[9] Cannon et al. JAMA (2000) 283: 2941.

[10] Whitbread et al. Emerg Med J (2002) 19: 66–67.

[11] Pedley et al. BMJ (2003) 327: 22–26.

[12] Bonnefay et al. Lancet (2002) 360: 825–832.

inappropriate is not a terribly fashionable one. It is, however, a very reasonable one. The additional cost of prehospital thrombolysis is small. Best estimates, although no more than estimates, put the cost at around £4000 per life saved.[13] The costs of maintaining a 24-h primary angioplasty service (particularly in the days of the European Working Time Directive) are high. On account of these costs and other hurdles, only 1647 patients underwent primary angioplasty in the UK in 2005–2006, a modest number, given the incidence of ST elevation MI (2231 patients had out-of-hospital thrombolysis over the same period).[14] Perhaps a combination of public education and prehospital thrombolysis, in an effort to cut symptom-to-needle times, would be the best place to invest a limited sum. Life is difficult for new therapies wishing to establish their place in ischaemic heart disease, in part because aspirin is a top-class drug. It is important to remember that the impact of a single dose of aspirin on mortality is substantial and approximately equivalent to that of reperfusion therapy of any sort.

Ultimately it may transpire that the optimal approach for the treatment of STEMI is a combination of prehospital thrombolysis and routine post-thrombolysis angioplasty (within 24 h). The results of the GRACIA-1 trial, taken together with the consistent observation that outcomes from out-of-hours angioplasty are relatively poor (just as they are for out-of-hours surgical procedures) may prove pivotal to our future approach.[15] Studies looking specifically at the combination of prehospital thrombolysis followed by routine angioplasty are awaited with interest. If all hospitals performing angioplasty were simply to reserve a slot on each list for primary angioplasty or acute post-thrombolysis intervention, the cost implications would be far less than those of a 24-h catheter suite. One might anticipate that cost savings (through reduced length of stay) would also be forthcoming through use of the more interventionalist approaches.

Other significant developments in the management of STEMI that may be approaching over the horizon include the use of stem cell therapy. One trial of modest size has looked at the infusion of autologous bone marrow stem cells 24 h following infarction. It would appear that such treatment reduces infarct size and may have a beneficial effect on remodelling.[16]

[13] Briefing paper for the NHS in Scotland No.9 (www.adbn.ac.uk/heru/pdfs/bptext9/pdf)

[14] 'How the NHS manages heart attacks' (www.rcplondon.ac.uk/pubs/books/minap06)

[15] Fernandez-Aviles et al. Lancet (2004) 364: 1045–1053.

[16] Janssens et al. Lancet (2006) 367: 113–121.

A thrombolytic chaser?

Another difficult question often faced when treating STEMI is, what to do when the ECG suggests a failure to reperfuse: a thrombolytic chaser, angioplasty or neither? Until recently, this question has remained unanswered. Two trials were undertaken in the UK during 2004, attempting to provide some evidence in this area. MERLIN and REACT both looked at patients given thrombolysis (generally streptokinase) for STEMI.[17,18] Failure of the maximally elevated ST segment to fall by at least 50% after 60 min of the onset of thrombolysis was taken to indicate failure to reperfuse.

In the MERLIN trial, patients were randomized to either conservative treatment or immediate coronary angiography, with intervention as necessary, in the event of nonresolution of the ST elevation. Thirty-day mortality was similar in the two groups but the composite endpoint (death, reinfarction, stroke, heart failure, or need for revascularization) was significantly higher in the conservative arm. However, almost all of this effect was due to differences in the need for subsequent 'clinically driven revascularization'. MERLIN only seems to demonstrate that the invasive arm brings forward angioplasty that would have otherwise occurred later in the admission, simply lending a little further weight to the economic (as opposed to outcome-based) argument for routine post-thrombolysis angioplasty. However, as is often the case in trial literature, the landscape had changed by the time of publication in that the rate of utilization of stents and GpIIb/IIIa antagonists was low in MERLIN compared to contemporary practice.

Results from the REACT trial are rather more helpful in suggesting a course of action. In REACT, patients were randomized to conservative treatment, repeat thrombolysis (generally with plasminogen activator) or immediate coronary angiography with intervention as necessary (where the use of stents or GpIIb/IIIa antagonists was much higher than in MERLIN). The composite endpoint was one of death, further MI, stroke or heart failure at 6 months. On an intention-to-treat basis, the invasive strategy was clearly superior to either repeat thrombolysis or conservative treatment with a halving in the composite endpoint. These results were achieved despite a greater delay in the provision of angioplasty than in MERLIN. Of note, repeat thrombolysis (a strategy much favoured in some centres but based on remarkably little evidence) seemed to offer no benefit at all over conservative treatment.

---

[17] Sutton *et al.* J Am Coll Cardiol (2004) 44: 287–296.

[18] Gershlick *et al.* NEJM (2005) 353: 2758–2768.

Testing times

When a patient is diagnosed with ischaemic heart disease, either putatively on the basis of the history or with supporting evidence from initial investigations, a process of risk stratification then needs to take place to guide ongoing management. There are a multitude of tests in the cardiologic armoury, including exercise testing on treadmill or bicycle, the stress echo, the thallium (myoview) scan and, of course, coronary angiography. Each has their place in both acute inpatient investigation and in the outpatient setting.

Following STEMI with successful reperfusion after thrombolysis, opinion and practice differs widely. Many centres now automatically offer angiography on initial admission. Others undertake exercise stress tests, usually on the fifth or sixth day to determine the need for and urgency of angiography. The choice of the fifth or sixth day is historical and somewhat arbitrary as the risk of dangerous arrhythmias plateaus around 72 h after infarction. Moreover, many hospitals employ modified Bruce protocol tests when the full protocol is likely to be more informative. Although both invasive and conservative approaches to angiography post-MI have their advocates, the conservative approach may serve to both increase initial length of stay and simply delay the inevitable femoral puncture. It is also worth noting that exercising the very elderly is not rewarding. If they are to progress to have angioplasty or surgical revascularization, it will be performed on symptomatic and not prognostic grounds. Accepting this, a gentle wander to the League of Friends café gives as much information as a formal exercise test and is probably more acceptable to the patient!

In patients with non-ST elevation acute coronary syndromes, great emphasis has been placed on the importance of a positive troponin in determining risk. This is supported by numerous clinical trials. The importance of this investigation has been enhanced further by the results of subgroup analysis of trials looking at the use of low-molecular-weight heparin, GpIIb/IIIa antagonists and, importantly, early intervention (automatic angiography) rather than conservative management plans. These trials indicate that the prognostic benefits of these therapeutic strategies are largely restricted to troponin-positive patients. Hence, the recommendation that angiography and intervention should be planned in all troponin-positive, non-ST elevation acute coronary syndrome (i.e. NSTEMI) patients on the basis not only of their high risk but also the proven benefit of intervention. Prognostic benefit, however, is less meaningful (and, for that matter, less established) to those over 75 years of age than it is to the younger patient, and continuing symptoms will always remain the main driver to further investigation in the elderly. Furthermore, many centres can and do fail to meet the demand generated by the recommendation of coronary angiography for all troponin-positive patients, due to limited resources and lack of immediate access. A more pragmatic approach is to set a level of risk at which patients can reliably be offered intervention with the available resources. For this, the troponin alone is too blunt a tool, and the more conscientious physician might attempt to work out the TIMI risk score.[19] There are seven questions to pose in relation to the patient and their presentation, illustrated in the following table. Patients with three or more of these risk factors have a very substantial risk of infarction or death (at least 1 in 7) over a 2-week period. Provided there is no coexistent pathology that would give rise to a very poor short-term prognosis, these patients should be offered angiography and intervention.

TIMI Risk Score[19]

Age over 65	0 or 1
Recent aspirin use	0 or 1
Severe angina in previous 24 h	0 or 1
≥3 conventional cardiac risk factors (↑ BP/↑ Cholesterol/DM/Smoking)	0 or 1
ST segment deviation of > 0.5 mm	0 or 1
Known coronary artery stenosis of > 50%	0 or 1
Raised cardiac enzymes	0 or 1
Total TIMI Risk Score	0 to 7

A rather more challenging situation is that of the troponin-negative case of acute coronary syndrome. Where there is no history of ischaemic heart disease, one is eager to reach a diagnosis. Where there is a previous history, one is quite reasonably suspicious of a now critical stenosis. In each case, exercise testing is entirely appropriate unless chest pain (which clinically sounds to be cardiac) persists, dynamic ST segment changes are observed or exercise is not viable for some other reason. A normal exercise test is of enormous, although not total, reassurance. Where questions still remain, the patient usually requires another test. According to the current setup in the UK, angiography is often most easily arranged for inpatients. Exercise or pharmacological (dobutamine) stress echocardiography and thallium scanning might be fair alternatives, if readily available.

When, one might ask, should the initial exercise test take place for the troponin-negative patient first presenting with possible angina on exertion?

---

[19] Antman *et al.* JAMA (2000) 284: 876–878.

In an ideal world, instantaneous exercise testing would be a reality. Few of us inhabit such a world. A reasonable and pragmatic approach is to hold on to patients already taking beta-blockers and aspirin for inpatient testing. Drug-naïve patients can potentially be allowed home for prompt outpatient assessment, having been commenced on cardioprotective therapy.

It is in the outpatient clinic where stress echo and myoview (thallium) scanning come into their own. The urgency of the decision-making process is rather less in this environment as chest pain at rest usually prompts referral as an inpatient. If, following clinical assessment and perhaps an equivocal exercise test, significant doubt remains as to the aetiology of symptoms, stress echo or a trip to the nuclear medicine department is called for. If the clinical suspicion of coronary disease is higher, then direct passage to angiography is justified. Noninvasive tests (of any type) may be able to demonstrate the region of myocardium responsible for symptoms and thus suggest the appropriate target lesions for subsequent angioplasty. Stress echo and thallium scanning also get around the age-old difficulties of exercising patients with right or, particularly, left bundle branch block on the resting ECG. On occasion, stress echo and thallium scanning can also be helpful in patients with angiographically demonstrated lesions that do not (angiographically) appear to be flow limiting. If the presence of symptoms is corroborated by the finding of a reversible defect, an invasive rather than conservative approach may be prompted.

More money than sense?

There has been no shortage of novel pharmacological and percutaneous therapies for the management of acute coronary syndromes in the last 20 years. All are based on plaque stabilization by preventing platelet aggregation and/or treating the culprit lesion through endovascular intervention. The assessment of clinical trials in this setting is easier when the therapies arrive on the scene in an orderly sequence (preferably separated by 4–5 years to allow trials to be performed, analysed and digested). The standard therapy can then be easily compared with a regimen based on a new therapy. In contrast, where numerous therapies arrive virtually simultaneously, sorting out the trial results presents a problem akin to a Rubik's cube. By the time a trial is published, the conventional therapy upon which it based its placebo arm is already outdated. There is a natural reluctance for the manufacturer of a given drug to repeat the trial with an updated placebo arm (which by definition is less likely to produce a favourable conclusion). As a result, the data are incomplete and comparisons are difficult. Only those well versed in the intricacies of these trials can try to piece together a coherent strategy and, even then, this has to be based to a greater or lesser extent on subgroup analysis. The unfortunate consequence of taking these trials at face value is that drug therapies are literally piled on top of one another with the attendant dangers of adverse interactions, complications and poor patient compliance. It is with some reason that the gastroenterologist engaged in acute general medicine serves up the increasingly exotic anti-platelet cocktail with a heavy heart.

It is not just the addition of new medications that produces this staggering complexity but also the reevaluation of older, established therapies. One example would be the recent fall from grace of the β-blocker as a first-line antihypertensive. This ongoing debate serves to illustrate a state of permanent evolution in pharmacological opinion, although it should of course be noted that β-blockers remain highly appropriate in patients with symptomatic ischaemic heart disease or a history of either myocardial infarction or heart failure.[20,21] The use of β-blockers elsewhere is also being questioned, with the COMMIT trial arguing against their use immediately following diagnosis of STEMI. Instead, it is argued that one ought to be more leisurely, introducing them a few hours down the line when those with severe infarct-related left ventricular failure will have had full opportunity to declare themselves.[22]

Up to the point of the introduction of low-molecular-weight heparin in unstable angina, the situation was relatively straightforward. The virtually simultaneous analysis of the introduction of three major GpIIb/IIIa antagonists with differing properties, the ADP receptor blocker clopidogrel, an early interventional strategy with angioplasty (again with rapidly changing techniques – particularly the introduction of stents), has however produced a bewildering number of possible therapeutic combinations, all of which have not been assessed with formal clinical trials (and nor will they be).

The evidence for the use of clopidogrel comes from two key trials – CAPRIE and CURE.[23,24] CAPRIE compared the impact of clopidogrel to that of aspirin in 20,000 patients who had experienced ischaemic events of one sort or another. CAPRIE suggested that clopidogrel alone was marginally better than aspirin alone in preventing further events over a 3-year follow up. Most of this marginal benefit seemed to arise from the lower number of patients in the clopidogrel arm who went on to have a myocardial infarction, a relative risk

[20] Lindholm *et al.* Lancet (2005) 366: 1545–1553.

[21] Kaplan *et al.* Lancet (2006) 367: 168–176.

[22] COMMIT Collaborative Group, Lancet (2005) 366: 1622–1632.

[23] CAPRIE Steering Committee, Lancet (1996) 348: 1329–1339.

[24] CURE Investigators, NEJM (2001) 345: 494–502.

reduction of around 20%. On subgroup analysis, it also appeared that the effect of clopidogrel may be a touch more powerful in diabetics and those who had had previous cardiac surgery. The next logical step was to examine the impact of the addition of clopidogrel to aspirin in the treatment of unstable angina. In the CURE trial, clopidogrel was given to patients presenting with unstable angina in addition to aspirin for a period of up to 12 months. Of the patients entered in the trial, 94% had an abnormal ECG. A quarter went on to have a troponin rise (therefore being recategorized as NSTEMI). There was a relative risk reduction of a fifth in the primary endpoint (cardiovascular death, myocardial infarction or stroke) at 12 months in the clopidogrel arm. The absolute risk reduction was around 2%. Unfortunately, there was a significant increase in bleeding with clopidogrel. When analysed again (on a *post-hoc* basis) to look just at the subgroup of 'potentially fatal' bleeds, the significance of this increase conveniently disappeared.

The manufacturers of clopidogrel were pleased with the results of CURE, and the drug has been heavily promoted. While a 20% relative risk reduction is impressive, the cost effectiveness of clopidogrel is worthy of comment. When used in the trial population at standard NHS price, around 50 patients need to be treated to prevent one primary endpoint, costing in excess of £20,000 (excluding the cost of the additional 'major bleed' in 1% of those treated). If one uses the broader indications for clopidogrel endorsed by the European Society of Cardiology, focusing more on history than on ECG abnormalities, costs will escalate dramatically. Clopidogrel may well be a fine drug, just as Dom Perignon '59 is a fine wine. The National Institute for Health and Clinical Excellence (NICE) has approved the use of clopidogrel in acute coronary syndrome.

Eager to consolidate clopidogrel's place in the CCU drug trolley, the manufacturers sought to generate evidence supporting the use of their medication in STEMI too. In the world's largest-ever clinical study involving almost 46,000 patients, clopidogrel was shown to bring about a 7% reduction in the relative risk of death, when given for a mean of 15 days immediately following STEMI (COMMIT).[25] Clopidogrel may also offer markedly better value for money in this setting.

The GpIIb/IIIa antagonists are used very sparingly in some institutions and with gay abandon in others. If nothing else, this serves to demonstrate the confusing data regarding these drugs. The GpIIb/IIIa receptor on the activated platelet binds fibrinogen and allows it to act as a bridge between the platelets. There are several intravenous agents that block the receptor and prevent this

---

[25] COMMIT Collaborative Group, Lancet (2005) 366: 1607–1621.

cross-linkage, including abciximab, a monoclonal antibody. The various agents differ in their selectivity and, importantly, their half lives following cessation.

A number of trials looking at the administration of GpIIb/IIIa antagonists around the time of angioplasty demonstrate a reduction in thrombotic complications, notably peri-procedural MI. Indeed, if continued for a period of 12 h following angioplasty, it would seem that abciximab may confer a mortality benefit. The sum of the data surrounding the use of GpIIb/IIIa antagonists suggests that benefits are modest but real. Cost effectiveness is again an issue. The European Society of Cardiology recommends the use of these agents in all troponin positive patients scheduled to undergo early revascularization.[26] Many institutions take this to mean any such patient scheduled to undergo angiography; others wait until they have the pictures to prove that revascularization is indeed required and yet others reserve the use of abciximab for high-risk angioplasties only. The European Society of Cardiology guidelines also highlight the heightened benefit of GpIIb/IIIa blockade in diabetics.

Movers and shakers

Cardiology has moved on apace in the last decade or so, as percutaneous coronary intervention has grown hugely in stature and volume. One almost feels sorry for the cardiothoracic surgeon who, having completed one of the most demanding and onerous training programmes around, is now rather less the NHS lynchpin than they may have anticipated. Not only are cardiothoracic surgeons constantly asked to divulge the finer details of their performance to the popular press but both their NHS and private practices are drying up due to a combination of herds of interventional cardiologists stepping heavily on their toes and Government waiting list targets. In recent years, it has come to be widely accepted (at least by physicians) that coronary artery bypass grafting (CABG) and angioplasty offer similar prognostic and symptomatic benefit in multivessel disease. Although high levels of restenosis have been a problem in percutaneous intervention, the arrival of drug-eluting stents has markedly reduced rates. However, the cardiothoracic surgeons are fighting back on several fronts.[27] Firstly, the charge is made that the majority of patients involved in randomized controlled trials comparing the two techniques have had single- or double-vessel disease, falling into a group previously known not to benefit from CABG. By extension, therefore, the group of 'sicker' patients with

26 European Society of Cardiology, Eur Heart J (2002) 23: 1809–1840.

27 Taggart, BMJ (2005) 330: 785–786.

multivessel disease and perhaps poorer left ventricular function (who are known to have the most to gain from surgery) are significantly (and unacceptably) diluted in the trial populations. Secondly, it is noted that the in-hospital mortality following CABG has remained constant in the UK over the last decade, despite a very much older and sicker substrate. Thirdly, the potential for a degree of bias in the presentation of clinical trial results is highlighted, with key facts hiding in the small print and paired editorials generally being penned by enthusiasts. Registry data from New York State also offers some solace to the cardiothoracic surgeon, reaffirming that those with the conventional indications for surgical bypass appear to do better with CABG than with angioplasty – likely because in addition to dealing with current target lesions, future targets are also bypassed.[28] In the absence of a consensus, the call for patients with multivessel disease to be discussed at multidisciplinary meetings seems reasonable.

What then have been the drivers to the rapid development of cardiology in recent years? A major impetus for change in the UK has perhaps been the political establishment. It is now acknowledged by most (and welcomed by some) that a paternalistic 'doctor knows best' system is not sustainable. Spurred on by a revolution in access to information, the patient now holds the levers. Waiting is regarded as passé, and cardiology was the first field, in the UK, to feel the pinch of government edicts with the introduction of door-to-needle target times for thrombolysis. The onward march of the relevant technologies has of course been pivotal too, facilitating change.

In the UK, there is an additional agent of change in the shape of the myocardial infarction national audit project (MINAP).[29] MINAP was set up by enthusiastic clinicians in part to monitor progress against the thrombolysis target. Another objective was to highlight discrepancies in acute cardiological care around the country and hopefully encourage the dissemination of good practice in so doing. The success of MINAP has been extraordinary. Despite being a voluntary audit, participation has reached (and remains at) 100% in England and Wales. Having measured (and perhaps contributed to) the achievement of the thrombolysis target, MINAP has now gone on to hold a spotlight up to the treatment of NSTEMI and highlight gross inequalities in access to angiography across the population.

[28] Hannan *et al.* NEJM (2005) 352: 2174–2183.

[29] 'How the NHS manages heart attacks' (www.rcplondon.ac.uk/pubs/books/minap06)

A trip to the theatre

Not infrequently, physicians, both cardiologists and generalists, may be asked by surgical colleagues to assess the suitability of a patient with a history of ischaemic heart disease, for elective noncardiac surgery. This is an activity that perhaps generates an amount of unnecessary anxiety and also some guesswork that might generously be described as educated. The essential messages are two: firstly, patients ought not to have special coronary investigation or invasive treatment prior to an elective operation unless symptoms would themselves have justified that course of action, and, secondly, β-blockade helps the ischaemic heart defend itself from the assault of anaesthesia. A recent study randomized over 500 patients with clinically significant coronary artery disease to receive, or not receive, revascularization (percutaneous or surgical) prior to their semi-elective surgery for aortic aneurysm or distal arterial bypass. There was no discernable difference in outcome at 2 years.[30] There are a number of tools that help an assessor predict the risk of a major cardiac event at the time of elective surgery, although predicting risk in itself is of little use other than to better inform both surgeon and patient regarding the risk–benefit balance of the proposed exercise.

Something for the weekend?

As a species, physicians fall woefully short when it comes to discussing matters of a sexual nature with their patients. Even in today's open and liberal society, over two-thirds of men with erectile dysfunction who were surveyed felt that they would avoid bringing the subject to the attention of their doctor for fear of causing embarrassment to them. A similar proportion believed that erectile dysfunction was not a 'medical problem'.[31] Fortunately, as a by-product of the advent of the specialist nurse in cardiac rehabilitation, the general physician has been spared some blushes. Patients with ischaemic heart disease, be that stable angina or indeed a recent acute infarct, may have a number of queries about the activities in which they are 'allowed' to engage.

While the thin curtains of the coronary care unit may make it a suboptimal place to bring up the intricate details of sexual function, the physician ought at the very least have some answers prepared, should the patient seek specific advice during the course of a ward round. Generally, patients should refrain from full intercourse for a month or so following an infarct and then gradually

[30] McFalls *et al.* NEJM (2004) 351: 2795–2804.

[31] Marwick, JAMA (1999) 281: 2173–2174.

build back up to previous levels of exertion. The idea that a patient's partner could perhaps take the physical lead might also be floated. Those with stable angina can be reassured, assuming that their levels of routine physical activity seem approximately proportionate. More specifically, sexual intercourse has been compared to walking a mile on the flat over 20 min, or briskly walking up and down a couple of flights of stairs. For those keen on even more objective measures, patients who cope with 4 min of a standard Bruce protocol should safely manage sexual intercourse.[32] The energy consumed as a consequence of one couple's sexual relations may be rather different from others, and a degree of flexibility is required with these guidelines!

Men with coronary atherosclerosis are of course prone to the same pathology in other arteries. Unfortunately, the drugs used in patients with atherosclerosis, notably β-blockers and thiazide diuretics, are also prone to dampen sexual prowess. When the anxiety generated by ischaemic heart disease is superimposed, it is not surprising that erectile dysfunction is a common problem. It is important to recognize that men with ischaemic heart disease are therefore at increased risk from the psychosocial causes of impotence, just as they are from the physical. It is worth bearing in mind too that a primary presentation with erectile dysfunction may be a marker of occult atherosclerosis elsewhere (or indeed of undiagnosed diabetes).

The outlook for men with erectile dysfunction has been revolutionized by the advent of the oral phosphodiesterase (type V) inhibitors such as sildenafil. However, it is important to remember that sildenafil and similar products (which potentiate vasodilatory nitric oxide pathways) are contraindicated in those taking nitrates on account of the risk of profound hypotension. An expert committee of the American Heart Association recommended that this contraindication is absolute. Furthermore, where patients have taken sildenafil in the 24 h prior to presentation with an acute ischaemic episode, nitrates ought not to be used in its treatment.[33] Others recommend that oral nicorandil and long-acting nitrates should be stopped 5 days prior to sildenafil use and that sublingual nitrate preparations ought be avoided in the 12 h following use.

AORTIC DISSECTION AND AORTIC SYNDROMES

Among the many chest pain sufferers in the emergency department are a few who describe severe chest pain radiating through to the back; in some, a diligent nurse may have identified a difference in blood pressure between the arms and, in a rather larger number, the radiographic appearance of the mediastinum

---

[32] Jackson, Int J Clin Practice (2004) 58: 358–362.

[33] Cheitlin *et al.* Circulation (1999) 99: 168–177.

(often on a film of questionable quality) may have been interpreted as being widened. All three of these features have a rather poor specificity for aortic dissection. Nonetheless, many of these patients will find themselves whisked round to the CT scan room. The difficult cases are those who, in addition to these features, also have evidence of ST elevation on their ECG. Unfortunately, thrombolysis is denied to many of these patients while awaiting a scan. Involvement of the coronary arteries in aortic dissection is very rare and nearly always involves the right coronary artery. If there is a good history and accompanying clinical signs for dissection, it is probably reasonable to delay thrombolysis for an inferior infarct (a group with a relatively good prognosis without thrombolysis in any case). With anterior ST elevation, it is reasonable to proceed with thrombolysis if a CXR is normal (even though 10% are normal in proven dissection); a patient presenting with a combination of an aortic dissection, a normal CXR and an anterior infarction (the territory of the left coronary artery) would be considered unlucky indeed! If the CXR is of poor quality, excluding aortic root dilatation and aortic regurgitation with a good transthoracic echo would be a reasonable next step.

Once diagnosed, those patients with dissection involving the aortic root (type A) need to be treated surgically, and the rest are treated medically. While waiting for the surgeon, delicate control of blood pressure is the order of the day, usually using intravenous labetalol. In the patient with acute left ventricular failure secondary to severe acute aortic regurgitation, intravenous nitrates or nitroprusside are alternatives.

Other mischief, short of proper dissection, can also occur within the aorta. An intramural haematoma, perhaps due to the rupture of the aortic vasa vasorum, may form. In this situation, the intima is intact; this finding, on CT or MR imaging, differentiates the condition from frank aortic dissection. Such differentiation is largely academic, as intramural haematoma may be a precursor to dissection and the treatment of the two is identical! Penetrating atherosclerotic ulcers can occur in the wall of the descending aorta, most often in elderly smokers. Erosion through to the adventitia is a prelude to transmural rupture. Such ulcers, which present in a similar fashion to aortic dissection, can be diagnosed on aortography. Traditionally, operative intervention (with the high risk that it carries for this patient group) was the only available treatment, although more recently, endovascular aortic stenting has begun to be offered.

CARDIAC FAILURE

Sudden breakdown

Acute heart failure remains one of the most dramatic presentations of all for the admitting doctor. Few graduates of the emergency department will have failed to note the reliability of the influx of patients with 'crashing LVF' at the tail end of the night shift. On occasion, patients may exhibit left ventricular failure *de novo*, perhaps as a result of a silent or ignored ischaemic event. More often though, symptoms will either have built up gradually (as in the case of a cardiomyopathy) or will be superimposed on a background of chronic compensated cardiac failure. Although physical examination may help in establishing chronicity, peeking at the patient's medication list is of course equally fruitful! While the presentation of acute heart failure can be sufficiently distinctive as to make its diagnosis relatively easy, this is not always the case. In those with coexistent lung disease, the primary problem on presentation is often extremely difficult to decipher. Enthusiasts may offer up hand-held echocardiography and fancy biochemistry (BNP measurement) to confirm one's clinical impression, and these tests will be vying to become established in emergency departments over the coming years.

Although a common presentation, acute heart failure is in itself a symptom complex rather than a diagnosis. These patients are not a homogenous mass and should not be treated as such. There are essentially two clinical questions to address: are there signs of fluid overload (is the patient wet or dry), and are there signs of low output (is the patient warm or cold)? The most common presentation is the most rewarding to treat. The patient who is wet and warm essentially requires the offloading of fluids, and diuretics followed by nitrates are the order of the day. Where the patient is wet and cold, the situation is more challenging to remedy. In general, vasodilatation followed by diuresis is indicated. Inotropes may well be required. When the patient appears to be dry and cold at presentation, things are often rather dire. Inotropes and cautious filling may be attempted but the prognosis is rarely good.

Circulatory support, by itself, rarely alters prognosis in those patients with cardiogenic shock and pulmonary oedema. The use of inotropes (and indeed balloon counterpulsation) is best viewed as a bridging mechanism to definitive therapy. This applies particularly in ischaemic heart disease where support may be required prior to revascularization. Circulatory support can also be helpful pending surgical repair in cases of left ventricular failure precipitated by an acquired VSD or papillary muscle rupture following an infarct.

It should of course be remembered that pulmonary oedema and left ventricular failure are by no means synonymous. The lungs function best when they look rather like a 'dry sponge'. When they are waterlogged and looking like a 'wet sponge', gas exchange suffers. Whether the lungs are dry or wet depends on a fine balancing of oncotic and hydrostatic forces across the exquisitely delicate alveolar membrane. Although pump failure is a frequent cause of raised pulmonary hydrostatic pressure and therefore increased alveolar fluid, there are also many other mechanisms of pulmonary oedema. On Everest or in the rainforest, high altitude or coral snake venom may be causal. In the Western hospital, there are a number of more likely suspects. Drugs including diltiazem, opioids, ciprofloxacin and nitrofurantoin can cause increased membrane permeability. Neurogenic pulmonary oedema can occur as a consequence of intracranial upset. A number of cases of dramatic pulmonary oedema following extubation have also been reported, perhaps on account of a monumental momentary fall in intrathoracic pressure as patients struggle heroically with their artificial airway upon awakening.[34] In the presence of severe mitral valve disease, pulmonary oedema can occur in the context of a left ventricle that continues to work valiantly.

Pharmacology aside, another useful tool in the treatment of acute left ventricular failure is continuous positive airways pressure (CPAP). Where the patient remains significantly hypoxic despite initial drug treatment or where the blood pressure struggles to tolerate generous doses of nitrates, CPAP can be extremely helpful. The treatment is surprisingly well tolerated when explained to the patient in a calm and rational manner. Alternatives to the traditional masks include transparent 'whole-face' masks, which patients often prefer. CPAP also seems the physiologically rational, although not firmly evidence-based, strategy when treating patients with some forms of noncardiogenic pulmonary oedema, when intubation is not judged necessary. Access to CPAP varies widely between hospitals and can be a particular issue on sites without formal high-dependency areas. Intensivists may be reluctant to take on patients with severe cardiac failure but ought to be encouraged to provide a time-limited trial of CPAP if that is within their gift.

The struggling pump

Acute heart failure is often a rewarding problem to treat. The patient with established chronic heart failure is less inclined to engender much excitement. Chronic heart failure does however account for a vast swathe of the collective NHS workload. Patients are numerous, and they attend relatively frequently, both for scheduled outpatient review and for unannounced visits for inpatient assessment. There are a number of reasons for this. A heart that struggles to perform is clearly bad news. Our treatments, when applied appropriately, offer modest survival benefit but there is no magic wand. Poor prescribing and low patient adherence further limit effectiveness. The medications that we do dispense are by no means harmless. Furthermore, patients with failing hearts

---

[34] Oswalt et al. JAMA (1977) 238: 1833–1835.

may well have an assortment of other problems – failing lungs, failing brains and perhaps even failing care packages.

Given the burden of disease and the position of chronic heart failure as something of a 'Cinderella' subspecialty, the attention paid to the condition by NICE was timely and welcome.[35] NICE has produced a comprehensive evidence-based guide to the treatment of chronic heart failure and has highlighted a number of key messages. Perhaps the most striking data expressed in the guideline are epidemiological. It is reckoned that just shy of a million people in the UK live with symptomatic heart failure. About 40% of patients diagnosed with heart failure are said to be dead in a year, although the annual mortality of survivors from that point onwards is much lower. Importantly, NICE estimates (and it can only be an estimate on account of the imperfect quality of the data collected in our health service) that heart failure accounts for a million inpatient days in the NHS each year. Roughly, 1 in 20 admissions to the acute medical take is due to heart failure, and this figure is set to rise as the pool of elderly patients most prone to the condition grows in size. The annual bill for treating heart failure (mostly the costs of hospitalization) will soon top £1 billion.

The NICE guidance is thorough, with algorithms offered for various diagnostic and therapeutic scenarios. In particular, assuming the absence of a clinical suspicion of valvular troubles, it is suggested that a normal ECG together with a normal brain natriuretic peptide (BNP) measurement is sufficient to exclude a diagnosis of heart failure in the primary care or outpatient setting, without recourse to an echocardiogram. With regard to treatment, the guidelines emphasize the importance of commencing (and gradually – fortnightly – titrating to maximum tolerated dose) therapy with ACE inhibitors and β-blockers in that order, irrespective of the presence or absence of symptoms at the time. Physicians in secondary care will often adjust doses more rapidly, which seems reasonable in the inpatient setting. Only if the patient remains symptomatic after these measures, should spironolactone and digoxin (in sinus rhythm) be considered. In this setting, digoxin may reduce the likelihood of hospitalization, whereas spironolactone does this and increases longevity. It stands to reason that drugs given for prognostic improvement ought to be given in maximum tolerable dose (within the recommended limits), irrespective of symptoms, while drugs given for symptomatic relief ought to be adjusted according to need. NICE assumes that ACE inhibitor effects are class effects and, although recognizing that only a limited

---

[35] CG005 (July 2003) (www.nice.org.uk)

number of β-blockers are specifically licensed for use in heart failure, condones the practice of continuing a different β-blocker in a patient already taking it. The potential dangers of sudden β-blocker cessation are also highlighted. Specific aetiological factors and significant fluid retention should of course be addressed appropriately from the outset.

NICE also arrived at the consensus view that influenza and pneumococcal vaccination should be offered to those with heart failure. The monitoring of patients having therapy for heart failure is important, and useful guidance is offered, particularly with regard to deteriorating renal function. NICE recommends that an increase in creatinine of 50% or to 200 μmol/l (whichever is lower) is acceptable. Likewise, serum potassium of less than 6 mmol/l is tolerable. Where increases are more dramatic (doubling in creatinine, creatinine of over 350 μmol/l or potassium over 6 mmol/l), ACE inhibitors should be stopped. Where increases in creatinine are between these levels, it is felt reasonable to halve the dose of ACE inhibitor and recheck the biochemistry.

The NICE guidelines direct the reader to a number of trials, in progress at the time they were written, which were felt likely to be of potential significance. Among these trials were VALIANT and Val-HEFT.[36,37] VALIANT aimed to assess any additive benefit of valsartan, an angiotensin receptor blocker (ARB), when given in combination with an ACE inhibitor to those with left ventricular dysfunction following an MI. There was none. Given this negative result, VALIANT was rather more interesting in terms of its construction.

As a trial, VALIANT was also designed to illustrate the similarities in outcome with ACE inhibitor and ARB monotherapy. The trial was put together such that the 'noninferiority' of the ARB could be demonstrated. Essentially, as long as valsartan appeared to have at least 55% of the impact of captopril, it would be 'noninferior'. Valsartan did manage this – the hazard ratio for patients on valsartan as opposed to captopril being 1.13. Patients taking valsartan suffered an excess of hypotension and renal dysfunction compared to those taking captopril. Those with a healthy degree of cynicism criticize such trials. If something is proven to work, why replace it? When buying a new car for instance, most of us would prefer the new vehicle to be superior to the forerunner rather than just a 'non-inferior' model. The choice of comparator for valsartan is also interesting. Why did the investigators choose captopril, a relatively elderly ACE inhibitor with a short half-life?

[36] Pfeffer *et al.* NEJM (2003) 349: 1893–1906.

[37] Cohn *et al.* NEJM (2001) 345: 1667–1675.

A finding of noninferiority is generally used by manufacturers in an attempt to 'takeover' all the licensed indications of the older drug, and captopril is relatively well endowed with regard to licensed indications.

Val-HEFT evaluated the addition of valsartan to standard therapy (often including a β-blocker and/or ACE inhibitor). The addition of valsartan did result in an overall reduction of the primary composite end-point (mortality plus hospitalization for heart failure). This effect was almost entirely driven by levels of hospitalization. When subgroup analyses were carried out (without prespecification or indeed appropriate power), it seemed that the addition of the ARB was beneficial to those taking either a β-blocker or an ACE inhibitor but not both. Indeed, when patients took all three drugs together, there appeared to be an excess of mortality (although arguments about the value of post-hoc analyses are equally applicable here).

The CHARM study also reported following the publication of the NICE guidance. CHARM had several arms, and one of them (CHARM-Added) examined the effect of adding the ARB candesartan to ACE inhibitor therapy in patients with congestive cardiac failure (LVEF < 40%). The addition of candesartan resulted in a reduction in the incidence of cardiovascular death or hospitalization for congestive cardiac failure (hazard ratio 0.85). Set against this was a modest increase in renal dysfunction and hypotension.[38]

The NICE guidance perhaps fails to focus sufficiently on the importance of fluid restriction in the treatment of severe heart failure, other than to point out that dehydration and confusion may be so precipitated. It seems glaringly obvious to the preclinical student that a good diuresis will be followed, as night follows day, by an equally impressive thirst. Few doctors think about informing their patients of this. Unless the patient with severe disease limits their fluid intake to some degree, doctors do nothing more than chase their tails, having little impact on the symptoms of heart failure. Indeed, the patient's quality of life will usually have been lessened, as much of their time will now be spent in the toilet! Many elderly patients with diminished mobility readily admit to nonadherence with prescribed loop diuretic therapy.

Six of one and half a dozen of the other

One of the most challenging scenarios in general medicine is that of the patient with the dual pathology of chronic cardiac and fairly severe renal failure, often with a common aetiology. Although perhaps rare in general practice, this population will be over-represented in those requiring hospitalization.

[38] CHARM Investigators, Lancet (2003) 362: 759–766.

Understandably, doctors become nervous when prescribing diuretics to this group, concerned that tipping a patient into a degree of acute prerenal failure will do them no favours. Although there is certainly room for caution, it also needs to be borne in mind that where there is evidence of fluid overload, this needs to be addressed. It is also crucial to remember that low doses of a loop diuretic will do the patient with established chronic renal failure neither good nor harm. With sluggish glomerular filtration and a creatinine of 400, 40 mg of furosemide will never have the chance to get to work in the renal tubules. The key to the treatment of this challenging dual pathology is to use the usual drugs in appropriate doses, monitoring the patient very closely both clinically and with blood tests. A peripatetic clinical nurse specialist may be key here. Perhaps the most important clinical measure of progress is the patient's weight, which is likely more reliable than the average doctor's assessment of fluid status. Identifying a patient's ideal dry weight is as important in the treatment of chronic heart failure as it is on the dialysis unit. Patients usually understand this and will often be keen to participate and take back some control.

On occasion, despite prudent drug choice and careful monitoring, one aspect of the patient's disease may improve at the expense of the other. Although breathlessness may get better, the creatinine might head onwards and upwards. When the kidneys are clearly not appreciating one's efforts to improve cardiac failure, a rather more traditional treatment may be attempted. If diuretic- and ACE-inhibitor-based therapy is neither tolerated nor successful, a trial of hydralazine and nitrates may be sensible. Instead of attempting to offload excess fluid, vasodilatation aims to make more room in the circulation for it. Although this may seem intuitively like a mere holding measure, results can be impressive. In black patients, the addition of nitrates and hydralazine to standard therapy for advanced heart failure is particularly effective, with significant reductions in rates of death and hospitalization.[39]

At the end of the day, it is important to remember that the combination of severe cardiac and renal failure is likely to be a lethal one. Treatment will not cure, but rather aims to prolong quality survival. Severe LV impairment is a far more significant diagnosis than many forms of cancer. Long-term survival is poor. The stereotypes of cardiologist and palliative physician may appear to have relatively little in common but patients with heart failure deserve the same level of information and support regarding their prognosis as individuals with motor neurone disease or cancer. Physicians ought to consider the role that they can play in achieving this goal.

---

[39] Taylor *et al.* NEJM (2004) 351: 2049–2057.

Difficulty relaxing?

The symptoms generated by the failing heart have long been a little difficult to explain. A patient's clinical presentation may seem to be out of kilter with their echocardiographic indices. It is worthy of note that left ventricular ejection fraction is a normally distributed variable in the population and that a combination of an individual's general physiological reserve and other factors will dictate whether or not there are symptoms of heart failure.[40] Indeed, population screening has shown that 3% of individuals have an ejection fraction on the wrong side of 30 % but around half of them have no attributable symptoms whatsoever. About 40% of incident cases of clinical heart failure in the Framingham study had ostensibly normal systolic function on echo.[41] Why then can there be such a mismatch between symptoms and echo findings? Over the last decade or so, one potential explanation – diastolic heart failure (or more broadly 'heart failure with preserved systolic function') – has gained rather greater (although by no means universal) credence. When a water pump fails, its feeble output is immediately noticed. In the case of the human heart, the lack of output may be a problem but more often, the inability of a poorly compliant left ventricle to 'pull' blood through the pulmonary vasculature may be the cause of the first outward sign of trouble, as left ventricular end diastolic pressure increases to supranormal levels.

In systolic heart failure, as the left ventricle fails and the ejection fraction falls, a larger end diastolic volume (EDV) is required in order to maintain the same stroke volume and cardiac output (for a given heart rate). In the normal heart, pressure in the left ventricle continues to fall in early diastole even after LV filling commences. There is essentially a vacuum effect, sucking blood from the atrium through to the ventricle. Therefore, early ventricular filling is an active and significant process. Only the final component of LV filling relies on atrial contraction. The 'active process of ventricular relaxation' is crucial, and this process itself can fail — diastolic heart failure. If there is a degree of systolic pump failure too (and some deny the existence of isolated diastolic failure as an entity), the situation is worsened, as the heart's response to systolic failure is dependent, to a degree, on enhanced ventricular filling.

Therefore, the heart can fail in systole or indeed in diastole. When there is systolic failure, the impact of diastolic dysfunction will be magnified. The mismatch between echo findings and symptoms may in part be explained by the fact that most of the measurements routinely reported concern systolic

[40] McDonagh et al. Lancet (1997) 350: 829.

[41] Vasan et al. J Am Coll Cardiol (1999) 33: 1948–1955.

function and the vigour of LV emptying. There are a number of indices that reflect the performance of the left ventricle in 'actively relaxing' and therefore performing the work of diastole. The most frequently used measure is that of the E/A ratio (or gradient). The E/A ratio reflects flow velocities measured by cardiac Doppler in early (E) and late/atrial (A) phases of ventricular filling, respectively. In athletes, there may be an increase in the E/A ratio in order to maximize LV EDV, delivering larger volumes of blood for systole. Where there is diastolic failure, the ratio is reversed as the early filling phase becomes ineffectual and more emphasis is placed upon the atrial contribution. Where there is isolated early diastolic failure, pulmonary venous pressure does not increase in the resting state. However, with arrhythmias and exercise, pulmonary pressures rise and symptoms ensue. Tachycardia reduces the time available in the cardiac cycle for early ventricular filling and thus exacerbates any problem with this phase.

The prevalence of predominant diastolic heart failure is uncertain. Powerful risk factors include hypertension (especially when associated with left ventricular hypertrophy) and COPD. When these conditions are excluded, incidence is estimated at around 1%.[42] Women (and notably larger women) seem particularly prone to diastolic heart failure. Given the mechanism of diastolic failure, it stands to reason that the onset of an atrial arrhythmia could precipitate dramatic clinical decompensation. This may account for a number of patients who are unable to tolerate such dysrhythmias but then go on to have apparently normal echocardiograms when in sinus rhythm. One of the pitfalls of using the E/A ratio as a measure of diastolic function is of course that there is no E/A ratio to measure in atrial fibrillation. Another is the poorly understood 'pseudonormalization' of the E/A ratio in patients with increasingly severe diastolic heart failure! The ratio is also an unreliable measure in the elderly.

Diastolic heart failure is undoubtedly a significant and under-recognized phenomenon, but some words of caution: although diastolic dysfunction can on occasion account for breathlessness, it is important to consider other potential causes that may coexist, including COPD and obesity. In addition, there is no defined and proven approach to the treatment of diastolic heart failure. One assumes that many of the drugs used in the treatment of systolic dysfunction will be helpful, but a literature search for supporting evidence is likely to disappoint. In particular, the angiotensin receptor blocker, candesartan, failed to demonstrate any mortality benefit against placebo in patients with symptomatic heart failure but with an LV ejection fraction of over 40% (CHARM-Preserved).[43]

[42] Fischer *et al.* Eur Heart J (2003) 24: 320–328.

[43] Yusef *et al.* Lancet (2003) 362: 777–781.

Phlebotomy for heart failure?

Venesection is perhaps the oldest of all treatments for heart failure and, in the acute setting, removing a unit of blood can be very effective in the relief of symptoms. Despite this, more modern, effective (and expensive) therapies have largely superseded bloodletting! However, blood tests are presently attempting to establish their role in the diagnosis of heart failure and indeed in the monitoring of treatment. BNP is a natriuretic peptide produced by the cardiac ventricles, and it is released into the circulation in response to ventricular stretch. Multiple studies have demonstrated that BNP levels increase sequentially in groups of patients with worsening degrees of clinical heart failure. BNP levels also increase on exercise, and this increase is exaggerated in those with LV dysfunction, even if it is asymptomatic. As always, there are confounding factors, and renal failure, hypertension and drugs may all alter BNP levels to a degree.

It is unlikely that the measurement of BNP will ever be desperately helpful with patients presenting acutely where traditional clinical skills will hopefully be employed to make a diagnosis (although there is a small but growing literature concerning the use of BNP in the emergency department setting, which is said to shorten hospital stay). In the community, however, the BNP assay may find a very useful niche. For the patient presenting with nonspecific breathlessness or swollen ankles, which may or may not be due to cardiac failure, a blood test is likely to be preferable to a referral for echocardiography. In patients presenting with symptoms and signs suggestive of heart failure, a BNP cut-off level has been identified, which gives the test a very respectable positive predictive value of 70% and (more importantly) a negative predictive value of 98%.[44] A simple blood test will not only prove very acceptable to patients but it may help to cut down on the large crowds congregating near the hospital echo suite. Indeed, in hospitals where there is no direct access to echo for the family physician, the cost savings may be very substantial. A recent systematic review has suggested that BNP measurement is a strong prognostic indicator for patients with heart failure. An increase in BNP by 100 pg/ml confers a 35% increase in the relative risk of death. Moreover, the measurement of BNP adds further prognostic information over and above an echo report. It may be that BNP levels after clinical stabilization on therapy are the best prognostic indicator of all.[45] It would seem that BNP is also elevated in

---

[44] Cowie *et al.* Lancet (1997) 350: 1347–1351.

[45] Doust *et al.* BMJ (2005) 330: 625–627.

diastolic heart failure although not to the same extent. The utility of the test in screening for and diagnosing diastolic failure is therefore much less clear.

It has also been suggested that the measurement of the n-terminal of pro-BNP may be useful in predicting the long-term survival of patients with stable coronary disease, giving further information even after assessment of the traditional cardiac risk factors and echocardiographic findings.[46] Time will tell.

Resynchronization

The onset of a dysrhythmia or impaired intraventricular conduction frequently causes problems for the patient with heart failure. When physiological reserve is already substantially reduced, a further loss in efficiency through rhythm disturbance can prove costly. Atrial fibrillation, for instance, will result in the loss of around 20% of the work of the cardiac cycle (perhaps more in those with significant diastolic failure). Furthermore, the factors causing heart failure are very likely to contribute also to the development of arrhythmia. Up to half of all deaths in those with heart failure are probably due to ventricular dysrhythmia. It is therefore crucial that rhythm abnormalities in general be spotted and dealt with.

In addition to the standard indications for permanent pacing, cardiac resynchronization therapy in heart failure is now of proven benefit.[47,48] For those patients with cardiac failure and a broad QRS (> 120 ms) with left bundle branch block morphology, attempting to recreate the physiological timetable for myocyte depolarization by bypassing malfunctioning conducting tissue now has a sound evidence base. Three pacing leads are placed, one in each of the two ventricles and one in the right atrium. The left ventricular lead is placed transvenously, making use of the coronary sinus. The technique of cardiac resynchronization is thought to be particularly effective where the QRS duration is over 150 ms. At best, the relative risk of death in patients with advanced heart failure can be reduced by up to a half with biventricular pacing. There is also good evidence for symptomatic relief in a subgroup of patients. Unfortunately, there is, as of yet, no reliable way of discerning responders from nonresponders. In addition, the successful placement of three leads can be complicated, and complications are naturally not tolerated well by this patient group. The COMPANION-HF trial has confirmed the benefits

---

[46] Kragelund et al. NEJM (2005) 352: 666–675.

[47] Abraham et al. NEJM (2002) 346: 1845–1858.

[48] CARE-HF Investigators, NEJM (2005) 352: 1539–1549.

of resynchronization therapy in patients with NYHA Class III or IV heart failure (of whatever cause) and intraventricular conduction delay. In addition, a hint of reduction in all cause mortality was observed for patients fitted with a pacemaker/defibrillator combination as opposed to a pacemaker alone.[49] This potential survival benefit would obviously not come cheap.

RHYTHM DISTURBANCE

Fibrillation, fibrillation, fibrillation...

Atrial fibrillation (AF) is surely one of the most common presentations to the general medical take. For those eager to keep up to date with the latest classifications, the terms paroxysmal, persistent (requiring exogenous cardioversion) or permanent should now be used. Around 10% of people over the age of 80 years have permanent AF. Despite its frequency on the post-take ward round, the acute treatment of atrial fibrillation is rather varied, and it is unusual to find two patients who have been managed in precisely the same way. Patients may be offered digoxin, β-blockade, amiodarone, a calcium channel blocker, a class 1c agent or, often, some combination of these. At times, these drugs seem to be given in a random order. What then would constitute the optimal therapy for new AF?

There are two relatively pressing questions to address when first seeing a patient with 'new' AF. The first concerns haemodynamic stability, and the second concerns chronicity. In the unstable patient, the treatment of new onset AF is of course urgent DC cardioversion. There will be times when the haemodynamic stability of a patient falls in a rather grey area. For instance, the systolic blood pressure may hover around 90 mm of mercury. Is this patient unstable by definition? It seems reasonable in such a case to look for evidence of end-organ performance: is the patient thinking clearly, reasonably well perfused and making adequate volumes of urine? If the answer to these enquiries is in the affirmative, one probably has a few hours in which to offer pharmacotherapy. The second question is one of chronicity. Is this definitely new AF with a distinct symptomatic onset, or might this simply be previously undiagnosed chronic AF? Only in the first case should one entertain the possibility of inpatient electrical cardioversion with its incumbent risks. In the acute situation, it seems sensible to offer anticoagulation to most patients presenting with new AF, where there is no contraindication. Anticoagulation needs to be started within 48 h of onset in order to minimize the risks of

---

[49] Bristow *et al.* NEJM (2004) 350: 2140–2150.

embolism at the time of any iatrogenic cardioversion. Once beyond this 48-h window, 4 to 5 weeks of anticoagulation is required, the only safe way around this being to establish that there is no atrial thrombus using transoesophageal echocardiography.

In the patient who does not clearly require immediate cardioversion, what are the treatment options? Frequently, the knee jerk reaction in the admissions unit is to commence digoxin for rate control. Another option of course is to do nothing for 24 h in anticipation of spontaneous cardioversion. In patients where one suspects that the AF represents the first presentation of chronic arrhythmia, perhaps on account of a history of hypertension and cardiomegaly on the chest X-ray, digoxin may be a reasonable choice. However, this is often an unreliable clinical impression, and thought ought to be given to the acute use of β-blockade or amiodarone. In the absence of cardiac failure, simple β-blockade may accomplish the rate control that one seeks and potentially help to tackle coexistent hypertension and ischaemic heart disease. Sotalol, with its combined Vaughan-Williams class two and three effects, has theoretical advantages over standard β-blockade but few patients ever achieve the high doses necessary to have any class-three impact, either through side effects or inadequate prescribing. Amiodarone is the drug that deserves most serious consideration in this situation. Although amiodarone's information leaflet is a particularly lengthy and depressing one, it has an impressive effect on rate and may facilitate 'spontaneous' cardioversion. Furthermore, patients who later find themselves being invited for interval cardioversion do significantly better when they are fully loaded with amiodarone, both in terms of version rates and maintenance of sinus rhythm.[50] The success rate of electrical cardioversion has been further boosted by the advent of biphasic defibrillators. Amiodarone is often a very appropriate choice of drug in the short and medium term, although caution (and careful monitoring) is certainly called for in those cases where it is then continued: indeed, the rationale for continuance ought to be frequently revisited so as to avoid generating work for colleagues in endocrinology, respiratory medicine and ophthalmology.

It is important to consider and investigate the reversible causes of atrial arrhythmia at the time of diagnosis, rather than embark on a lengthy and potentially unsuccessful pharmacological treatment plan. Clinical signs of infection, hyperthyroidism and alcoholism ought to be sought. Electrolytes and thyroid status should both be sent. An echocardiogram is a very reasonable

[50] Chun *et al.* Am J Cardiol (1995) 76: 47–50.

investigation to request at the time of presentation with AF but it is important to remember that the value of this test (in the assessment of left ventricular function) is much reduced when the heart rate is excessive. The echo should therefore be deferred until rate control is established, where possible. An additional difficulty in patients presenting with atrial arrhythmias is the decision as to whether or not one needs to check for myocardial damage, either causal or consequent to the tachyarrhythmia. There is no hard and fast rule but, in general, this test will probably not alter management. A mildly raised troponin in the context of a dramatic tachycardia is unlikely to have quite the same prognostic value as in other circumstances.

There are of course other approaches and other drugs that can be used in the treatment of AF. In patients with frequent paroxysms, it may be acceptable to provide drug packs containing oral flecainide and propofenone for use in the home at the time of symptom onset. This has been demonstrated to be a safe strategy, cutting down substantially on emergency department attendances.[51] It may of course be that individuals having frequent paroxysms, not held in check by simple drug therapy, would be better off being assessed for an ablation. It has been shown that paroxysmal atrial fibrillation is often triggered by foci within the pulmonary veins as they enter the left atrium.[52] Radiofrequency ablation, using a transeptal approach allowing access from the systemic veins, has been used to good effect.[53]

To anticoagulate or not to anticoagulate?

Where the intention is to invite a patient back to hospital for elective cardioversion following rate control, formal anticoagulation is essential. Both warfarin and amiodarone should be given prior to attempted cardioversion and continued for a period thereafter. However, whereas one's gut instinct may be that sinus rhythm is preferable to atrial fibrillation, this assumption has been revisited in recent years. In trials where patients with largely symptomatic atrial fibrillation have been randomized to receive primary rate control or aggressive pursuit and maintenance of sinus rhythm, results have been mixed. Overall, no difference in survival rates has been demonstrated, although a strategy of aggressive rhythm control would appear to result in more hospitalization and more adverse drug

[51] Alboni et al. NEJM (2004) 351: 2384–2391.

[52] Haïssaguerre et al. NEJM (1998) 339: 659–666.

[53] Jaïs et al. Eur Heart J (2003) 5: H34–H39.

effects but, paradoxically, perhaps better exercise tolerance.[54,55,56] Single-mindedly pursuing the achievement and maintenance of sinus rhythm is likely to be a laborious and ultimately thankless task for both the patient and physician. Rather than assuming that cardioversion ought to be attempted for all, it is now widely accepted that the indication is stronger for patients who are young or symptomatic and in those with aortic stenosis or HOCM. With regard to cardioversion, it is important to know when to give up!

If we are to accept therefore that a patient has permanent AF, we need to assess the appropriateness of formal anticoagulation to reduce the chance of embolic stroke. It has been estimated that one-sixth of all ischaemic strokes in those aged over 60 years can be attributed to AF.[57] The side effects of lifelong warfarin are real and potentially deadly. We worry particularly about the possibility of harming the frail and elderly patient through warfarin use, although it is of course this group that also has the most to gain. A recent paper has elegantly demonstrated that a physician's prescribing habits in this area are likely to be affected by the adverse haemorrhagic events experienced (although not by the preventable ischaemic strokes witnessed), rather than by any objective evidence.[58] The SPAF-III investigators identified a number of factors, in addition to a previous cerebrovascular event, any one of which signifies a 'high' risk of thromboembolic stroke for those in AF.[59] These risk factors are systolic blood pressure greater than 160 mmHg, being a female over 75 years of age and congestive cardiac failure. For those with adequately treated hypertension alone, the risk of stroke is classified as 'moderate'. Following stratification, the SPAF-III investigators calculated annual risks of ischaemic stroke and, based on this, recommended levels of anticoagulation (see the table on page 32).

Echocardiographic findings, although not essential, can also help to inform the anticoagulation decision. Poor left ventricular function will confirm a clinical suspicion of cardiac failure, and left atrial enlargement will further favour anticoagulation. Set against the benefit of warfarin is the risk

54 AFFIRM Investigators, NEJM (2002) 347: 1825–1833.

55 Hohnloser et al. Lancet (2000) 356: 1789–1794.

56 Nattel et al. Lancet (2006) 367: 262–272.

57 Wolf et al. Stroke (1991) 22: 983.

58 Choudhry et al. BMJ (2006) 332: 141–143.

59 SPAF-III Investigators, Lancet (1996) 348: 633–638.

of major haemorrhage. This risk increases with the age of the patient. For the general population, warfarin has a serious adverse event rate of 1–2% per year. In patients in their eighties, outside the confines of a trial, this risk is likely 3 or 4% per annum. It should be noted that atrial fibrillation is not one of the situations in which aspirin and warfarin have additive benefit (those situations being prosthetic valves and acute coronary syndrome).

Risk of embolic stroke in atrial fibrillation

Level of Risk	% CVA per annum	NNT*	Recommended treatment
Previous CVA/TIA	10	14	Warfarin
High	6	33	Warfarin
Moderate	3	66	Either
Low	1	200	Aspirin

* NNT refers to the number treated for 1 year to prevent an event, if warfarin therapy is used in place of aspirin (adapted from SPAF-III).

Syncope and the resting ECG

'Collapse query cause' is the bane of the general physician's life — seemingly endless streams of people experiencing poorly characterized episodes with innumerable possible causes. Emergency departments seem reluctant to discharge and, at worst, a failed occupational therapy assessment may be the sole reason for admission. Searching for the specific cause may feel like searching for the proverbial needle in the haystack. There are, however, a number of cardiological causes to be on the look out for, particularly in the younger patient. Although they will present only rarely, picking them up tends to impress colleagues and (more importantly) may substantially improve a patient's prognosis! Some of the rather more esoteric aetiologies of syncope can be discerned from the resting ECG. Such causes include Brugada syndrome, Wollf–Parkinson–White, long QT and right ventricular dysplasia. Although all are pretty rare, they are important to identify and a highly detailed, even pedantic, history is essential.

Brugada syndrome, of which there are three subtypes, has a prevalence of somewhere between 1 in 150 and 1 in 2000. The syndrome, first described in 1992, involves the malfunctioning of the alpha subunit of the sodium channel. Although inherited as an autosomal dominant, there is incomplete penetrance with a marked male preponderance clinically. Up to 60% of cases are thought to be sporadic. The malfunctioning sodium channel predisposes to the development of ventricular tachycardia or fibrillation in a significant proportion of patients, usually when at rest. The ECG may well demonstrate a number of abnormalities including high take-off of the ST segment anteriorly, right bundle branch block morphology and left axis deviation. Curiously, these abnormalities may be fleeting. When observed, these ECG features alone warrant referral to an electrophysiology specialist for consideration of stimulation studies. Where combined with a history of unexplained collapse, an implantable defibrillator will usually be indicated. The mean age at diagnosis is around forty years.

Arrhythmogenic right ventricular dysplasia (ARVD) is a variety of cardiomyopathy localized to parts of the right ventricular myocardium. The muscle becomes necrosed and is replaced by fibrofatty tissue that acts as a focus for ventricular arrhythmias. Untreated, excess mortality runs at around 1% per year, and ARVD accounts for a significant proportion of sudden cardiac deaths in the young. Diagnosis involves identifying structural RV abnormalities (segmental RV dilatation or RV aneurysm) and characteristic ECG changes including an epsilon wave in lead one with T wave inversion and prolongation of the QRS complex localized to the anterior leads. Symptoms (syncope) or sudden deaths tend to occur with exertion and perhaps with emotional stress. Treatment centres on the use of amiodarone and β-blockers, including sotalol. In patients with sustained symptomatic dysrhythmias, an implantable cardioverter–defibrillator (ICD) is indicated.

The electrical barrier between atria and ventricles, with the AV node as the only point of communication between the two, develops *in-utero*. On occasion, development of this cardiological equivalent of the Berlin wall may be incomplete, with accessory pathways allowing conduction, perhaps in either direction. Such abnormal conduction is prone to lead to the development of atrioventricular reentrant tachycardias (AVRT). If such an accessory pathway is capable of anterograde conduction, there may be an initial slow phase of ventricular activation via this abnormal route: hence, a reduced PR interval and a slurred upstroke to the QRS complex, the delta wave. Such an abnormality is found in around 3 per 1000 resting ECGs. The presence of such a resting ECG abnormality, along with tachyarrhythmias, is termed Wolff–Parkinson–White syndrome. Where the accessory pathway is only capable of retrograde conduction, the resting ECG is likely to be normal, although AVRT can still occur. For obvious reasons, the development of AF in patients with an accessory pathway capable of anterograde conduction can be particularly troublesome with ventricular response proceeding at a similar rate. The incidence of atrial flutter and atrial fibrillation is significantly increased in WPW and, although the initial presentation may be with a narrow complex reentrant tachycardia, this may not be the only dysrhythmia to which the patient is susceptible.

During an episode of AVRT, it may be difficult to distinguish WPW from an AV nodal reentrant tachycardia (AVNRT). The distinction, however, is an important one, as the use of AV nodal blocking drugs (such as digoxin and verapamil) may cause preferential activation of the ventricle via the accessory pathway in WPW when the patient develops an atrial dysrhythmia. The use of adenosine acutely in SVT is generally safe, although it is contraindicated in patients known to have WPW, as blockade may precipitate ventricular fibrillation in those presenting with AF.

One of the hallmark features of AVRT or AVNRT to look for is the presence of inverted P waves shortly following the QRS complexes, as abnormal atrial depolarization occurs. The R-P interval is short in AVNRT and long in AVRT (although this is of limited clinical value). Where the accessory pathway is left-sided (as is usually the case), the QRS deflection is likely to be predominantly positive in the anterior leads, which is unusual in other causes of SVT. The drug of choice for the acute treatment of likely AVRT is flecainide. Ablation of the accessory pathway is curative and therefore attractive in those with a history of frequent symptomatic or life-threatening episodes. For the asymptomatic patient, optimal care is rather more difficult to define.

Elongation of the QT interval above the upper limit of the normal range (460 ms) may predispose to VT, which may be polymorphic (*Torsades de Pointes*). The longer the QT interval, the greater is the chance of VT. The core problem in cases of long QT is malfunctioning of the ion channels controlling the speed of repolarization. These ion channels may be inherently abnormal or may have impaired performance due to drugs or electrolyte abnormalities. The congenital types are extremely rare, although a number of genetic irregularities have now been identified, opening up the possibility of specific therapy in the future. Once recognized, treatment is likely to involve β-blockers. On occasion, cardiac sympathectomy may be indicated, although implantable defibrillators have largely superseded this technique. Acquired long QT may be due to deficiencies of calcium, potassium or magnesium. A multitude of drugs prolong the QT interval, including the class-three Vaughan-Williams antiarrhythmics (which rarely induce VT). Among the commoner drugs that may precipitate VT through QT prolongation are the tricyclics, haloperidol, lithium, erythromycin, quinine and the ill-fated antihistamine terfenadine. Treatment involves correction of the electrolyte abnormality or cessation of the incriminated drug.

When to pace

Quite who should and who should not be considered for temporary or permanent pacing is a topic of frequent discussion between on-take physician and cardiologist. Certainly, the number of patients having temporary wires placed has declined in recent decades. There are some good reasons for this, including the reduced burden from peri-infarct ischaemic arrhythmias now that thrombolysis tends to concertina the period of risk. Cutaneous temporary pacing pads are also much more widely available, perhaps reducing the perceived need for 'just-in-case' temporary wires. However, it may be that fewer doctors now feel adequately skilled to carry out this procedure and perhaps, appropriately (assuming an altered risk–benefit), there is more reluctance to proceed.

The broad reasons for cardiac pacing, be it temporary or permanent, are three: for the relief of symptoms, for prognostic benefit and where the reliability of the escape rhythm is felt to be unsound. There are several categories of indication for permanent pacing. Strong indications include third-degree heart block where there is symptomatic bradycardia, an underlying requirement for negatively chronotropic drugs, documented pauses of over 3 s and a resting heart rate below forty when awake or in association with neuromuscular disease. In addition, pacing will be required following AV nodal ablation. Pacing is indicated for second-degree heart block of any type where there is associated symptomatic bradycardia. 'Weaker' indications include patients with first-degree heart block and cardiac failure. Assuming permanent pacing can be carried out within a few days, temporary wires are only required where the bradyarrhythmia is associated (or is likely to become associated) with symptoms of circulatory inadequacy in the resting bed-bound patient. In the case of acute MI, such situations would include symptomatic bradycardia unresponsive to atropine, Mobitz type-2 second-degree block, alternating right and left bundle branch block and trifascicular block (unless it was known to have been present prior to presentation).

The nomenclature of the permanent pacemaker has become increasingly complex as the technology has marched on. In essence, a pacemaker will be ascribed three, four or perhaps more letters. The first two letters refer to the chamber or chambers being paced and being sensed. The third letter describes the pacemaker's response to the sensed impulse (for instance, does the sensed impulse trigger or inhibit a response). The fourth letter denotes whether or not the pacemaker is able to alter its behaviour to suit the underlying heart rate and the extent to which it is programmable. A fifth letter describes the possible response of the unit (if any) to tachyarrhythmia. DDD pacemakers are most frequently implanted at present. In patients with atrial activity, attempts at 'physiological pacing' with dual-chamber systems have become more commonplace. Although intuitive, there is currently little data to suggest any significant benefit in terms of morbidity or mortality.

Jump start

Sudden cardiac death frequently features in the news — promising young athletes suddenly no more. It is important to remember that the local newspaper will have rather less to say about 70-year-old Mr. Smith, an invalid following several infarcts and an amputation, who may also have died rather unexpectedly. Although clearly an extremely important group to address, representing a large slice of total sudden deaths, the incidence of sudden cardiac death in the 'fit' is clearly much lower than in other populations. Now that we have tools with which to treat patients at demonstrably increased risk of sudden cardiac death, difficult and interesting questions arise as to how best to identify such individuals and how much money ought to be spent on this exercise. Although those with a family history of sudden death are an obvious first port of call, most young people dying suddenly have no such history. In around 90%, death unfortunately represents the first and only clinical presentation. Clearly, it is important that appropriate actions are taken to safeguard those who are incidentally discovered to have Brugada, or who have a worrisome ECG when assessed in the light of a relative's sudden death. This is a challenging and controversial area. There is no consensus as to the correct treatment protocol for relatives of young victims of sudden death. Given this situation, decisions are rightly left to electrophysiology subspecialists.

A substantial body of evidence has however been built up as to the benefits that can be accrued through the use of implantable cardioverter-defibrillators (ICD) in patients with poor cardiac function. For secondary prevention (where there is a history of unstable arrhythmias or indeed averted sudden death), the AVID trial demonstrated a 50% reduction in the relative risk of death.[60] In the MADIT-1 trial, patients with a history of nonsustained VT, a low ejection fraction and inducible nonsuppressible ventricular arrhythmia at the time of electrophysiological studies were offered implantable defibrillators. The relative risk of death was reduced by over 60%.[61] In combination, studies suggest that in order to keep an extra person alive 2 years hence, 4 implants need to be used in the secondary prevention population and around 18 for primary prevention. SCD-HEFT demonstrated a 23% reduction in the relative risk of death in patients from Class II or III of the NYHA classification with an ejection fraction of less that 35%, when fitted with an ICD in addition to optimal therapy.[62] It should be noted that the cost of such a device (and its fitting) is in the region of $50,000 US.

[60] AVID Investigators, NEJM (1997) 337: 1576–1583.

[61] Moss *et al.* NEJM (1996) 335: 1933–1948.

[62] SCD-HEFT Investigators, NEJM (2005) 352: 225–237.

The MADIT-2 trial enrolled patients with prior myocardial infarction and an ejection fraction below 30% and randomly offered ICD placement. The trial was stopped early because one-third fewer people died in the treated group.[63] Nothing in medicine is simple though, and another trial reported no survival benefit in a similar group of patients (enrolled very soon after their myocardial infarct).[64] Commentators have proposed that risk stratification and prophylaxis against ventricular dysrhythmias following MI ought wait a while after myocardial perfusion has been restored. Quite how long it should wait remains an unanswered question but, for the moment, MADIT-2 is the guide.

MODERN MANAGEMENT OF VALVULAR HEART DISEASE

As the decades have passed and cardiothoracic experience has been assimilated, the risks of cardiopulmonary bypass and valve replacement have fallen. Over the same period though, the interventional cardiologist has become skilled in various techniques of percutaneous valvuloplasty, in some cases offering a viable alternative to sternotomy and all that it entails. And for those patients undergoing valve replacement, technology has also moved on. The Starr-Edwards (ball and cage) valve introduced in 1960 has now been largely superseded by the Bjork-Shiley (tilting disc) and St. Jude (double-tilting disc) valves as the favoured prostheses. In addition, xenografts and cadaveric valves are becoming more commonplace. Indeed, for some patients, the homograft is very definitely the optimal choice. In the young drug addict, for instance, the ability to avoid warfarin and the reduced risks of recurrent endocarditis make a cadaveric valve ideal. Helpfully, cadaveric valves can be kept on ice for a number of years. Porcine xenografts (Carpentier-Edwards) also have their place and remove the need for anticoagulation. Unfortunately, however, their life expectancy is typically limited to less than 10 years (about right for a pig), and even less when asked to cope with the rigours of the younger adult's circulation. Given all these advances, the indications for valve replacement have altered over the years.

Rheumatic fever is rare now in the West, and mitral stenosis is therefore declining in incidence. It is important to recall some of the less common causes of mitral stenosis, including carcinoid and, of course, the mimics — left atrial myxoma or thrombus (which can coexist with stenosis). In addition to the typical symptoms, it is worth remembering that mitral stenosis can cause

63 Moss *et al.* NEJM (2002) 346: 877–883.
64 Hohnloser *et al.* NEJM (2004) 351: 2481–2488.

right ventricular hypertrophy and angina, even with normal coronaries. The clinical signs of mitral stenosis are of particular interest to the physician as this is the only 'common' valvular disease where the auscultatory findings are likely to reflect the severity of the lesion. In particular, a loud S1 implies that the leaflets are still mobile, and a long murmur in diastole reflects severe stenosis. In general, symptomatic deterioration in mitral stenosis is gradual, although the onset of AF is likely to result in a dramatic decline. Specific treatment is due when symptomatic heart failure develops or the valve area falls to less than 1 cm^2 (the normal being around 5 cm^2). Wherever possible, the native valve should be kept and valvuloplasty or open valvotomy are favoured, assuming there is no left atrial thrombus. Valvuloplasty is performed from the right side of the heart, and the interatrial septum is punctured. A mitral valve replacement is indicated where there is coexistent mitral regurgitation, atrial thrombus, valve calcification or another indication for sternotomy (such as a need for revascularization). Often, a younger patient would undergo 1 or 2 valvuloplasties before proceeding to mitral valve replacement.

The regurgitant mitral valve is now more common than its stenotic brother due to the decline in incidence of rheumatic fever. The severity of mitral regurgitation is sometimes difficult to assess, both clinically and with echocardiography. In acute mitral regurgitation, the murmur may be quiet or absent. In the context of a myocardial infarction, urgent valve repair or replacement is the treatment of choice, as these patients do not respond well to medical therapy.

The spectrum of chronic mitral regurgitation runs from asymptomatic mitral valve prolapse to chronic severe mitral regurgitation with impaired left ventricular function. Prolapse occurs in up to 6% of the population and causes much undue anxiety. Minor degrees of prolapse have no prognostic significance and do not need regular follow-up. High-risk patients are men over 45 years of age and those patients with evidence of leaflet redundancy and significant mitral regurgitation: these patients should be followed up with regular echocardiography. Most patients will require endocarditis prophylaxis, with the exception being those with isolated mid-systolic clicks. Much play has been made of the slight increase in the incidence of sudden death (due to ventricular dysrhythmias) in this condition but there is debate on how this should be assessed and treated: the best guide is to treat just as one would normally manage such ventricular ectopic activity, with reassurance or where there are symptomatic palpitations, β-blockade. Syncope should be taken seriously and investigated accordingly.

Because the left ventricle offloads into a low pressure system in MR, left ventricular dysfunction occurs late. Unfortunately by the time significant left ventricular impairment has occurred, the outcome from repair or replacement is modest: when the ejection fraction falls below 30%, there is little benefit from surgery over medical therapy. The echocardiographic criteria for repair or replacement in patients who are asymptomatic are an ejection fraction of < 60%, an end systolic diameter of over 45 mm or, in the absence of these features, the development of pulmonary hypertension or AF. Decisions are easier when the patient with severe MR becomes symptomatic with breathlessness — referral for surgery is appropriate. Repair is preferable to replacement and the posterior leaflet is easier to repair than the anterior.

Stenosed aortic valves are becoming more commonplace as the population ages and congenitally bicuspid valves have the opportunity to mature and present problems. Indeed, the sclerosed valve is also being diagnosed more frequently. Sclerosis implies thickening and calcification of the aortic valve without significant obstruction to flow and is not entirely benign. There is an excess of cardiac events in patients with aortic sclerosis although it is possible that the calcification is simply a marker of atherosclerosis and calcification in the nearby coronaries. If one chooses to watch a narrowed and stenotic aortic valve, it is likely that the gradient will increase by 5–10 mm of mercury each year. It is usual to recommend replacement of the valve as soon as any attributable symptoms develop or there is any evidence of left ventricular impairment, as untreated, life expectancy in this situation is only around 2 years. In the patient completely free of symptoms, an echocardiogram is due twice yearly at review. Although exercise testing has traditionally been frowned upon in aortic stenosis, it can sometimes be useful in determining the timing of valve replacement: a reduced exercise tolerance or a fall in blood pressure being useful indicators.

If symptoms have appeared, or if the peak velocity across the valve has reached 4 m/s (corresponding to a valve area of less than 0.6 cm^2), surgery beckons. The pressure gradient is not useful in the presence of significant ventricular impairment and the echo technician will assess the valve area in another way. Aortic valve replacement is not to be undertaken lightly in the elderly and consideration of the risk–benefit in the light of comorbidities should be made. However, nor should one be readily put off valve replacement (certainly not on the basis of age alone) as impaired left ventricles can and do recover – sometimes spectacularly. Previously, if the risks of surgery were judged too high, aortic valvuloplasty was occasionally offered, although the results were neither brilliant nor long-lasting and this procedure has been abandoned. Traditionally, ACE inhibitors have been regarded as contraindicated in significant aortic stenosis on the grounds that vasodilatation is potentially dangerous when the left ventricle is unable to respond by increasing cardiac output on account of obstruction to flow. In recent years, a debate has developed around this view.[65] A more moderate stance is now taken and in all but the most severe cases of aortic stenosis, it is recognized that ACE inhibition may in fact delay the progression of aortic valve calcification and perhaps even the development of left ventricular hypertrophy and haemodynamic deterioration. Other pharmacological advances include the proposition that statin therapy may delay the progression of aortic stenosis, independent of cholesterol effects. A modestly sized retrospective analysis of patients with nonrheumatic aortic stenosis certainly provides promising data on statin use, although other studies have been negative.[66] For the moment, surgery is the only therapy for aortic stenosis with a firm footing in evidence.

The words 'aortic regurgitation' are likely to unleash the names of multiple eponymous signs from the brain's archive. It is perhaps more useful however to remember that surgery is again indicated just ahead of irreversible left ventricular damage. Patients with moderate to severe aortic regurgitation should avoid anaerobic exercise. The patient with aortic regurgitation should also be reviewed twice yearly. The onset of symptoms, objective evidence of an enlarging heart or a decline in left ventricular function, is a ticket for theatre. Other sinister signs include a widening of the pulse pressure and the appearance of lateral T wave changes on the ECG.

[65] Cox *et al.* Lancet (1998) 352: 111–112.

[66] Rosenhek *et al.* Circulation (2004) 110: 1291–1295.

Chapter 2

Razeen Mahroof and Jonathan Salmon

HIGH-DEPENDENCY MEDICINE

High-dependency medicine occupies a rather uncertain territory between the general medical ward and intensive care unit (ICU). In the UK, it is conventionally defined by the need to support one failing organ system (other than by intubation and ventilation, which is an intensive care activity) or by a requirement for close monitoring. Historically, many hospitals have had departments that practised a form of high-dependency medicine without ever having defined it as such. They often did an excellent job but were heavily dependent on a local culture that viewed their activities as 'normal'.

At the lowest level, a high-dependency unit (HDU) can be part of a general ward where a few monitors have been added as an afterthought. At the other extreme are purpose-built mini ICUs, distinguishable from their parents only by an absence of ventilators. Superficially, having one's HDU attached to the ICU is attractive. However, transferring all one's sick patients to a separate department risks de-skilling general nursing and medical staff. Demand for intensive care increases by approximately 5% per year and an adjacent HDU is a convenient target for a territorially ambitious ICU director.

The evidence for most HDU treatment is extrapolated from that which appears to work in ICU (which tends to have the slightly unambitious endpoint of survival to 28 days): this may not always be appropriate. An example is the use of activated protein C in sepsis. In patients who are extremely sick it reduces mortality (absolute risk reduction of 7%). In a less sick cohort, the effect is lost.[1,2] Conversely, patients in the very early stages of sepsis may benefit from treatments aimed at increasing cardiac output and tissue oxygen

---

[1] Bernard *et al*. NEJM (2001) 344: 699–709.

[2] Abraham *et al*. NEJM (2001) 353: 1332–1341.

delivery, an approach that also appears to work in pre-operative patients but which does not have the same impact in those with established critical illness.[3]

In ICU, robust outcome studies are a recent development. These have generally been elaborate and expensive multi-centre studies and have, universally, been difficult to organize and administer. In HDU, where mortality is significantly lower, even larger studies will be required to show smaller benefits. These will be time consuming, expensive and hard to perform.

Recognizing the sick patient

Sometimes attributed to Osler, the statement 'patients do not die of their disease, they die of the physiologic consequences of their disease' is particularly pertinent in high dependency medicine. These physiological alterations are often clinically obvious but go unrecognized. Most disease processes will affect the circulation, respiratory or renal function, or level of consciousness, en-route to becoming life threatening. However, in some cases these changes may be subtle or the time period in which intervention may be effective is short.

Monitoring of simple variables such as respiratory and heart rate, blood pressure and level of consciousness can identify patients at increased risk of death. In one study, if two of these were abnormal, patients had a mortality of 9% whereas when three were abnormal, mortality rose to 21%.[4] The majority of patients who suffer a cardiopulmonary arrest in hospital have abnormal vital signs many hours before the event. It has been suggested that at any given time, over 10% of patients in general wards are at risk or have deteriorated to a point where they need care beyond that which can be provided in a normal ward setting. In the UK, where nurse to patient ratios on general wards are low, the presence of a sick patient may consume disproportionate amounts of nursing time and jeopardize the care of other patients. Transferring such patients to an HDU may allow better care of the remaining ward patients.

Several studies have shown that doctors of different grades fail to identify patients who have started to deteriorate or, if they do recognize them to be ill, act inappropriately. On root cause analysis, such failings are often found to be due to long-standing systemic problems, rather than individual error.

If we are going to manage these patients better, we must first identify them and then provide appropriate treatment by the right people in the

---

[3] Rivers et al. NEJM (2001) 345: 1368–1377.

[4] Department of Health, Critical Care Outreach: progress in developing services. Crown, 2003.

right environment. Several systems have been developed to improve identification of patients at risk, including that taught in the ALERT course.[5] Most rely on various combinations of simple clinical observations (such as temperature, heart rate, blood pressure, respiratory rate and conscious level). These systems seem to work well for surgical patients but are harder to calibrate for medical patients who more frequently have multiple co-morbidities and thus higher baseline scores.

Having identified the sick patient and trained a pool of staff to deal with such problems, how does one guarantee a proper and timely response? Approaches vary, from merely informing a passing junior doctor to activating a full-fledged medical emergency team (MET). When these teams were initially introduced, those hospitals that implemented them reported impressive reductions in cardiac arrests, ICU admissions and mortality. However, a recent multi-centre trial in Australia, comparing hospitals where a MET was introduced with those where it was not, has failed to show benefit.[6] This may reflect baseline drift: the MET philosophy is now widely accepted in Australia and it is possible that informal behaviour by individuals has changed such that introducing a formal MET now confers little additional benefit. In the NHS where limited resources require patients to compete for available beds, a MET may allow more timely assessment and risk stratification of sick patients and could therefore be beneficial. This needs to be properly studied.

The clients

The range of possible diagnoses that can lead a patient to HDU is enormous. However, all tend to produce one or more of a limited number of organ failures of which circulatory, respiratory and renal failure are the most important to a general physician. Disorders of other organ systems sufficient to cause referral to critical care rarely exist in isolation – as such, they are more likely to require intensive care admission.

Pump failure

The simplest definition of shock is failure to deliver sufficient oxygen to mitochondria. Causes include sepsis, hypovolaemia, anaphylaxis and cardiac failure as well as spinal injury and cellular poisoning. Shock may be clinically obvious (decompensated) in which the patient is hypotensive, or compensated

---

[5] www.port.ac.uk/special/alert

[6] Hillman *et al.* Lancet (2005) 365: 2091–2097.

where the blood pressure is maintained. Compensated shock may be described as overt if there are clinically obvious features of circulatory embarrassment (including oliguria and tachycardia) or covert if the only abnormalities are biochemical (such as a high lactate). Alternatively, it may require invasive monitoring to identify. There are numerous physiological responses to early shock, including diversion of blood away from the splanchnic circulation leading to failure of gut mucosal barrier function.

Translocation of bacteria across the gut mucosa is one of several possible mechanisms by which shock can produce a systemic inflammatory response: the important aspect of these phenomena is that they can occur before shock becomes overt. This has two major clinical consequences. First, patients may develop organ failure without ever showing unequivocal evidence of shock. Second, although overt, decompensated shock is easy to recognize, it is more difficult to be certain that a patient has been fully resuscitated.

Assessing the circulation

Ideally, one would like a monitor that can recognize changes in regional perfusion of vulnerable tissues reproducibly, non-invasively and cheaply. In the absence of such a device, a simple, pragmatic approach involves asking five questions of the circulation: are the heart rate and rhythm efficient; is the blood pressure sufficient to perfuse the brain, heart and kidneys; is tissue perfusion adequate; is there evidence of hypovolaemia and is the cardiac output (and hence tissue oxygen delivery) appropriate for tissue requirements?

Which pressure should one measure? In ICU, it is conventional to focus on the mean arterial pressure (diastolic BP + 1/3 pulse pressure) and this is also the most appropriate pressure to monitor in HDU, particularly if invasive monitoring is being used. The usual target pressure in an ICU patient is between 60 and 80 mmHg. Chronically hypertensive patients and those with cerebrovascular disease or raised intracranial pressure may require higher mean arterial pressures to maintain cerebral perfusion.

Diastolic blood pressure determines coronary perfusion. Patients with normal mean but low diastolic pressures are at risk of myocardial ischaemia, particularly if they have hypertrophied ventricles. Arbitrarily, a diastolic pressure above 35 mmHg seems a reasonable target. The most effective and controllable way to raise the diastolic pressure is by norepinephrine infusion. Systolic pressure is probably the least important as far as organ perfusion is concerned but is the most reproducible measurement, without recourse to invasive monitoring.

Where a major arterial dissection or rupture is a possibility, one should also take account of pulse pressure. If this is wide, shear stress on the vessel wall is increased. The rate of change of pressure is also important. This is the rationale for using β-blockers as part of one's initial conservative treatment for dissection as negative inotropy slows the rate of rise of aortic pressure and so reduces wall stress. Vasodilators alone may reduce mean arterial pressure without affecting pulse pressure. Whichever drug is used initially, it should be short-acting – distinguishing between hypotension due to aortic rupture and iatrogenic drug overdose can otherwise be difficult.

Capillary refill time is a crude but traditional measure of tissue perfusion and is perhaps more useful for initial assessment than for continuous monitoring. Hourly urine output provides a convenient assessment of changing renal function – the ideal of 0.5 ml/kg/h works well for normal-sized patients but needs adaptation towards ideal body weight in the very obese, most of whose excess weight should be regarded as metabolically redundant. Blood gases provide a convenient way to detect and follow metabolic acidosis (and for this purpose, central venous samples are as useful as arterial samples).

The base excess/deficit (normal range 0 ± 2 mmol/l) is a convenient thought-free way of assessing the metabolic component of a pH disturbance but cannot be interpreted in isolation. Traditionally, a base deficit (negative base excess) worse than 5 mmol/l is regarded as 'worrying' and worse than 10 as 'dire'. However, this assumes lactic acidosis as the cause.

The four most common causes of a metabolic acidosis in clinical practice are lactic acidosis (most commonly due to circulatory failure), diabetic keto-acidosis, renal dysfunction and hyperchloraemia – usually iatrogenic due to sodium chloride administration. The other important source of confusion is the patient with a pre-existing acid–base disorder. In this context, hypoalbuminaemia, hypochloraemia, potassium depletion and chronic hyper-capnia all produce metabolic alkaloses and can lead one to underestimate the severity of a subsequent metabolic acidosis. Blood lactate concentration is commonly assumed to reflect the degree of tissue hypoxia or failure of peripheral conversion of lactate to bicarbonate. High blood lactate concentrations may be seen in any shock state, in liver dysfunction and a variety of metabolic disorders. Iatrogenic causes include metformin in patients with renal dysfunction, theophylline infusions and epinephrine infusions in patients with limited cardiac output. Generous infusion of Hartmann's solution can also lead to modest increases in blood lactate.

Very few sick patients escape hypovolaemia, the usual question is: 'how bad is it'? If volume depletion did not cause the problem in the first place, inflam-mation and capillary leak will produce tissue oedema at the expense of circu-lating volume. In turn, oedema tends to stimulate an inappropriate diuretic response from the attending physician. There is no evidence that crystalloid is better or worse than colloid, and no basis for choosing a specific fluid other than its side effect profile, its cost and one's own prejudices. Colloids are very expensive and crystalloids are cheap. Whichever replacement fluid is used, there is general agreement that one should give 'enough' – though everybody seems to define this differently. The traditional belief has been that one needs to give only one-third as much colloid as crystalloid (because colloid is confined to the vascular compartment while crystalloid diffuses throughout the extracellular space). Like many traditional beliefs, this has been questioned. A recent, very large multi-centre Australian study compared albumin and saline in acute fluid resuscitation.[7] During the study period, the ratio of saline to albumin administered was approximately three to two. However, this reflects total fluid administration during the study period. In the very short-term (during resuscitation), colloids are probably retained in the circulation sufficiently well that our traditional beliefs remain valid. In practice, there seems little reason for continuing to use colloids such as gelatins, which have similar physical properties to albumin. Hydroxyethyl starches, which contain significantly larger molecules, may still have a limited place but are relatively expensive.

Judging when a patient has received 'enough' fluid is difficult without some form of invasive monitoring. The most convenient approach is to give fluid challenges guided by a central venous catheter. There are two important principles behind this. The first is that the static central venous pressure (CVP) is a poor guide to intravascular volume and it is difficult to predict what the optimal pressure is for any individual, particularly as most shocked or septic patients develop a degree of diastolic dysfunction and require higher ventricular filling pressures than their healthy counterparts. The second is that if one gives a short-lived fluid infusion into an empty circulation, the pressure will rise transiently then fall again. If the circulation is full the rise in pressure will be sustained. One can give 500 ml of crystalloid over 15 min and then stop infusing for a further 15 min to observe the response (250 ml of crystalloid can be given if the patient is particularly frail). If the circulation is full, the CVP will rise by 2 mmHg (3 cm H_2O) or more during the infusion and will remain more than 2 mmHg higher than the starting pressure 15 min after the infusion has stopped. Failure of the CVP to rise during the infusion implies that the circulation is empty. Exaggerated rises may reflect oddities in the function of the right ventricular or pulmonary vessels, or simply suggest that the circulation is full.

....

[7] SAFE Investigators, NEJM (2004) 350: 2247–2256.

Much of the mystique surrounding the ICU is based on complex monitoring of cardiac output and subsequent manipulation of the circulation. Strategies to increase tissue perfusion (by increasing cardiac output) have been shown to improve mortality in peri-operative patients but using inotropes to increase cardiac output in the patient with well-established critical illness has been shown to be ineffective. These studies used cardiac output (or surrogates) as their endpoints rather than assessing the adequacy of tissue perfusion. However, one study has shown that very early treatment to improve cardiac output (started in the emergency department) may reduce mortality in severe sepsis from 46 to 31%.[8] This study used central venous oxygen saturation ($S_{cv}O_2$) as a surrogate for cardiac output. If $S_{cv}O_2$ appeared inadequate, cardiac output and tissue oxygen delivery were increased using blood, fluids and dobutamine infusions. This study has yet to be repeated.

Mixed venous and central venous oxygen saturation

The true mixed venous oxygen saturation (S_vO_2) is measured in the pulmonary artery and provides an estimate of how well-matched cardiac output is to global tissue oxygen utilization. If demand exceeds supply, a greater proportion of the delivered oxygen is extracted and the venous oxygen content falls. The normal O_2 saturation is 75%; low levels (below 60%) imply minimal cardiac reserve and carry a poor prognosis, particularly in cardiogenic shock. To measure S_vO_2 requires a pulmonary artery catheter, a device which is unfashionable in many ICUs and unwelcome in most HDUs. $S_{cv}O_2$, the central venous saturation, is a reasonable surrogate and can be obtained by taking a blood gas sample from the superior vena cava (though not the IVC or right atrium) where the saturation is 5–10% higher and an arbitrary value of 70% can be taken as a threshold below which oxygen delivery may be critically low and intervention may be useful. This can be measured continuously and expensively using a catheter designed for the purpose or intermittently and cheaply by taking samples from a conventional central venous catheter.

Vasoactive drugs

Vasoactive drugs can most easily be classified by their main effects. Effectively there are four categories of drug to consider: 'pure' vasoconstrictors (norepinephrine); ino-constrictors (epinephrine and dopamine); ino-dilators (dobutamine) and vasodilators (glyceryl trinitrate). In addition, there are drugs with inotropic

----

8 Rivers *et al.* NEJM (2001) 345: 1368–1377.

properties that may be useful occasionally (e.g. glucagon and digoxin). These drugs are fairly well understood, inexpensive and will cover most situations. Levosimendan, a new inotrope that acts by calcium sensitization is promising. Patients with poor perfusion and low blood pressure may be treated with dopamine or epinephrine infusions. An alternative is to combine norepinephrine and dobutamine (though preferably via separate lumina on the central venous cannula).

General approach to overt, decompensated shock

Distinguishing between causes of shock can be surprisingly difficult in the early stages and a clear diagnosis may only become apparent after resuscitation. The immediate priorities are airway, breathing and blood pressure followed by general circulatory resuscitation. At the bedside, there is usually time to administer a fluid challenge while someone is preparing a vasoactive infusion and, in most cases, this will be appropriate. If the blood pressure is frighteningly low, small boluses of epinephrine from a minijet (0.25–0.5 ml of 1:10,000 solution, flushed with saline) repeated as required may salvage the situation. Bear in mind that the circulation time is likely to be prolonged and one may not see an effect for 60 s or so (it will feel longer). Thereafter, the choice of drugs depends upon the likely cause.

In all except cardiogenic and spinal shock, the most important aspect of resuscitation is to provide an adequate circulating volume. Large volumes of fluid may be required. Enough has probably been given if a fluid challenge produces a sustained rise in CVP and the $S_{cv}O_2$ does not increase further. If the circulation remains inadequate, and is not restored with vasoactive drugs, there is little else to be done.

In cardiogenic shock, norepinephrine is probably the most effective drug to support the blood pressure. If perfusion remains inadequate ($S_{cv}O_2$ and serum lactate provide the most convenient initial estimates – both can be obtained from the same central venous sample), adding dobutamine in low doses may be useful. Dopamine or epinephrine are viable alternatives to norepinephrine but will tend to increase myocardial oxygen consumption. Mechanical assistance (e.g. intra-aortic balloon counterpulsation) should be considered as a bridge to definitive treatment in acute coronary syndromes. Similarly, mechanical ventilation may be life saving. If diastolic dysfunction seems likely, maintaining diastolic blood pressure and controlling heart rate are critical. If, in addition, left ventricular outflow is impaired (aortic stenosis, classical HOCM) one should avoid vasodilators: using norepinephrine, epinephrine or dopamine. One must remember that pulmonary embolus, pericardial tamponade and tension pneumothorax can produce apparent cardiogenic shock and require rather different treatment. Cardiogenic shock due to drug overdose (β-blockers, some calcium antagonists and tricyclic antidepressants) may be better treated with glucagon – in the last case, very high doses have been reported to work when conventional doses have failed.[9]

Spinal shock can be regarded as extreme vasodilatation without a compensatory increase in heart rate. Vasopressors are most effective. Atropine or glycopyrrolate may be useful if heart rate is very low.

Respiratory inadequacy

The conventional classification of respiratory failure into types 1 and 2 is of limited value. The more important questions are: how severe is the oxygenation deficit, is ventilation compromised, does the patient need ventilatory support and, finally, what type of support would be appropriate?

Type 1 respiratory failure is defined as a $P_aO_2 < 8$ kPa when breathing air but, as most breathless patients are given oxygen, this may not be particularly helpful. One could remove the oxygen mask and measure arterial blood gases sometime later, but not all patients will survive this manoeuvre. An alternative is to work out how much lower the P_aO_2 is than one would expect for a given FiO_2. This can be done accurately using the simplified alveolar gas equation which allows one to calculate the alveolar partial pressure of oxygen (P_aO_2) and then applying a small correction for physiological shunt. However, it is almost as accurate to assume that if the patient's lungs were perfect, the P_aO_2 would be approximately 10 kPa less than the inspired percentage of oxygen (8 kPa less if the FiO_2 is less than 0.35). If the actual P_aO_2 is less than a third of the predicted value, the patient has severe respiratory failure and should be watched closely. Most such patients do not require ventilatory support (any patient receiving 50% oxygen with a P_aO_2 of 13 kPa falls into this category) but they do have limited reserve and may deteriorate rapidly.

Although usually obvious, the diagnosis of ventilatory failure can be difficult. The question should not be, is the P_aCO_2 elevated, but rather, is it higher than one would expect? A high P_aCO_2 indicates hypoventilation but this may be a physiological response to a profound metabolic alkalosis. Similarly, a 'normal' P_aCO_2 is inappropriate in a patient with a metabolic acidosis and should also be regarded as constituting ventilatory failure. Far too frequently, people assume that hypercapnia implies chronic CO_2 retention, hypoxic drive and turn the inspired oxygen down. However, hypercapnia occurs as a pre-terminal event in almost all cases of respiratory and cardiac failure. Therapeutic hypoxia may be

---

[9] Sensky *et al.* Postgrad Med J (1999) 75: 611–612.

appropriate in the patient with end-stage respiratory disease who will not tolerate non-invasive ventilation. In all others, one should use oxygen to correct hypoxia and ventilation to control CO_2.

It is important to distinguish between intubation and ventilatory support. Intubation is required to bypass airway obstruction, to defend the airway if the patient's own protective reflexes are not working or to assist in clearance of secretions.

Patients who do not need intubation may be managed, at least temporarily, with non-invasive mask ventilation (NIV) or continuous positive airway pressure (CPAP). Both require a co-operative patient and neither is easy to tolerate for prolonged periods though improvements in mask design and regular changes of mask (such as nasal to full-face) can be helpful.

CPAP

In addition to its well-established effects on the upper airway in obstructive sleep apnoea, CPAP has pulmonary and cardiovascular effects. If positive pressure is applied to the airway, expiration ends at a higher lung volume. This increases the effective alveolar volume, increasing the surface area available for gas exchange and tends to improve oxygenation. In most cases, particularly if the lungs are oedematous, the increased volume reduces the effects of surface tension and also reduces work of breathing. However, if the lungs are hyper-inflated or if the chest wall is abnormal, work of breathing may be increased. Similarly, over-distension of alveoli may jeopardize alveolar perfusion and increase dead-space, causing P_aCO_2 to rise. The main cardiovascular effect is to increase intrathoracic pressure, reducing venous return and thus right and left ventricular diastolic filling. This may be particularly useful in acute left ventricular failure.

CPAP has been shown to improve oxygenation in hypoxic patients and to improve outcome in acute severe left ventricular failure. In the latter context, it may also reduce hypercapnia when this occurs as part of terminal ventilatory failure. It is potentially hazardous in airway obstruction. In most patients with primary lung pathology, improvements in oxygenation are not matched by a reduction in the need for intubation and ventilation. It should, therefore, be regarded as a holding measure, whilst anaesthetic help is sought, rather than a definitive treatment.

NIV

Non-invasive ventilation (NIV) is usually taken to mean positive pressure ventilation via a face mask. The haemodynamic and respiratory effects are similar to CPAP but, because it assists inspiration, work of breathing should be further reduced. In practice, this depends upon reasonable synchronization between the ventilator and the patient's own ventilatory efforts. It is of unequivocal benefit in patients with infective exacerbations of COPD where early (and perhaps intermittent) use can reduce fatigue and prevent further deterioration.[10] In patients with advanced exacerbations, it is less successful (though still worth trying if intubation is not an option).

Use of NIV in other situations is controversial. Although it may reduce work of breathing, aid CO_2 clearance and improve oxygenation, it does not help and may even hinder secretion clearance. There is no evidence that it reduces intubation rates in patients with pneumonia. In theory it should be effective in left ventricular failure but the evidence is contradictory. This may be because most of the early studies used relatively unsophisticated ventilators and synchronization between patient and machine was poor. Anecdotal ICU experience is that NIV can be highly effective in LVF: an up-to-date trial is needed.

COPD apart, NIV is best regarded as a technique to be used in an ICU setting where there are very good reasons for avoiding intubation (e.g. the immunosuppressed patient) rather than as an HDU technique. Side effects include gastric distension due to swallowed air. This may interfere with ventilation and, in any patient undergoing prolonged CPAP or NIV, it is sensible to place a nasogastric tube.

Renal failure

From an HDU perspective, the key questions are, is there a pre-renal (circulatory) problem, is there an obstructive component and can the patient be managed conservatively or is artificial support required? Many patients have multiple contributory causes: it is sensible to ensure the circulation is fully resuscitated and it is embarrassing not to have checked that the urinary catheter is patent and all nephrotoxic drugs have been stopped. Indications that help should be sought sooner rather than later are: high potassium levels, fluid overload, severe metabolic acidosis and hypercatabolic states (e.g. creatinine concentration rising by more than 150 µmol/day). Renal failure in the context of sepsis or other organ dysfunction should usually be referred to the ICU rather than a renal unit unless the two units are co-located. If the patient is producing some urine, there is a temptation to encourage a little more with furosemide: this may make one feel better but probably will not make much difference to the patient.

---

[10] Kinnear *et al.* Thorax (2002) 57: 192–211.

If the kidneys have failed, options for support include haemofiltration and haemodialysis. Haemofiltration is less efficient at solute removal than dialysis but it has the advantages of simplicity and less haemodynamic disturbance. Both techniques allow precise control of fluid balance and can usually control most metabolic disturbances (including hypo- and hyperthermia). Dialysis is more effective in drug overdose and is more convenient for stable patients with isolated renal dysfunction. It may also be safer in patients with bleeding disorders in whom one wishes to avoid systemic anticoagulation.

Sepsis

Sepsis is the most common reason to admit a medical patient to HDU and is associated with a high rate of progression to ICU and subsequent mortality. The basics of treatment have not changed for many years: source control (removal, where possible, of infected material), appropriate use of broad-spectrum antibiotics and adequate (i.e. enthusiastic) fluid resuscitation. It is probably reasonable to try to optimize the circulation (i.e. use fluids and dobutamine to raise the $S_{cv}O_2$ above 70%) if treatment can be started in the first few hours, otherwise a more conservative approach may be sensible. Other treatments, such as activated protein C (drotrecogin alpha), are applicable only to intensive care patients with multiple organ failure. Current evidence suggests it has a modest effect in the critically ill but no effect in less severe illness, where harms may outweigh benefits. It is not a relevant treatment for HDU patients.

Recently, a large series of evidence-based guidelines, termed the 'surviving sepsis campaign' has been produced.[11] This has been widely adopted in many ICUs. The document provides an excellent synthesis of treatments that may help in sepsis and is worth reading. However, much of the evidence is weak. Whether the recommendations should be applied to all ICU patients is questionable; further generalization to HDU may be naïve.

Treatment limitation

Traditionally, for a patient to be admitted to ICU, the implications were that the disease process was fully reversible and no prior restrictions were placed on the treatment offered. As the population ages and attitudes change, more patients with major co-morbidities are accepted by ICUs. Many of these patients are admitted with limited treatment goals and an understanding that

---

[11] Surviving Sepsis Campaign Guidelines, Crit Care Med (2004) 32: 858–872.

failure to respond to treatment in an appropriate timescale or development of new organ failures should lead to palliation rather than escalation.

A similar philosophy may be even more appropriate in HDU. It is probably better to offer a short, sharp course of aggressive HDU treatment to frail patients with single organ failure (e.g. sepsis and circulatory embarrassment or exacerbations of COPD) rather than exposing them to a prolonged 'trial of survival' on a general ward. Those who fail to respond are unlikely to survive ICU admission and it may be appropriate to limit treatment in these cases. Such decisions should be taken early and proactively to avoid misunderstandings. Similarly, terminal illness should not be an absolute contraindication to HDU admission. Patients with severe pain or distress can be difficult to manage on a busy general ward and an HDU may provide an environment where regional anaesthesia and intravenous analgesics and sedatives can be provided safely.

Chapter 3

Jamie Coleman and Robin Ferner

POISONING

Many are called but few are chosen

While overdose and poisoning are very common reasons for acute admission
to hospital in the United Kingdom, death after reaching hospital is thankfully
rare. Most deaths occur in adults who intend to kill themselves. They take large
overdoses and shun medical assistance, presenting late. A few deaths occur
from the delayed effects of poisoning or due to the inadequate treatment
of poisoned patients. The role of the admitting physician is to avoid this,
so one is wise to treat all poisoned patients as if they have taken a potentially
life-threatening intoxication until proven otherwise.

What's your poison?

So what is a poison? This question was answered by Paracelsus who coined the
catchy phrase 'Dosis sola facit venenum' – only the dose makes it a poison.[1]
In other words, everything is poisonous in high enough doses. Think of oxygen
toxicity, poisoning with table salt and water intoxication. All drugs have
adverse effects, and toxic adverse effects are simply those that appear at doses
or concentrations higher than those normally used for therapy.

The commonest drugs taken in overdose are paracetamol, benzodiazepines
and antidepressants. In some parts of the country, heroin and other opioids are
catching up. Guidance concerning the diagnosis, treatment and management of
most poisons can be found on the internet from the primary clinical toxicology
database in the UK, TOXBASE.[2] The UK National Poisons Information Service
(NPIS), which directs callers to the appropriate regional clinical toxicology centre,

---

[1] Borzelleca, Toxicol Sci (2000) 53: 2–4.

[2] www.spib.axl.co.uk

can help with specialist medical advice on unfamiliar poisons, cases of life-threatening poisoning and special patient groups (e.g. children and pregnancy).

Identification of the poison may be straightforward if the history is complete and further management can then be guided by the drug, dose, formulation and timing. Where one does not know exactly what was taken, a collateral history can sometimes be obtained from the patient's significant other or rescuer. Here the 'Sherlock Holmes' approach can help establish a diagnosis; a search may yield empty drug containers, tablets, capsules, or other clues.

Drug poisoning can present as unconsciousness, drowsiness or bizarre behaviour. Put another way, any unconscious or drowsy patient and any patient behaving bizarrely could be poisoned. When in doubt, rule it out.

Mixed poisonings are quite common. They can arise either from co-ingestion (for example, taking alcohol and a benzodiazepine) or from compound preparations such as co-codamol (paracetamol is contained in more than 100 over-the-counter drug preparations). The assessment and management of patients who have taken a mixture of drugs (especially with alcohol) can be challenging.

The long and the short of it

Most poisoning we see is the result of a single large exposure and the effects appear within minutes to hours. There are some poisons that accumulate and cause problems only after long-term ingestion. Effects may not become manifest for months or years after exposure begins. Chronic poisoning can produce smouldering symptoms and signs that can be misinterpreted as natural disease before the diagnosis becomes apparent. Heavy metal poisoning from mercury and lead are classic examples. Some poisoning is both inadvertent and indolent – for example, the poorly maintained gas flue.

How bad is it, Doc?

Risk is the probability that some hazard will cause harm. In cases of poisoning there are risks of injury to staff as well as patients; although usually small, staff risks are not negligible. Injudicious management of patients attacked with tear gas, for example, can disrupt the whole Emergency Department and beyond. Life-threatening hazards include the management of patients poisoned with the most potent organophosphorus war agents, such as Sarin, and with cyanides (mouth-to-mouth resuscitation is a poor idea). If chemical contamination is a potential risk, the Regional Chemical Hazards Centres of the Health Protection Agency (in the UK) can help.[3] In response to current

---

[3] The Health Protection Agency also has special Chemical Hazards and Poisons Divisions, for details see their website www.hpa.org.uk

perceived terrorist threats, many more emergency departments now have decontamination units.

In, out, swirl it all about

Some revision of pharmacokinetics, often called toxicokinetics in the context of poisoning, may help clinicians understand the principles of managing poisoning and treat individual patients. The basic pharmacological principles are the same as with any drug. First, the drug must get into the system (absorption); then it must go to the organs, tissues and cells (distribution) to reach the site of action; then it undergoes chemical transformation in the body (metabolism) and finally it leaves the body, usually via the kidneys (elimination). The effects of a drug are in part determined by each of these four processes.

Most poisons are taken by mouth, but toxic effects can occur after inhalation (e.g. carbon monoxide), injection (e.g. intravenous opiates) or absorption through the skin (e.g. fluoric acid). When tablets are taken by mouth, they must dissolve before they can be absorbed from the gastrointestinal tract. Enteric-coated tablets and modified-release formulations may delay absorption and hence the onset of poisoning. Also, in a large overdose, partially dissolved tablets (e.g. aspirin) can coalesce to form tablet bezoars (concretions) in the stomach, again delaying the absorption of the drug. Some drugs, for example, those with anticholinergic effects and opioids, slow gastric emptying, and so also delay absorption. In all these cases of potentially slow absorption, one has to anticipate that poisoning will be delayed, and ask for adequate observations and laboratory monitoring, for an appropriate time.

The process of drug movement through the body is termed distribution. For those substances that remain in the bloodstream (such as heparin), their volume of distribution (V_d) is equivalent to the blood volume. Some substances, such as alcohol, are distributed in total body water ($V_d \sim 50$ l). Where the substance leaves the bloodstream and is preferentially bound in deep body tissues such as fat, the volume of distribution can be much greater. The V_d for amitriptyline is about 1000 l. This is important if one considers 'purifying the blood,' for example, by haemodialysis. This only removes the drug from circulating blood. If the drug is only being extracted from 5 l out of a 1000, there is no hope of removing worthwhile amounts.

Gut decontamination – vomiting is messy (and unhelpful)

Gut decontamination attempts to prevent a drug being absorbed after it has been swallowed. While gut decontamination sounds like a good idea and the popular image of 'pumping out the stomach' persists, there is very little evidence that induced vomiting or gastric lavage will remove appreciable quantities of poison and abundant evidence that both procedures can cause harm. Ipecacuanha, a potent emetic that can cause vomiting in 20 min, is no longer recommended because it can cause central nervous system depression and also delay more effective treatments.[4] Gastric lavage can result in aspiration, laryngospasm and arrhythmia. There is some evidence that it can make poisoning worse by washing drugs into the small intestine. Given these limitations, it is probably best to avoid the procedure unless persuasively recommended by an expert.

Activated charcoal has largely replaced other decontamination techniques and is used as first-line treatment to adsorb many poisons. It is a fine, black powder produced by burning organic materials and treating the residue with chemicals or steam to remove impurities and increase its available surface area. A standard dose of 50 g has the surface area of 50,000–100,000 m^2 (the average on-call room has a floor area of under 10 m^2). It only adsorbs those poisons that can be held in its many pores and therefore, it is ineffective for small ions such as lithium and potassium, or for some organic compounds such as alcohol and paraffin. The charcoal is not absorbed into the body, it passes through the gastrointestinal system and is eliminated with the bound substance in the faeces.

Get rid quick – active elimination techniques

Multiple-dose activated charcoal can enhance the elimination of drug already absorbed, either by acting as a sink for drugs drawn into the gut (if there is a concentration gradient across the gut wall) or by interrupting entero-hepatic recirculation. It can enhance the elimination of several drugs, including tricyclic antidepressants and carbamazepine. Despite the theory, it has not been demonstrated to improve clinical outcomes.

'Dialysis techniques' are used to clear those drugs that have a small V_d from the plasma. Haemodialysis works by passing blood across a semi-permeable membrane. It is most useful where there is severe metabolic disturbance (for example, in the treatment of poisoning with salicylates or metformin) or where the poison can itself affect renal function, as with lithium. Haemofiltration is more widely available than haemodialysis and is effective at removing some drugs. There are reported successes of its use in lithium poisoning as well as in removing iron and digoxin complexes. Haemoperfusion, where blood is passed across an absorptive charcoal column, is now rarely used.

---

[4] The root of Cephaëlis ipecacuanha, a South American small shrubby plant, which possesses emetic, diaphoretic and purgative properties. Oxford English Dictionary. 2nd Ed, Oxford University Press, Oxford, 1989.

Toxidromes – pictures of poisoning

When a reliable history is not available, the presence of symptoms and signs characteristic of a particular group of poisons, the toxidrome, allows the astute physician to impress onlookers by confidently pronouncing on the most likely cause and instituting the correct treatment. The most telling clues come from a small number of observations that can become routine: What is the patient's general state (so agitated that the hospital's security staff cannot hold him down or so deeply unconscious that the anaesthetist is already there)? Is the pulse fast or slow? What is the respiratory rate? What is the pupil size? Are the tendon reflexes brisk or depressed? What are the temperature and blood pressure?

It is sometimes difficult to be sure whether a patient has taken an anticholinergic drug rather than a sympathatomimetic, since both can cause agitation, pupillary dilatation and tachycardia. In this situation, a normal blood pressure, absence of sweating and urinary retention point towards the former, while hypertension, sweating and normal micturition suggest the latter. When multiple drugs are involved, there are often mixed features with no identifiable toxidrome.

GENERAL PRINCIPLES

Careful observation and supportive care are the mainstays of management for many poisons. Any patient who has taken a potentially serious overdose should be observed for at least 6 h before discharge from medical care. A dramatic collapse can be rather satisfying to deal with under the bright lights of the resus room; less so in the corner of the outlying gynaecology ward. All patients who have required resuscitation, those who develop complications during admission and those who need active elimination techniques, need intensive care or high dependency observation.

Anti-this and anti-that (antidotes and antibodies)

Sometimes one can use specific treatments – antidotes – to counter-act the poison. Different antidotes work in different ways, including antagonism at receptor level (naloxone), enzyme inhibition (fomepizole), binding the toxic substance (desferrioxamine) and other collateral effects (preventing cellular damage with acetylcysteine). Beware! Randomized controlled trials are lacking for many of the treatments used in poisoning. As a result, there are different 'vogues' of management and today's treatment may itself be tomorrow's poison. Hot coffee enemas are no longer recommended to treat opioid poisoning.

The decision to use an antidote may not be straightforward, even where the poison is known and an antidote exists. For example, as many as 15% of patients treated with acetylcysteine for paracetamol poisoning may develop anaphylactoid reactions. Cobalt edetate (used as an antidote in cyanide poisoning) is itself cardiotoxic if there is insufficient cyanide present to bind the cobalt.

The appropriate use of the laboratory in managing poisoned patients

There is an old adage that one should not ask for a test if the result will not change management. This is especially true in managing poisoned patients, so consider carefully what tests should be requested and how they could help. Often, no tests will be necessary. Sometimes, qualitative tests – for example, for the presence of opioids in urine – will suffice and no quantitative tests are needed.

While many junior doctors and nurses request salicylate concentrations as well as paracetamol levels when they send samples on poisoned patients, there is little justification for this, since symptoms, signs and disturbances of acid-base balance will reveal significant salicylate poisoning in adults. 'Toxicology screens' are not very helpful.

Quantitative results help in some cases of acute poisoning

Paracetamol	Guide to antidotal therapy
Anticonvulsants: carbamazepine, phenytoin and sodium valproate	Especially important if the patient is epileptic and may develop status with low concentrations
Lithium	Guide to dialysis (remember not to use a lithium-heparin tube)
Carbon monoxide (HbCO)	Guide to continuing oxygen therapy
Iron	Guide to antidotal therapy
Digoxin	Guide to dosage of digoxin-binding antibodies
Methanol and ethylene glycol	Guide to antidotal therapy or dialysis
Salicylate	Guide to dialysis

Adapted from Olson.[5]

If there is doubt as to whether toxicology tests might be helpful, samples of heparinized blood, serum and urine should be taken and kept refrigerated. It is better to discard an unused sample in a recovered patient than to never have taken it, only to regret it later.

X-ray screening can be useful to confirm ingestion of radio-opaque tablets (such as ferrous sulphate) and can show packages of cocaine, heroin or other drugs swallowed or 'packed' by smugglers ('mules').

Electrocardiography is important in assessing cardiovascular risks of drugs that can cause ventricular arrhythmia (e.g. tricyclic antidepressants); QT-prolongation

[5] Olson, Poisoning & Drug Overdose. 4th Ed, McGraw-Hill, New York, 2004.

(e.g. chloroquine) and bradycardia and complete heart block (e.g. calcium antagonists).

SPECIFIC POISONS

Paracetamol

Paracetamol poisoning is common. As little as 7.5 g can cause toxicity and greater than 10 g is potentially fatal in an adult. While morbidity and mortality from paracetamol poisoning has fallen in the UK in recent years, this is most likely due to the restriction in 1998 of pack sizes available for public sale, rather than any change in medical management.

Untreated patients are at first asymptomatic, with biochemical evidence of hepatotoxicity developing 24–48 h after ingestion and peak signs of liver failure occurring 72–96 h after exposure. In the most severe cases, there can be an early and severe lactic acidosis, so measurement of venous bicarbonate concentration can guide the need for urgent assistance in management.[6] Drugs that induce liver metabolism increase the amount of toxic paracetamol metabolite (N-acetyl-p-benzoquinoneimine) produced and malnutrition reduces the amount of sulphur-containing amino acid available to mop it up. It follows that drugs that induce hepatic metabolism, for example, carbamazepine, phenytoin and alcohol ingested chronically increase the risk of severe liver damage. So too do HIV, anorexia nervosa, repeated overdose and other conditions that deplete stores of sulphur-containing amino acids.

Acetylcysteine, which provides exogenous sulphydryl groups, prevents serious liver damage in patients with potentially severe poisoning provided that it is given within 8 h of ingestion. The longer the treatment is delayed after 8 h, the more likely it is that some damage will occur. It should still be given as fears that it might make matters worse in late paracetamol poisoning are ungrounded. It is of demonstrated value in patients who present so late that they already have hepatic encephalopathy. The decision to treat is based upon the paracetamol level taken within a 4- to 16-h window, guided by the familiar nomogram.

The first part of the acetylcysteine treatment course is given to increase plasma concentrations rapidly and replenish liver sulphydryl groups before the damage is done. However, it is also prone to cause the release of histamine and other mediators from mast cells, and it may therefore provoke urticaria, wheeze and hypotension. This anaphylactoid reaction usually occurs early in

[6] Volans *et al.* Clin Med (2003) 3: 119–123.

treatment when the infusion rate is highest. If the reaction does occur, the infusion ought to be stopped and chlorphenamine (chlorpheniramine) given. Salbutamol may also be helpful. Once the reaction has subsided, the treatment can be recommenced at half the previous infusion rate. One must then ensure that the whole dose is given (over a longer timeframe than originally planned).

When patients present late with high paracetamol concentrations or when they have abnormal liver function, a raised creatinine level, severe acidosis or a raised and increasing prothrombin time despite treatment, it is best to seek specialist advice sooner rather than later for consideration of transplantation.

Salicylates

Serious salicylate poisoning is now rather rare in the UK. Poisoned patients usually have gastrointestinal upset but tinnitus is the cardinal symptom. This can lead to deafness and a rather distracted patient. Epigastric tenderness, tachypnoea and sweating can be present but are non-specific. Occasionally, patients develop non-cardiogenic pulmonary oedema, or hypoglycaemia with convulsions.

One should also suspect salicylate poisoning in a patient who has an otherwise unexplained metabolic acidosis with a high anion gap. These biochemical findings narrow the toxicological differential diagnosis considerably although methanol, ethylene glycol and isoniazid poisoning can also be responsible.

The management is not straightforward. Some patients will have few symptoms and no biochemical disturbance with plasma salicylate concentrations within the therapeutic range (up to 250 mg/l). They can be given repeated doses of activated charcoal to prevent further absorption and only require rehydration, potassium replacement and supportive treatment. Others will have very severe acid–base disturbance. If, in addition, the plasma salicylate concentration is very high (over 700 mg/l), then haemodialysis is usually the treatment of choice since it allows correction of the acid–base disturbance and removal of salicylate. In the remainder, with moderate biochemical disturbance and intermediate values of plasma salicylate concentration, infusion of dilute (1.26%) sodium bicarbonate solution can help to correct acidosis and to increase urinary excretion of salicylate. There is no direct evidence that bicarbonate infusion improves clinical outcome.

SSRIs

SSRIs are less dangerous in overdose than older antidepressants but their toxicity can be significantly enhanced by co-ingestion with other drugs such as monoamine oxidase inhibitors, tricyclics or lithium. While many patients may exhibit no specific clinical features after ingestion, nausea and vomiting, agitation, incoordination and drowsiness can ensue. Seizures also occur even late after presentation and if recurrent, should be treated with benzodiazepines.

Rarely, features of the 'serotonin syndrome' manifest. This is characterized by some or all of hyperpyrexia, neurological disturbance (drowsiness/confusion), autonomic instability and an elevation in serum creatine kinase. The patient's temperature should be measured and if greater than 38°C, this should prompt the clinician into measuring the creatine kinase and monitoring the renal function carefully. Patients suffering from the serotonin syndrome can be difficult to manage because of agitation and delirium. Autonomic instability with tachycardia and labile blood pressure can be challenging to treat effectively. The control of hyperthermia, a bad prognostic sign, may require intensive care with neuromuscular paralysis and intubation, as well as traditional cooling methods. Intravenous dantrolene is sometimes used as the paralysing agent but there is little supporting evidence for its particular use. Similarly, therapy with serotonin receptor ($5HT_{2A}$) antagonists such as cyproheptadine has been used but its efficacy has not been rigorously established.[7]

TCAs

Tricyclic antidepressant poisoning is still seen. The classic picture is of coma and signs of anticholinergic poisoning, with dilated pupils, tachycardia and hyperreflexia. It is worth considering the diagnosis in any patient who is unconscious and has dilated pupils. There are catches: dosulepin (dothiepin), while otherwise typical, tends not to cause very marked dilation of the pupils and patients who are deeply unconscious can have hyporeflexia. Seizures and myoclonus are common but usually short-lasting and not in themselves life-threatening. Death is usually due to malignant ventricular arrhythmia. Laboratory tests can show the presence of tricyclic antidepressant if there is doubt over the diagnosis.

Management is mainly supportive although activated charcoal can be given by mouth or nasogastric tube if the airway is protected. The most important question is whether the patient has, or is at risk of, serious tachyarrhythmia, which is a fatal complication of tricyclic poisoning. This makes a twelve-lead ECG (in addition to continuous rhythm monitoring) essential to manage tricyclic poisoning safely. Prolongation of the corrected QT-interval, broadening of the QRS and any form of supra-ventricular or ventricular tachycardia should act as warning signs. Any broad-complex tachycardia, even in sinus rhythm,

7   Boyer et al. NEJM (2005) 352: 1112–1120.

is an indication for the specific antidote – an infusion of 50 mmol of sodium bicarbonate (as 100 ml 4.2% solution over 15–20 min), repeated if necessary. Whilst not widely known, sodium bicarbonate is potentially life-saving, even in the absence of frank acidosis, as both the alkalinization and the increase in serum sodium concentration contribute to the anti-arrhythmic effect. Conventional anti-arrhythmic agents are potentially dangerous, and should be avoided.

One aspect of management that causes difficulty is recovery from tricyclic poisoning, since patients who have been in tricyclic-induced coma are commonly very agitated during this phase. Firm and persistent nursing care are then preferable to further poisoning the patient with psychoactive agents.

Alcohol

The signs of alcohol intoxication are evident to anybody who has spent time in an emergency department (or indeed a Pub) on a Saturday night. Unfortunately, the signs are not specific. Doctors tend to forget the difference between a sufficient explanation and a necessary one: while alcohol ingestion may be sufficient to explain unconsciousness in an unshaven man admitted to casualty, it is not necessarily the explanation and he may still have had a treatable intracranial haemorrhage.

Less commonly, signs of alcohol intoxication are due to other alcohols, such as methanol or ethylene glycol. The history and biochemical results showing renal impairment or a low venous bicarbonate concentration, should prompt formal measurement of the acid–base status and anion gap. If these show a metabolic acidosis with a high anion gap and normal lactate (when salicylate is absent), then the laboratory will need to be persuaded to measure methanol and ethylene glycol concentrations.

Opioids

Even those who have led a sheltered life will know that skinny patients with tattoos and 'track marks,' admitted with coma, respiratory depression and pin-point pupils are likely to be poisoned with an opioid. The general principles of management apply but artificial ventilation can be avoided if judicious quantities of naloxone are administered.

The key issue is to give the correct dose. Too little antidote, and the patient remains unconscious, requiring intensive support; too much and the patient wakes up, offers expletives and leaves before treatment is complete. Self-discharge is potentially dangerous for the patient because the half-life of naloxone is only around 20 min. Morphine has a half-life of about 3 h. Some advocate an intramuscular injection of a larger amount of naloxone but this practice is really treating the clinician rather than the patient. It is better to titrate the initial dose of naloxone to restore respiratory drive; if the patient again lapses into unconsciousness or respiratory failure, a continuous infusion of naloxone should be given (at an initial hourly rate of two-thirds of the dose required to wake the patient up). Rarer complications of opioid overdose include non-cardiogenic pulmonary oedema, even after naloxone has been given, and rhabdomyolysis.

Organophosphorous agents

Organophosphorous agents are used as pesticides; the most toxic compounds can be used for chemical warfare and terrorism. They poison the nervous system by inhibiting acetylcholinesterase, resulting in sustained cholinergic activity. This causes the characteristic signs of miosis, rhinorrhoea, hypersalivation, sweating, diarrhoea, vomiting and urinary incontinence. At neuromuscular junctions, stimulation initially causes twitching, then muscle weakness. Central nervous system involvement leads to convulsions, respiratory failure and death.

The first priorities in management are to protect the attending physician and other health workers, then to limit further absorption: contaminated clothing should be removed and the patient thoroughly washed, as the agents are absorbed through the skin as well as by inhalation and oral ingestion.

In symptomatic patients, supportive care is required and this can include artificial ventilation. The specific treatment to overcome the cholinergic stimulation is to give atropine, often in heroic doses repeatedly (every 10–30 min) until secretions have dried up and the patient becomes cool and dry. Several hundred milligrams of atropine may be needed to treat one patient and the average hospital's stock will soon be depleted. The duty pharmacist should be activated sooner rather than later! Intravenous diazepam may be needed to control agitation, muscular twitching and convulsions. There is debate about the use of oximes which work by reactivating a proportion of the acetylcholinesterase, but in the UK, current recommendations are to give pralidoxime in cases of moderate or severe poisoning. All suspected or confirmed cases of organophosphorus pesticide poisoning in the UK should be discussed with the NPIS. All suspected or confirmed terrorist attacks or releases of organophosphorus nerve agents should be discussed with the Health Protection Agency: the police may also have a passing interest!

PSYCHIATRIC INPUT

In patients who have taken an overdose with the intention of suicide or indeed those where genuine intent to cause personal injury is suspected, an assessment of further intent to self-harm is usually required. Neurological abnormalities and inebriation make any further appraisal almost impossible, and a premature request for a psychiatric assessment in such patients may make the general physician unpopular with their colleagues in liaison psychiatry.

Chapter 4

Paul Newey and John Reckless

ENDOCRINOLOGY AND LIPIDS

ENDOCRINOLOGY

The majority of endocrine problems do not present initially to the endocrinologist. Rather, they appear via a host of referral pathways: the general practitioner, the general physician, the neurologist or the ophthalmologist, to name a few. This accords a rather privileged position to the endocrinologist, who is able to investigate and diagnose potential problems at someone else's suggestion. Almost all diagnoses are perhaps obvious in retrospect. One of the great challenges is to identify those patients who warrant investigation from the larger pool in whom serious pathology is unlikely. In addition, the nonspecificity of many of the clinical presentations coupled with their relative scarcity ensures that some diagnoses are frequently overlooked or dismissed: it should be noted that it is both inevitable and necessary that there will be a considerable volume of negative investigation to ensure an appropriately high pickup rate.

Endocrinology manifests itself to the physician in a number of guises, and generalists need to be familiar with the correct management of the more common endocrine presentations (such as thyrotoxicosis), as well as the initial management of the more dramatic manifestations of endocrine disease (including thyroid storm and pituitary apoplexy). Appropriate interpretation of laboratory results, particularly when unexpected, is also crucial (e.g. hypercalcaemia, hyponatraemia). Additionally, it is important that where more complex endocrine disease is suspected, initial investigation is performed rationally and early specialist referral made.

Thyroid dysfunction

Overactivity, underactivity or a mass in the neck may be classical presentations, but the almost ubiquitous (and perhaps overdone) measurement of thyroid-stimulating hormone (TSH) in the acute-take and outpatient settings makes appropriate interpretation essential. The clinician should commit to a reason for measurement (and not just "to see") and respond to the result in that light. Thus, if the test was done to exclude hypothyroidism, then a suppressed TSH should not lead to immediate antithyroid treatment, as if the patient had been thyrotoxic. Some presenting symptoms occur in both over- and underactivity, but some, such as tiredness, are so common in the general population that they are poor discriminators. Routine testing may have limited the dramatic presentations of thyroid disease, but it has increased the detection of mild or subclinical disease. In addition, it is important to recognize the occasional oddity requiring specialist input.

Biochemical screening is usually performed with a single measurement of TSH. If the TSH is abnormal, free thyroxine and/or free triiodothyronine (fT4, fT3) levels are measured and will clarify most cases. However, interpretation of thyroid function tests in the hospital setting comes with a health warning: almost any pattern of thyroid test abnormality may be seen in the severely ill patient and may be attributable to nonthyroidal illness. Commonly, in acute illness, TSH is suppressed and free hormone levels are low, a homoeostatic reflection of a cata-bolic state. In some severely ill patients with underlying mild untreated hypothy-roidism, this may appear as an inappropriately normal TSH, while there may occasionally be a temporary compensatory rise in TSH in recovery from acute illness. Unless there is strong clinical suspicion of overt thyroid disease (perhaps associated with an atrial arrhythmia) or figures are strikingly abnormal, it is wise to treat results with caution, and if possible to repeat measurement after 6 weeks without intervention. However, there are clearly occasions when abnormal results are pertinent and require immediate action.

The overactive thyroid[1]

While thyroid disease is the commonest endocrine disorder after diabetes, only rarely does hyperthyroidism present dramatically to the hospital general physi-cian. However, it may play a part in admission to the medical take, reflecting a diversity of features, including atrial fibrillation and other tachycardias. Confirmation of the diagnosis is usually straightforward with elevated fT3 and/or fT4 and suppressed TSH. Thereafter, the question arises as to whether the aetiology is autoimmune (Graves' disease), multinodular or due to a solitary toxic nodule. Other causes are exceedingly rare and the province of the specialist, but factitious thyrotoxicosis may occasionally present on-take, and mild

---

[1] Cooper *et al.* Lancet (2003) 362: 459-468.

thyrotoxicosis may rarely be exacerbated by excess iodine consumption (such as with seaweed (kelp) supplements).

Presenting features may be diverse. Typically, patients present with weight loss, palpitations, anxiety, sweats or heat intolerance and fatigue. Examination usually demonstrates a tachycardia, fine tremor and warm, moist extremities. Such features may be less apparent in the elderly, where atrial fibrillation is more frequent and where 'apathetic' thyrotoxicosis may occur. Examination may reveal goitre (diffusely enlarged, solitary or multinodular). Goitre may sometimes be painful and tender, suggesting an acute thyroiditis. Alternatively, the thyroid may not be palpable. Diffuse symmetrical enlargement, with or without a bruit, indicates active Graves' disease. Dysthyroid eye disease (and the rarities of pretibial myxoedema and thyroid acropachy) is virtually diagnostic of Graves' disease. Dysthyroid eye disease is more common and more severe in smokers. It should be recognized that while active eye disease is most often associated with active thyroid disease, eye changes may occur independently and may be asymmetrical. However, such eye changes can also be due to rare orbital tumours.

In marked thyrotoxicosis, the alkaline phosphatase may be elevated, and temporary mild hypercalcaemia occurs occasionally. The diagnosis of autoimmune (Graves') disease is usually clear on clinical grounds but thyroid peroxisome antibodies are present in 70–80% and TSH-receptor antibodies in greater than 90%. However, antibodies are present in some individuals (female more than male) who never manifest thyroid disease. Thyroid ultrasound rarely makes a significant contribution to the management of the straightforward thyrotoxic patient unless there is a substantial goitre. Radio-nucleotide uptake scans (usually technetium) have a limited role; they can contribute to the diagnosis of a solitary toxic nodule (nodule uptake with suppression of uptake in the normal gland), or of subacute thyroiditis (where generalized reduced uptake may be seen).

The treatment modalities of antithyroid drugs, radioiodine (I^{131}) and surgery have changed little. Surgery and I^{131} are irreversible, but drug treatment has high relapse rates. For those presenting with marked symptoms and confirmatory biochemistry, initial treatment and symptom control with a combination of antithyroid drugs and beta-blockers is standard practice, and a euthyroid state is required prior to surgery. Rate control in atrial fibrillation may be difficult until the patient is euthyroid, and cardioversion in suitable individuals needs to be postponed until euthyroid and stable.

Antithyroid drugs

In the UK, younger patients are typically treated with antithyroid drugs, in contrast with the US, where radioiodine is frequently first-line therapy.

High rates of post-radioiodine hypothyroidism require lifelong thyroxine therapy and this, coupled with radioactivity issues in women of child-bearing age, are the reasons for the more conservative approach in the UK. Carbimazole and propylthiouracil are the most widely used agents. Local policy will dictate whether a 'dose titration' or 'block and replace' regimen is employed, as well as the length of treatment. The starting dose of carbimazole is usually 20–40 mg (the equivalent propylthiouracil dose being 200–400 mg). As the thyroid settles, the drug dose is titrated, initially at intervals of 4–6 (and later 8–10) weeks to keep a normal fT3, the maintenance dose usually being 5–20 mg daily. In the 'block and replace' regimen, as fT3 becomes normal, 75–100 mcg of thyroxine is added, and the high initial dose of the antithyroid drug is continued. In the situation of a changing thyroid status, the TSH lags behind fT3 and fT4 levels by a number of weeks, and the free hormones should be used to inform treatment adjustment. It is essential that the patient is fully aware of the uncommon drug side effects of rash, and most importantly of agranulocytosis. It is also good practice to clearly document discussion of the latter in the notes and in communication with the general practitioner. A sore throat (with or without aphthae) and fever for more than a day requires an immediate neutrophil count, even though intercurrent upper respiratory tract viral infections are almost always the cause. Agranulocytosis is commonest at high dose and in the initial 3 months of treatment, but can occur at any stage. An individual allergic to one of the drugs can be exposed to the second but, as perhaps 10% will have a similar response, an alternative treatment should be considered: after agranulocytosis with one agent, the second is also best avoided. Occasionally, these drugs may disturb liver function. Beta-blockade is helpful in the initial few weeks in the significantly symptomatic individual (using propranolol 40–80 mg three times daily).

In Graves' disease, the shorter the treatment duration, the greater is the relapse rate. Typically, at least 12–18 months treatment is given. Failure to ensure good control is common, and the specialist or an interested GP should be responsible for supervision. Therapy will achieve long-term remission in approximately 50% of those with Graves' disease treated appropriately, and recurrence is most likely in the first 6 months after stopping treatment. Recurrence is unpredictable but is more common in males, smokers, those with a large goitre and where high maintenance doses are required. If recurrence occurs, more definitive treatment with either radioiodine or surgery is usually indicated.

Radioiodine

Radioiodine therapy is administered as a single dose, usually as a capsule, and needs to be prescribed by an endocrinologist, radiotherapist or nuclear medicine consultant holding an appropriate licence. Antithyroid drugs need to be stopped 2 weeks before treatment as radioiodine uptake into the gland is otherwise blocked. Radioiodine is usually the treatment of choice in the older patient, while younger females need counselling about deferring pregnancy for 3 months. Patients receiving radioiodine require counselling about avoiding close prolonged contact with pregnant women and prepubertal children for around 3 weeks after treatment. Some individuals will require further treatment. Radioiodine may exacerbate dysthyroid eye disease, and, if such treatment is essential in an individual with eye changes, this is likely to require steroid cover for several weeks. Patients need to be closely followed to identify the point at which hypothyroidism develops, beginning with fT3 measurements approximately 8 weeks after therapy, and, if biochemically euthyroid, around 6 months later. They should then have yearly TSH measurement. Patients need to be aware of the risk of early hypothyroidism and the very high lifetime risk for thyroxine replacement therapy. One exception to this may be the solitary toxic nodule, where the suppressed normal thyroid will not have taken up significant I^{131} and may function normally after obliteration of the overactive nodule.

Surgery

Surgery can be used for any patient, but is indicated for individuals with large goitres, with allergy to antithyroid drugs and more often in younger than elderly patients. Patients need to be rendered euthyroid prior to anaesthesia. While in decades past a subtotal (90%) thyroidectomy was common, frequent recurrent thyrotoxicosis years later in the remnant has now led to total thyroidectomy being usual. Patients need to be counselled as to the requirement for lifelong thyroxine replacement (and the potential risks of surgery). Occasionally, urgent surgery is indicated in the thyrotoxic patient. In such circumstances, rapid thyroid blockade may be required. Administering potassium iodide for 7–10 days will render most patients euthyroid. Surgery must be performed promptly on achieving euthyroidism, as the blocking effect of such iodinated compounds is short-lived.

Other situations

Temporary thyrotoxicosis may occur postpartum, when treatment may not be required or should be of limited duration. In rare patients, an acute thyroiditis may occur with an acutely painful inflamed goitre and temporary biochemical thyrotoxicosis (which may not be clinically apparent). Hypothyroidism may occur at a later stage. The acute episode may require treatment with high-dose prednisolone, and patients should be under specialist supervision.

Storms

Occasionally, thyrotoxicosis may present as a life-threatening emergency in the form of thyroid storm. This does not necessarily imply particularly excessive levels of thyroid hormone. Rather, it typically occurs in those who have established (but usually not fully treated) thyrotoxicosis, upon whom a further superimposed stress is placed. It may occasionally be the first presentation of thyrotoxicosis. Most frequently the precipitant is an acute infection but numerous other stressors may precipitate a crisis. These include the administration of radioiodine or radiographic contrast agents, sudden withdrawal of antithyroid medication, surgical interventions and childbirth. Taking (or having recently taken) antithyroid medication, an antecedent history suggestive of thyrotoxicosis or a strong family history of thyroid disease may be indicators, but such information may not be known to the clinician at presentation.

Cardinal features of thyroid storm include altered mental state (severe agitation, psychosis or coma), tachycardia or tachyarrhythmias, hyperpyrexia and marked vomiting and diarrhoea. There may be multi-organ decompensation including cardiac failure, respiratory distress and acute renal failure, and there is a high mortality (30–50%).

Management should take place in intensive care and may require the input of multiple specialties. Treatment is supportive, coupled with specific therapies to rapidly control both the release of thyroid hormones and their peripheral effects. High-dose propylthiouracil or carbimazole should be commenced immediately (liquid propylthiouracil via nasogastric tube if necessary), followed later by potassium iodide, which will inhibit further thyroid hormone release. High-dose glucocorticoids are usually given and may inhibit conversion of T4 to T3 to ameliorate peripheral effects. High-dose propranolol may control tachyarrhythmias (calcium channel blockers are an alternative in those with known bronchospasm) and limit symptoms. Other supportive measures include the administration of broad-spectrum antibiotics in those with likely infection, chlorpromazine for agitation and further anti-arrhythmics for resistant tachycardias.

Hypothyroidism[2]

Hypothyroidism is rarely the primary reason for acute admission, but it may be an unrecognized contributor in the elderly. In its severest form, the patient may present with profound compromise. The aetiology is usually primary

---

[2] Roberts *et al.* Lancet (2004) 363: 793–803.

autoimmune disease (Hashimoto's thyroiditis), but it may follow thyroidectomy, radioiodine or noncompliance with thyroid hormone replacement. Treatment is with thyroxine (most often 125 mcg daily), and there are very limited indications for triiodothyronine therapy. In patients with severe hypothyroidism a lower dose of 50 mcg daily may be given for a week, then 100 mcg daily, before a full dose is given (aiming to restore the TSH to the lower third of the normal range). TSH is an unreliable measure of status in the 1–2 months after a dose change. Once a stable full dose of thyroxine has been achieved, there is no strict justification for long-term routine monitoring of TSH, unless compliance is in doubt: on submaximal doses, there is a place for ongoing checks. In some patients it may be necessary to accept an fT4 that is somewhat high, even with a suppressed TSH, in order to achieve a midrange fT3 in individuals who are poor peripheral deiodinators. In such situations, referral to an endocrinologist is appropriate. Excess thyroid replacement, as with subclinical thyrotoxicosis, can increase long-term risk of atrial fibrillation and osteoporosis.

Asymptomatic individuals with borderline raised TSH values need to be watched and treated if TSH rises over subsequent months. Where individuals have high thyroid peroxisome antibody levels, treatment should be initiated early as the majority of these patients will progress to overt hypothyroidism. Patients euthyroid on submaximal thyroxine replacement (< 125 mcg daily) should have 6–12 monthly TSH monitoring, as residual endogenous hormone production will gradually fail.

Low fT3 and fT4 levels and a normal or low TSH may reflect acute illness, but it must be remembered that TSH alone as a screening test will also miss secondary hypothyroidism due to pituitary failure. The laboratory must be asked to measure fT3/fT4 in known or suspected pituitary disease. It is essential not to immediately replace thyroid hormones in potential pituitary disease until the hypothalamus–pituitary–adrenal axis is assessed. Giving thyroxine to a pan-hypopituitary patient risks an acute Addisonian crisis.

Myxoedema coma

Myxoedema coma is rare but frequently fatal. Marked impairment of neurological function is present leading to coma but severe widespread manifestations of hypothyroidism are usually found. It is most common in elderly women with long-standing thyroid disease, either unrecognized or inadequately treated, or in those who are noncompliant with replacement therapy. It is more frequent in winter, implying that hypothermia itself may act as a precipitant. Other triggers include severe infection, anaesthetic agents, sedatives and tranquilizers, β-blockers, cardiac failure and trauma.

Clinical manifestations are diverse. There may be cardiovascular compromise with bradycardia, conduction defects and impaired ventricular contraction, while profound hypoventilation may lead to hypercapnia and respiratory acidosis with coma due to reduced ventilatory response to rising CO_2. Hypothermia may be marked. Intestinal obstruction or paralytic ileus may occur with impaired peristalsis and bowel wall oedema. Confusion, depression, hallucinations and seizures may be features in the comatose patient. Hyponatraemia is common due to water retention rather than sodium depletion. Further blood abnormalities can include a raised lactate dehydrogenase and creatine kinase, hypercholesterolaemia and anaemia.

The general principles of treatment are to correct the correctable and commence thyroid hormone replacement. Unfortunately, there is little evidence to guide optimal treatment. Ventilatory support is frequently required, and early extubation should be avoided. Passive rewarming, aiming for a slow rise in core temperature, may be performed where hypothermia is marked. Hyponatraemia may respond to fluid restriction. Hypertonic saline is rarely indicated. There should be a low threshold for antibiotic and glucocorticoid therapy to treat possible infection and adrenal insufficiency, respectively.

The main area of controversy is how best to replace the thyroid hormone deficit. One opinion is that replacement should be gradual, to avoid precipitating myocardial ischaemia and tachyarrhythmias, using intravenous fT4. The other view suggests intravenous fT3 to rapidly correct the hormone deficit. Both have theoretical disadvantages, with the impaired conversion of fT4 to fT3 in severe illness on the one hand and the increased risks of acute adverse events with variable fT3 concentrations following intravenous administration on the other. Some use combination therapy.

Subclinical thyroid disease[3,4]

Screening frequently identifies asymptomatic individuals with normal fT3 and fT4 but an abnormal TSH. A suppressed TSH may indicate subclinical endogenous hyperthyroidism, but also the exogenous cause of over-replacement with thyroxine (which may be intentional in the management of patients with previous thyroid cancer). It should be distinguished from temporary TSH suppression in acute nonthyroidal illness. The natural history of persistently demonstrated subclinical thyroid overactivity is uncertain, with perhaps a 5–10% annual

[3] Surks *et al.* JAMA (2004) 291: 228–238.

[4] Papi *et al.* Am J Med (2005) 118: 349–361.

progression to overt disease. The potential increased risks of future atrial fibrillation and accelerated osteoporosis are arguments for treatment.

Moderate, persistent elevation of TSH with normal fT3 and fT4 describes subclinical hypothyroidism, found most frequently in women over 60 years of age. Overt hypothyroidism develops at around 5% per year, and there may be excess cardiovascular risk if untreated. Consensus for treatment exists when TSH levels are above 10 mU/l, and replacement therapy should be initiated. Treatment may be appropriate at lower elevations of TSH when thyroid antibodies are high or where pregnancy exists or is contemplated. Where symptoms are plausible but unconvincing, there may be a case for a trial of submaximal thyroxine replacement over 2–3 months, but placebo effects are difficult to exclude. These patients with subclinical thyroid disease may benefit from assessment by an endocrinologist.

Amiodarone, lithium and the thyroid

Amiodarone and lithium can induce significant thyroid disturbance, and thyroid tests should be measured prior to treatment and regularly at 3–6-month intervals during treatment. Abnormalities in thyroid function are seen in up to 50% of patients chronically receiving amiodarone, largely due to the high iodine content of the drug. For many, the thyroid dysfunction requires no treatment, but is dependent on the patient's iodine status, drug dose and length of treatment. Effects may be unpredictable, however, paradoxically leading to both under- and overactivity. Hypothyroidism is the most common abnormality in iodine-replete regions. Thyrotoxicosis occurs in ~2% of amiodarone-treated patients in the West (higher if iodine deficient) and presents a significant challenge to the endocrinologist. Stopping amiodarone may not be an option, and, even where possible, the thyroid dysfunction may last for many months due to the long half-life of the drug. Amiodarone-induced thyrotoxicosis (AIT) may occur by two mechanisms; from iodine excess in those with multinodular goitre or Graves' disease (Type 1 AIT), or from a direct cytotoxic effects leading to a destructive thyroiditis, which can occur rapidly and unpredictably at any stage of treatment (Type 2 AIT).

Diagnosis may be difficult and worsening of underlying cardiac disease or arrhythmias may be the first clue. Amiodarone's side effects may mimic the features of thyrotoxicosis (with weight loss and fatigue). A suppressed TSH and elevated fT3 and fT4 make the diagnosis straightforward, but more modest abnormalities may be seen in clinically euthyroid individuals. In particular, amiodarone may inhibit peripheral tissue conversion of fT4 to fT3, leading to elevations in fT4 in euthyroid individuals, and transient decreases in TSH may also occur.

When treating amiodarone-induced thyrotoxicosis, antithyroid drugs are usually initiated and amiodarone should be discontinued, or the dose reduced, wherever possible. Steroids may be effective in those not responding to antithyroid drugs (typically in those with a destructive thyroiditis). Occasionally, carbimazole, potassium chlorate and steroids may be needed in combination, and rarely one may need to resort to surgery. Some patients will become hypothyroid, requiring lifelong thyroxine therapy even if amiodarone has been long withdrawn. Specialist referral should be made early and although a number of tests may help to differentiate between type 1 and type 2 AIT, a pragmatic approach to treatment is usually taken. Treatment is usually best monitored by fT3 levels because of potential disruption of T4 to T3 conversion.

Amiodarone is important in treating malignant arrhythmias, but is too readily prescribed acutely by junior staff despite alternatives, often continued long-term without persisting indication, and often at excessive dose. Amiodarone-induced thyrotoxicosis challenges endocrinologists and cardiologists alike, and it may be fatal. Due consideration should be given before routine prescription.

Lithium is effective in recurrent affective disorders, especially manic-depressive illness, but interferes with thyroid metabolism. It is concentrated in the thyroid, and inhibits thyroid hormone production and release. There may be pituitary TSH compensation (with some elevation of TSH in perhaps 20% of patients), but lithium can be both goitreogenic and lead to hypothyroidism requiring thyroxine replacement.

Adrenal disease

Significant adrenal pathology is relatively uncommon but includes two of the most satisfying diagnoses to make in clinical medicine — those of Addison's disease and phaeochromocytoma. If left undiagnosed, both may be rapidly fatal but each is eminently treatable once recognized. Their rarity makes recognition challenging. This is particularly true on a busy medical take, where it may be difficult to identify those in whom alarm bells should sound, against the backdrop of common nonspecific symptoms.

Adrenal insufficiency[5,6]

The diagnosis of Addison's disease (adrenocortical insufficiency) is frequently obvious in retrospect, but unfortunately harder to make on first presentation.

[5] Oelkers, NEJM (1996) 335: 1206–1212.

[6] Ten et al. J Clin Endocrinol Met (2001) 86: 2909–2922.

Some patients will have sought medical advice on numerous occasions without the diagnosis being considered, before presenting severely ill in an Addisonian crisis. Death is likely if unrecognized, but treatment with hydrocortisone and fluids is simple and life-saving. Every physician dealing with acute medicine should be prepared to make the diagnosis and treat appropriately.

While tuberculosis was the most frequent cause in the nineteenth and early twentieth centuries, the commonest aetiology is now autoimmune, occasionally as part of a polyglandular syndrome. Auto-antibodies raised against the adrenal cortex may be identified in around 70%. Other causes include opportunistic infection secondary to AIDS or systemic fungal infections, or malignancy involving the adrenals due to metastatic carcinoma or lymphoma. Acute adrenal insufficiency is also uncommon and easily missed. Adrenal haemorrhage in meningococcal septicaemia leading to circulatory collapse is well-established, and immediate antibiotics and steroid replacement are life-saving. *Pseudomonas* infections, asplenia, warfarin therapy or other coagulopathies may also be implicated in adrenal haemorrhage.

Secondary adrenal insufficiency due to pituitary disease should also be considered. Visual-field defects, headaches, evidence of other pituitary dysfunction or a history of previous pituitary surgery or radiotherapy will strongly suggest a secondary cause. Differentiation may be achieved by absence of hyperpigmentation, low levels of ACTH, or clinical evidence of hypopituitarism. Sheehan's syndrome is due to acute postpartum pituitary infarction from hypotension, while pituitary apoplexy may occur from an acute bleed, usually into a pre-existing pituitary adenoma.

Symptoms and signs of chronic adrenal disease may vary. Fatigue, weight loss, dizziness, weakness and, importantly, postural hypotension are typical. Nausea, vomiting and diarrhoea may also be present. Hyperpigmentation is characteristic of primary adrenal insufficiency due to the high levels of ACTH and associated melanocyte-stimulating hormone. Evidence of other autoimmune diseases, such as vitiligo, may be evident. Addisonian crises typically present with hypovolaemia and hypotension associated with central nervous system depression. Clues to the diagnosis may be apparent from routine biochemistry, with hyponatraemia, hyperkalaemia, hypoglycaemia and a metabolic acidosis, although it is usual for such tests to be normal in all but the most advanced cases of Addison's disease. The white-cell differential may show lymphocytosis with eosinophilia.

The key to successful management is to consider the diagnosis early and adopt a low threshold for steroid treatment. Administering steroids is unlikely to be harmful even if the diagnosis is not substantiated. In the acutely unwell, a random cortisol should be sent prior to administration of intravenous hydrocortisone and normal saline. The diagnosis will be suggested by a low random cortisol and may be confirmed with a subsequent short synacthen test, which is best performed around 9 O'clock in the morning. Plasma cortisol is measured at the outset and again at 30 min following intravenous injection of synacthen. A normal response sees an increase in plasma cortisol by at least 200 nmol/l, to over 550 nmol/l. In some hospitals, an intramuscular protocol is preferred, and a 60-min sample will often be collected in addition. Primary adrenal insufficiency is likely in the presence of raised ACTH levels with a failure of cortisol levels to rise appropriately following administration of synacthen. An adrenal antibody test may support the diagnosis.

Patients on replacement hydrocortisone should delay their morning dose until after the SST. Patients who have been on steroid doses higher than replacement (> 7.5 mg prednisone daily) may not respond to the SST, but may do so after 3 days prior adrenal stimulation with 1 mg intramuscular synacthen daily. If chronic steroid therapy can be gradually reduced, adrenal recovery may occur in some patients. In chronic secondary adrenal insufficiency there will usually be a failure to respond to a SST, as low levels of ACTH may have lead to adrenal atrophy. This contrasts the situation in acute pituitary failure where the response to ACTH may be preserved despite acute cortisol deficiency. In secondary adrenal failure, as with exogenous adrenal suppression, adrenal function may be shown to be normal if there is prior chronic stimulation with ACTH (a 'depot synacthen' test).

The usual hydrocortisone replacement requirement is around 15–25 mg per day, given as 10–15 mg on waking, 5 mg at midday and 5 mg at about 4 pm. The endocrinologist may undertake plasma cortisol day curves in patients on higher doses or who are symptomatic to exclude undue peaks or troughs in the cortisol profile. In adrenal failure, around 90% of patients also need a mineralocorticoid, fludrocortisone, usually at 50–100 mcg daily. In secondary (pituitary) adrenal failure, only about 10% require fludrocortisone because the renin-aldosterone system remains intact.

Patients who have presented with adrenal insufficiency need education about 'sick day' rules. During an intercurrent illness, steroid dosages should be doubled for 2–3 days. If vomiting occurs, the previous dose should be taken again. If vomiting is repeated, urgent medical support is required for an antiemetic. Continued vomiting requires admission. A steroid card should be carried, and a 'MedicAlert' bracelet or necklace is advisable. An ampoule of hydrocortisone (along with a syringe and needle) can also be given to the patient to take with them on overseas trips.

Patients who are acutely sick or undergoing major surgery will need increased and often parenteral hydrocortisone. Postoperatively, patients will require 2–3 times their normal dose of hydrocortisone, for 48 h and until taking a light diet.

Phaeochromocytoma[7,8]

The diagnosis of phaeochromocytoma is important to make as these rare cate-cholamine-secreting tumours are frequently fatal if untreated. However, recognition, diagnosis and management may be extremely challenging. Their ability to present with diverse, episodic symptoms ensures that they are often overlooked by patients and physicians. In addition, their scarcity (~2 per million per year) means they are dismissed as too 'unlikely' to investigate. Phaeochromocytoma is not an infrequent postmortem diagnosis: it is paramount to remain vigilant and, once suspected, to arrange prompt and appropriate investigation.

Phaeochromocytomas arise from chromaffin cells, most frequently from within the adrenal medulla. While not entirely accurate, the approximate 'rule of 10' is helpful; that 10% are extra-adrenal, 10% bilateral, 10% familial, 10% malignant, 10% asymptomatic and 10% occur in children. Recently, up to 25% of apparently sporadic cases have been shown to have a germ-line mutation in one of the various susceptibility genes, whereas up to 20% of cases occur at extra-adrenal sites (paraganglionomas).[9] Although frequently abdominal, extra-adrenal disease may occur at diverse sites including cardiac, skull base and bladder. Such extra-adrenal disease may pose a particularly difficult challenge.

With diversity in presentation, phaeochromocytomas may mimic other diseases. Classically there is sustained hypertension often refractory to conventional treatment. Additionally, 'superimposed' short-lived crises consisting of headache, palpitations and sweating are frequently seen. Other manifestations include anxiety, tremor, chest and abdominal pain, nausea and vomiting as well as constipation. Rarely, the presentation may be more dramatic with acute coronary syndromes, arrhythmias, left ventricular failure, acute renal failure, stroke or seizures, all recognized. The extent to which an individual is affected will often correspond to the degree and type of catecholamine excess.

Who should be investigated? Groups of high priority include those with refractory hypertension, particularly identified at a young age; those with either a family history of phaeochromocytoma or one of the associated familial conditions; those identified to have an adrenal 'incidentaloma' on imaging;

[7] Lenders *et al.* Lancet (2005) 366: 665–675.

[8] Ilias *et al.* J Clin Endocrinol Metab (2004) 89: 479–491.

[9] Neumann *et al.* NEJM (2002) 346: 1459–1466.

and those who have cardiovascular instability perioperatively or following administration of intravenous contrast.

The diagnosis of phaeochromocytoma requires demonstration of catecholamine excess. In the UK, 24-h urinary fractionated catecholamines (noradrenaline, adrenaline) and metadrenalines (normetadrenaline, metadrenaline) are most frequently measured. Plasma catecholamines (or plasma-free metadrenalines) are used in some centres.[10]

Two normal 24-h urinary metadrenalines will usually be adequate to exclude the diagnosis as these have both high sensitivity and specificity. The urine collection bottle requires hydrochloric acid preservative. Males, particularly, need warning not to urinate directly into the container because of the risk of 'splash-back'. Numerous drugs may interfere with the assay, as may coexisting acute illness, when interpretation may be difficult and necessitate remeasurement after a time delay. The list of potential drugs interfering with the various assays is long, and local laboratory guidance should be sought. Where tests are abnormal, withdrawal of most drugs is suggested but hypertension may prevent this. In those with borderline results or a high pre-test probability, plasma metadrenalines may be useful, as their sensitivity is higher with a powerful negative predictive value. However, their reduced specificity largely precludes use for general screening.

Once biochemical excess has been demonstrated, tumour localization is required. Initial anatomical imaging with CT or MRI is mandatory. MRI is favoured as it tends to allow better adrenal tissue characterization. In addition, the absence of contrast allays fear of precipitating a crisis. Traditionally, patients are alpha- and beta-blocked prior to IV contrast for CT scanning, although newer contrast agents have been shown to be safe without such preparation. If an adrenal source is not identified, further imaging is required to locate the tumour.

There is debate over the optimal use of functional imaging in specialist circles. Isotope (mIBG) scanning is frequently employed to identify extra-adrenal, multifocal or metastatic disease. It may be useful if MRI imaging is negative, but appropriate expertise is required and availability may be limited. If imaging is negative or is inconclusive, adrenal vein sampling may be useful. Unlike mIBG this requires prior alpha and beta blockade and is based on finding a reversed noradrenaline: adrenaline ratio in the adrenal vein on the affected side.

Once identified, the goal should be surgical removal after patient preparation with alpha- and beta-adrenergic blockade to ameliorate effects of catecholamine excess. Alpha blockade with the noncompetitive phenoxybenzamine

10 Kudva *et al.* J Clin Endocrinol Met (2003) 88: 4533–4539.

is commenced first, followed by beta-blockade with propranolol. Isolated beta-blockade carries the theoretical risk of hypertensive crisis from unopposed alpha receptor stimulation. Doses should be titrated cautiously with clinical monitoring of plasma volume and blood pressure. Typically, several weeks of blockade should be employed. In addition, patients may be admitted immediately preoperatively for intravenous phenoxybenzamine. Suggestions that alternative alpha blockers or calcium channel blockers may be used in preparation remain debatable. Surgical removal should only be undertaken in experienced centres and may be laparoscopic where appropriate. The expertise of the anaesthetist is as important as that of the surgeon. Alpha and beta blockade may be discontinued postoperatively with repeat urine collections after a couple of weeks to confirm biochemical cure. Rarely, in the acute situation, intravenous alpha blockade may be needed, carefully titrated against intravenous fluids (because of the acute vasodilatation and hypotension that may occur).

Phaeochromocytoma may be associated with inherited syndromes, including multiple endocrine neoplasia type 2 (MEN-2) (with activation of the ret protooncogene), von Hippel Lindau (VHL) disease (with a loss of function mutation of a tumour suppressor gene) and in some cases of neurofibromatosis. More recently, mutations in the succinate dehydrogenase B and D genes have also been implicated.[11,12] Screening for mutations in the VHL and MEN-2 genes as well as in the SDHB and SDHD is recommended in those with apparently sporadic disease who are young (< 50 years), and in those with extra-adrenal disease. Patients with MEN syndromes need to be under regular specialist review (and to have their serum calcium watched).

Is it Cushing's?

Harvey Cushing described features of cortisol excess from adrenal hyperplasia due to a pituitary tumour producing excess ACTH (Cushing's disease). Cushing's syndrome encompasses other causes — a benign or malignant adrenal tumour, an ectopic source of ACTH (such as from a bronchial carcinoid or carcinoma), or from excess exogenous steroid usage. While the principles of localizing disease may be straightforward, considerable difficulty may be encountered in clinical practice. The realm of the general physician is thankfully limited to answering the more focused question: 'is it Cushing's'?

Symptoms of cortisol excess are myriad, with weight gain, altered mood and proximal weakness being characteristic, and the history may go back

---

11 Baysal *et al.* Science (2000) 287: 848–851.

12 Neumann *et al.* NEJM (2002) 346: 1459–1466.

several years. Signs include central obesity, striae, bruising, thin skin, 'buffalo' hump and typical facies. Whilst the 'full house' of features may make the diagnosis apparent, their presence may be variable (or hidden from view). Many features (such as obesity, hypertension, diabetes) are common in the general population, and deciding when to investigate may be difficult. Proximal myopathy, spontaneous bruising and purple striae have a higher predictive value, but may not be evident.

Once queried, prompt and appropriate investigation is required to confirm or (more often) refute the diagnosis. Two 24-h urinary free cortisol measurements should be performed along with an overnight dexamethasone suppression test. At 11 PM, 1 mg of dexamethasone is given orally, and plasma cortisol is taken at 9 AM the following morning. If the urine collections are within the normal range and the overnight dexamethasone test negative (9 AM cortisol less than 50 nmol/l), Cushing's is virtually excluded and further investigation is unlikely to be warranted (the rare case of cyclical Cushing's is an exception). If equivocal or overtly abnormal, more formal testing is required.

Cushing's syndrome is confirmed by the failure of cortisol to suppress (< 50 nmol/l) on a low-dose dexamethasone test (0.5 mg dexamethasone given orally every 6 h for 48 h). Cortisol and ACTH levels should be taken at the start and end of test. In addition, the loss of diurnal cortisol secretion is almost universal, and an elevated midnight cortisol substantiates the diagnosis, although it is often difficult to reliably obtain.

Once confirmed, localization is the remit of the specialist. A high dose dexamethasone suppression test (2 mg dexamethasone every 6 h for 48 h) may identify pituitary driven disease (a fall in cortisol of more than 50% from baseline). Failure to suppress implies adrenal or ectopic disease. Baseline ACTH levels contribute: undetectable ACTH suggests adrenal disease; moderate elevations imply pituitary disease, although higher levels may point towards an ectopic source. Doubt may remain, as considerable overlap may exist between tests results. Further specialist testing is sometimes employed (e.g. response to corticotrophin releasing hormone — the CRH test or inferior petrosal sinus sampling). Imaging is undertaken once localization is suggested. Pituitary MRI (gadolinium enhanced) or adrenal MRI/CT requires no explanation. Ectopic disease, if not immediately apparent, may prove difficult, if not impossible, to locate.

Ultimately, where possible, treatment is surgical. A degree of control should usually be achieved medically prior to surgery (or in the inoperable) with metyrapone or ketoconazole. Pituitary disease is usually tackled by selective transnasal or transsphenoidal hypophysectomy, although cure is not always achieved. Radiotherapy and/or bilateral adrenalectomy (now ideally laparoscopically) may also be required. Unilateral surgery is undertaken for an adrenal adenoma or carcinoma (10% of adrenal Cushing's). Subsequent replacement therapy is again the remit of the specialist but, initially, it is broadly as described earlier. Patients with Cushing's syndrome due to ectopic ACTH may have severe metabolic disturbance in the absence of typical clinical signs.

Adrenal 'incidentaloma'[13,14]

With modern imaging techniques, an adrenal mass may be an inadvertent finding, particularly in the older patient. Size is important, and larger lesions (> 4 cm) should be considered for surgery, as malignancy is more likely. Smaller lesions are generally benign. Imaging characteristics may help in identifying the likely benign adenoma (e.g. low attenuation on CT). Otherwise, investigation should aim to exclude a functioning mass. A 24-h urine measurement of metadrenalines and cortisol together with an overnight dexamethasone suppression test should be performed. In addition, in those with hypertension, plasma potassium (with renin–aldosterone level if appropriate) is required. Functioning tumours require surgery. Otherwise, some form of serial interval imaging is required, although protocols vary. If radiological appearances remain unchanged over time (typically between 6 and 24 months) and persistent hormonal inactivity is demonstrated, no further follow-up may be necessary.

Pituitary disease

Pituitary adenomas are uncommon, nearly always benign, and may be functioning or nonfunctioning. They present because of excess hormone production, hypopituitarism or local pressure effects from an enlarging gland. Hormonally active tumours may produce prolactin, growth hormone or ACTH (TSH- and gonadotrophin-secreting tumours are exceedingly rare), and clinical sequelae will depend on this.

Acromegaly (with possible gigantism if the disease develops before the end of adolescence and epiphyseal fusion) develops slowly, and looking at a patient's photographs over a decade or more can be illuminating. The classical features are a coarsening of facial features (with prominent supraorbital ridges, prognathism, macroglossia, large nose) and large spade-like hands and feet. Questions about shoe size and ring enlargement are standard. If acromegaly is suspected, exclusion is required. Insulin-like growth hormone (IGF1) is

[13] NIH Consen Statements (2002) 19: 1–25.

[14] Thompson *et al.* Curr Opin Oncol (2003) 15: 84–90.

an initial screening test, but if doubt persists, then a formal 75 g oral glucose tolerance test should be performed. A lack of appropriate growth hormone suppression (to < 2 mU/l) suggests disease.

Whatever the likely aetiology, the possible presence of a pituitary tumour should prompt imaging with MRI (CT only being used where MRI is contraindicated). There is no role for plain skull films. Formal peripheral visual-field tests are mandatory, as is a full assessment of pituitary function.

Functioning tumours are normally treated initially by transsphenoidal surgery, the exception being prolactinomas (see below). The use of long-acting somatostatin analogues (e.g. octreotide, lanreotide) has become commonplace in the management of acromegaly, although surgery remains ultimately central to treatment in most. Nonfunctioning adenomas not impinging on the visual fields may be managed conservatively over years, but must be followed at least annually as they may continue to enlarge and require subsequent intervention. Radiotherapy is used as a subsequent supplementary treatment but does not have a primary role. Typically, it is employed in the management of nonfunctioning tumours where there is either significant residual or recurrent disease after initial surgery. In addition, it may occasionally be used for functioning tumours, for example, in acromegaly where a combination of surgical and medical therapy fails to achieve biochemical cure. In Cushing's, radiotherapy is indicated where disease remains active following pituitary surgery or in those for whom bilateral adrenalectomy is being considered as either primary therapy (now rare) or where control has not been achieved by other means (to reduce risk of uncontrolled ACTH production leading to Nelson's syndrome). Radiotherapy only works slowly, over years, and long-term hypopituitarism is common. Annual assessment of pituitary function is obligatory.

Hyperprolactinaemia

The discovery of an elevated serum prolactin is a common clinical entity, prompting frequent endocrinological referral. It may elicit a certain amount of anxiety in the nonspecialist as it raises the possibility of underlying pituitary pathology. Minor elevations are also frequent, which may give rise to uncertainty. It may be difficult to know whether to dismiss such elevations as irrelevant or to pursue further investigation. Unfortunately, prolactin is often added to a 'hormone screen' in vaguely gynaecological presentations without a clear indication. Therefore, it is important that the general physician has awareness of causes of hyperprolactinaemia, an appropriate approach to assessment and a willingness to consider early specialist referral.

In females, the measurement of serum prolactin is most frequently prompted as part of routine investigation for amenorrhea, infertility or following the reporting of galactorrhoea. Although hyperprolactinaemia in men may result in impotence, infertility and reduced libido, these are rarely reported as initial symptoms, and routine prolactin measurement is relatively unusual. Prolactin measurement is also routine where pituitary pathology is suspected or demonstrated on imaging.

The extent to which the prolactin is elevated may provide a useful guide to the likely aetiology. Levels greater than 1000 mU/l (in the absence of pregnancy) require investigation. Although levels over 3000 mU/l usually represent prolactinomas – either micro- (< 1 cm) or macro- (> 1 cm) – more modest elevations are harder to interpret. They may represent a micropro-lactinoma; a nonfunctioning macroadenoma (or any other pituitary mass) compressing the pituitary stalk and leading to 'disconnection hyperpro-lactinaemia'; or a nonstructural cause. Still-higher elevations (> 6000 mU/l) are almost always macroprolactinomas. Elevations may be impressive (> 100,000 mU/l).

Other causes of raised prolactin should not be forgotten. Elevated prolactin can occur in primary hypothyroidism, whereas many psychotropic drugs (e.g. sulpiride, chlorpromazine, haloperidol) and antiemetic agents (e.g. metoclo-pramide, domperidone) will elevate prolactin through a dopamine-related central action. SSRIs can also raise prolactin, although the mechanism is unclear. Sometimes prolactin can be secreted in a polymeric form, called macroprolactin, which is picked up in the assay, but is biologically inactive and is not clinically significant. Modest elevation can also occur in stressed individuals, and repeat measurements should be made. Current or recent breast feeding should be remembered. Repetitive breast self-examination by the woman to see if galactor-rhoea persists stimulates the release of prolactin, thereby leading to persistence of the problem.

Management addresses the underlying cause and is the remit of the specialist. Pituitary imaging is inevitable where pituitary pathology is suspected. Hypothyroidism should be treated and implicated drugs withdrawn if clinically appropriate (although this is often not possible). Unlike other pituitary tumours, macroprolactinomas are treated with a dopamine agonist (cabergo-line, bromocriptine, quinagolide) in almost all circumstances, even with optic chiasm distortion. Over months to years, the tumour may regress and disappear, and when the dopamine agonist is withdrawn after several years, the tumour may not recur. Microprolactinomas are treated medically to restore fertility and, hence, the sex hormones necessary for bone health – their natural history is not one of progression even if left untreated.

Apoplexy and assessment of pituitary function in the acute setting

Pituitary apoplexy most commonly results from spontaneous haemorrhage into a pre-existing, albeit unknown, pituitary macroadenoma. It may present dramatically and be indistinguishable from other forms of intracranial haemorrhage. Acute severe headache, visual loss, cranial nerve damage or impaired consciousness may be the presenting features. Recognition of the syndrome is essential with appropriate assessment and implementation of hormone replacement. Early surgical intervention may preserve vision and improve outcome.[15]

If hypopituitarism is suspected acutely, then blood should be taken for fT3 or fT4 (TSH being normal or suppressed), random cortisol, electrolytes and prolactin. Resuscitation may include parenteral and then oral hydrocortisone, but a plasma cortisol should first be taken. It is dangerous to give thyroxine replacement alone, as increasing the metabolic rate may precipitate an Addisonian crisis. Clearly, in this situation, extensive investigation by the generalist is not appropriate.

Presentation of hypopituitarism may be subtle without classical Addisonian or hypothyroid signs. Thus, pigmentation will be absent, and hypothyroid-coarsened features will be replaced by a smoother, sallow skin.

Hyponatraemia[16]

Hyponatraemia is a frequently encountered problem for the general physician. Although the commonest causes of hyponatraemia are not strictly endocrinological (e.g. thiazide usage), it is a common reason for referral. Indeed, the incidence of hyponatraemia in the hospitalized patient may reach 15–30%. Although usually asymptomatic, it may be associated with significant morbidity and mortality. Inappropriate management of hyponatraemia is also frequent and may result in further morbidity.

How effectively hyponatraemia is managed is dependent on careful patient assessment and the ability to accurately assess an individual's volume status. Although it occurs as the endpoint of numerous pathophysiological processes, hyponatraemia almost always reflects an excess of water relative to sodium, be it due to overt water excess or disproportionate salt depletion. The commonest causes of water excess include the syndrome of inappropriate ADH secretion; the increased water reabsorption seen in CCF; nephrotic syndrome and

[15] Rendeva et al. Clin Endocrinol (1999) 51: 181–188.

[16] Reynolds et al. Clin Endocrinol (2005) 63: 366–374.

cirrhosis; and psychogenic polydipsia. Clearly, in the hospitalized patient, inappropriate fluid management is also a frequent cause. In terms of salt depletion, thiazide diuretics are by far the commonest cause of hyponatraemia, although various forms of renal disease as well as nonrenal loss may also be responsible. Although uncommon in those presenting with hyponatraemia, an Addisonian state must be considered, whether due to pituitary failure, primary adrenal failure or secondary adrenal failure associated with exogenous steroid use.

The ability to assess fluid status is central to making the appropriate diagnosis and instituting the correct management. This can be difficult and may require measurement of the central venous pressure. In addition, it is mandatory to measure the plasma and urinary osmolality, as well as urinary sodium. Taken together, this information should enable a diagnosis to be made. Where an individual is hypovolaemic, low urine sodium suggests a nonrenal cause (e.g. gastrointestinal). In patients with fluid overload (e.g. cardiac failure, cirrhosis), urinary sodium is normally low. Euvolaemic patients may be more difficult but high urinary sodium may suggest the syndrome of inappropriate antidiuretic hormone (SIADH), whereas low urinary sodium may suggest inappropriate fluid replacement.

SIADH is a frequent cause of hyponatraemia in the hospital setting, associated particularly with chest (malignancy, infection, pneumothorax) and CNS (head injury, subarachnoid haemorrhage, meningitis) disease and with many drugs (ecstasy, SSRIs and sulphonylureas to name but a few). Diagnosis is made in the presence of euvolaemic hyponatraemia, low plasma osmolality and inappropriate elevation of both urine osmolality and urinary sodium (after the exclusion of renal, thyroid and adrenal disorders). With treatment of the underlying cause, short-lived fluid restriction (500–1000 ml/24 h) is often all that is required. It is important to ensure that fluid restriction is enforced. When the cause is likely to be more longstanding, the use of demeclocycline may be indicated.

Only rarely is the correction of severe hyponatraemia with hypertonic saline indicated; typically when the fall in sodium has been rapid and severe clinical features are present (e.g. seizures, coma). Correction should be controlled (e.g. 0.5 mmol/l/h) to minimize risk of central pontine myelinolysis. Protocols exist for such replacement, and specialist advice should be sought.

Primary hyperparathyroidism[17]

Primary hyperparathyroidism (PHPT) is a common endocrine disorder, with hypercalcaemia frequently discovered coincidentally following 'routine'

[17] Bilezikian *et al.* NEJM (2004) 350: 1746–1751.

biochemical measurement of serum calcium (which should be corrected for serum albumin). It occurs most frequently in the postmenopausal woman (presentation in women exceeds that in men two- to threefold), although it may occur at any age. In almost all cases, PHPT is because of a benign adenoma (85% being a single adenoma). PHPT is typically sporadic but may be familial.[18] At a younger age, PHPT is a central feature of multiple endocrine neoplasia type 1 (MEN-1), occurring in over 90%. It also occurs in 30–40% of those with MEN-2, and multiple glands are frequently involved in both. PHPT almost always represents benign disease. Parathyroid carcinoma is a rare cause of PHPT and tends to be associated with very high levels of PTH and may manifest itself with a more severe presentation. A mass may also be identified.

The differential diagnosis of hypercalcaemia is important but few diagnoses will demonstrate a coexisting inappropriate elevation of plasma parathyroid hormone (PTH), being limited to PHPT, tertiary HPT in end-stage renal disease, thiazide and lithium therapy and familial hypocalciuric hypercalcaemia. The latter is suggested on the basis of mild hypercalcaemia, a low normal or reduced urinary calcium excretion and perhaps a family history. Humoral hypercalcaemia of malignancy does not fall into this differential as PTH-related peptide (PTH-rP) is not detected by the PTH assay. PHPT may occur with normal serum calcium, particularly with coexistent vitamin D deficiency. It is usual to exclude myeloma by protein electrophoresis and urinary Bence-Jones protein measurement.

Significant symptoms are frequently absent although, if specifically asked, symptoms such as fatigue, lassitude and lack of sexual interest may be more prevalent than in control groups. Evidence of end-organ damage should be sought. Skeletal involvement is uncommon on plain radiography (not indicated routinely), but assessment of bone mineral density is mandatory. Osteoporosis is common, most prominent at the distal radius and to a lesser degree at hip and lumbar spine. Renal stones or nephrocalcinosis is found in 15–20%.

When identified by routine calcium measurement, disease is frequently mild, asymptomatic and not causing end-organ damage. This leads to debate about when surgical intervention is appropriate. The NIH guidelines, upon which the following table is based, have been designed to help clarify matters.[19,20]

----

[18] Miedlich *et al.* Clin Endocrinol (2003) 59: 539–554.

[19] NIH Consen Statements (1990) 8: 1–18.

[20] Bilezikian *et al.* J Bone Miner Res (2002) 17: N2–N11.

Criteria for parathyroidectomy

Serum calcium > 0.25 mmol/l above upper end of the normal range
Creatinine clearance reduced by over 30%
Urinary calcium over 400 mg/day
BMD T score ≤ 2.5 SD at any site
Age under 50 years

Mild, asymptomatic disease may be nonprogressive and can be treated conservatively, but patients must be followed long term, since about a quarter will progress. These patients should also be encouraged to drink over 3 l fluid daily. Given this unpredictability, some advocate a more aggressive approach where surgical risk is low. Well-being may improve even when no specific symptoms were identified. Below the age of 70 years, surgery may increase life expectancy but, even in the older patient or in those with substantial comorbidities, surgery may improve symptoms and quality of life.

An experienced surgeon is essential. Modern ultrasound may help identify the adenoma site. Some will use intravenous methylene blue immediately prior to surgery to stain the glands. The traditional bilateral neck exploration achieves success rates approaching 95%. More recently, a minimally invasive, unilateral approach has been adopted by some, which does require preoperative sestamibi scanning and ultrasonography for localization. This approach is excellent when a single adenoma is identified, but fares less well if definitive identification fails. Where re-exploration is required, selective venous sampling may also be required.

The management of acute hypercalcaemia requires active fluid replacement. Where moderate primary hyperparathyroidism is being managed conservatively, patients need to be advised to maintain a high fluid intake, as admission with severe hypercalcaemia usually reflects poor fluid intake, perhaps with a precipitating intercurrent acute illness. Treatment with a bisphosphonate (intravenous pamidronate) or zolendronic acid may be needed either in the acute management of marked hypercalcaemia or where comorbidities or patient wishes preclude surgical intervention.

LIPID DISORDERS AND THE GENERAL PHYSICIAN

The main importance of lipids and dyslipidaemia for the acute physician is in relationship to primary or secondary prevention of macrovascular disease, but acute pancreatitis can be associated with severe hypertriglyceridaemia.

The causal relationship between low-density lipoprotein-cholesterol (LDL-C) and coronary heart disease (CHD) is clearly established, as is the inverse relationship between high-density lipoprotein-cholesterol (HDL-C) and CHD. An individual's global CHD risk relates to sex, age, smoking, hypertension, total (or LDL) cholesterol to HDL-C ratio, and diabetes. Dietary change, lifestyle modification and various drug groups can all reduce this global risk, but it was the advent in 1990 of the well-tolerated statins that changed the outlook. Further studies in the last 5 years have substantially extended the evidence base, and the guidelines of the Joint British Societies have now been updated.[21] Reduction in relative risk from LDL-C lowering is seen equally in different patient groups, in males and female, at ages up to at least 85 years, with and without diabetes, in hypertension and with other drug therapies. There currently does not seem to be a particular low level of LDL-C below which benefit ceases. Importantly, and despite the much flatter relationship between cholesterol and stroke, the statin studies have shown substantial reduction in thrombotic stroke with LDL-C lowering. Treatment for all risk factors should be undertaken for all at high risk. This includes those with clinical cardiovascular disease (CVD) in any territory, diabetes, familial hypercholesterolaemia and whose global CVD risk is ≥ 20% over 10 years (equivalent to 15%/10 years coronary heart disease risk). The charts from which to calculate absolute risk are available in the back of the British National Formulary, and the 20%/10 years threshold has been endorsed by NICE.[22]

It must be emphasised again that when an individual has sufficient risk to require intervention, all risk factors that contribute should be addressed. Thus, the blood pressure target is < 140/< 90 (< 130/< 80 in diabetes). However, focusing here on cholesterol, the target is < 4 mmol/l, and the target is < 2 mmol/l for the key LDL-C. The greater the reduction in LDL-C, the greater the relative risk reduction, and benefit is seen in those at both high and low absolute risk.

Patients presenting with an acute event should have a statin started after a random cholesterol is measured, and a fasting profile should be measured at subsequent specialist or primary care follow-up to ensure that targets are achieved and to assess triglycerides. In primary prevention patients, two separate measurements (at least one as a full fasting profile) should be assessed before treatment. Secondary causes of dyslipidaemia (such as hypothyroidism, uncontrolled diabetes, excess alcohol, obesity, certain drugs) should be addressed. Although there is not yet outcome data for ezetimibe, it will lower

---

[21] Joint British Societies' Guidelines, Heart (2005) 91: V1–V52.

[22] TA094 (January 2006) (www.nice.org.uk)

LDL-C by an additional 20% when added to other treatments. Patients with severe or poorly responsive dyslipidaemia should be referred for specialist advice. Where there is significant mixed dyslipidaemia, or hypertriglyceridaemia persists after LDL-C has reached target in high-risk patients, additional therapy with a fibrate, nicotinic acid or omega-3 fish oils can be considered, and again specialist advice may be appropriate.

Where an individual is identified with hypercholesterolaemia, and especially where there is a strong family history of CVD, it is mandatory for the clinician to identify first-degree relatives and to encourage their active screening, and support can be offered to the patient and family.[23]

Statin therapy has been very successful with a very low rate of serious side effects.[24] Approximately once in 30,000–50,000 patient-years of treatment, severe myositis and rhabdomyolysis may occur. Patients should be warned that if they get generalized muscle discomfort, pain, tenderness or weakness lasting more than a couple of days, they should have a creatine kinase checked, although the symptoms will very rarely be drug related. There is little to choose between the five statins available, with CVD outcome data for four (atorvastatin, fluvastatin, pravastatin, simvastatin). Many drugs are metabolized through the cytochrome P450 3A4 pathway, as are simvastatin and atorvastatin. Fluvastatin and pravastatin are metabolized via different routes and may therefore pose less risk of drug interactions: they may, for example, be safer in patients taking drugs such as ciclosporin or anti-retrovirals.

First-choice statin will now be determined largely by cost, for simvastatin is off patent (and also pravastatin) and costs have fallen to about 15% of the original value. Currently, simvastatin 40 mg is likely to be first choice before moving to alternatives. Most of a statin's effect is obtained with the low entry dose, and only about 6% extra LDL-C lowering is seen with each dose doubling. Very approximately for a given milligram dose of each statin, from pravastatin or fluvastatin, there is increased LDL-C lowering of about 6% moving to simvastatin, a further 6% to atorvastatin and 9% further again moving to rosuvastatin. Low-dose simvastatin (10 mg) is available for over-the-counter purchase on a pharmacist's advice for suitable middle–older age individuals with sufficient risk (10–20% CVD/10 year risk), below that qualifying for NHS prescription.

With severe hypertriglyceridaemia (> 10 mmol/l and especially > 20 mmol/l), pancreatitis can occur even in the absence of other causes. Individuals who are obese,

---

[23] www.heartuk.org.uk

[24] Ballantyne *et al.* Arch Int Med (2003) 163: 553–564.

diabetic or have taken excess alcohol are at high risk, usually in the context of an underlying mixed dyslipidaemia. Management in the acute situation is calorie restriction and IV fluids, and the triglycerides will tend to settle over 2–4 days. Statins are not of value in this situation of severe hypertriglyceridaemia, and fibrates or fish oils may be appropriate.

In individuals with more moderate hypertriglyceridaemia, the CVD risk is increased, especially if HDL-cholesterol is low. First-line management will still be to lower LDL-C to target, but fibrate treatment may be used alone or in combination with statins in the higher risk groups such as those with diabetes. Gemfibrozil should not be used with a statin, and fenofibrate would usually be the choice.

Chapter 5

Aparna Pal and David Matthews

DIABETES AND OBESITY

A big fat problem

Type 2 diabetes is fast becoming the scourge of the modern world. In parts, the prevalence is greater than 20%.[1] In general, governments and health care providers have watched the rise of this largely preventable disease with alarm but passivity. Only recently has there been a concerted burst of public health and research interest. This diabetes epidemic directly mirrors the worldwide surge in obesity, giving rise to terms such as 'diabesity' and 'globesity'.

The collection of alarming statistics gets larger by the month: global figures for the number of people with diabetes are projected to double by 2025, from the current estimate of 170 million, and type 2 diabetes increasingly occurs in children and adolescents (such that it may be the predominant form of the disease in this age group within 10 years).[2] The figures for obesity are sobering. Men and women in England are getting bigger: up to one-fifth of the adult population is now obese – not overweight – but obese.[3] If a baby born in the UK today becomes overweight or obese, it is estimated that its life expectancy will be shortened, on average, by 2.5 years. It is reckoned that by 2050 (if current trends continue), the same baby would be able to expect on average, 5.5 years less life than his or her peers (largely because general benefits predicted in health and life expectancy will bypass the obese and overweight).[4] We have not yet turned the corner. Our children are fat and they are getting fatter. Around 15% of children are now

---

[1] WHO, Preventing chronic diseases: a vital investment (2005) (www.who.int)

[2] IDF, World atlas of diabetes (2003) (www.idf.org)

[3] Health Survey for England, Department of Health (2002) (www.dh.gov.uk)

[4] Government Actuary's Department and Department of Health, England (unpublished), cited by Chief Medical Officer (29 September, 2005).

clinically obese, and a large number more are overweight. Fat parents tend to have fat children.[5]

The most serious problem with the epidemic of obesity is the associated epidemic of type 2 diabetes. With weight increase, the risk of developing diabetes rises logarithmically.[6] If this rising tide is to be halted, the changes that will need to be made are more than merely cosmetic: a wholesale shift in attitudes and culture will be required. The tragedy is that whilst obesity is reversible (at least in theory), the complications of diabetes are not. Whilst action will be necessary right across society, there is also an onus on doctors to coordinate the most effective attack on these diseases where they already exist. For type 2 diabetes, levels of morbidity and mortality are incontrovertibly reduced by aggressive control of glucose, blood pressure and lipids. There is ample opportunity to contain the damage caused by this disease.[7,8,9,10,11,12]

Bordering on diabetes

With diagnosed diabetes being the tip of the iceberg of impaired glucose tolerance (IGT), one will often encounter hyperglycaemia on the acute medical intake. The WHO diagnostic criteria are well-established. They reflect cardiovascular risk related to glycaemia, and the glycaemic criteria were lowered in the 1990s to ensure that those at risk because of fasting hyperglycaemia were diagnosed and treated. There has also been a shift away from the oral glucose tolerance test (OGTT) which, although sensitive, is time-consuming. A repeated fasting plasma glucose (FPG) is adequate, practical and preferable. Diabetes is currently defined as an FPG in excess of 7.0 mmol/l. In the absence of symptoms, two samples should be taken, at intervals. It is generally pointless doing an OGTT in the acute setting. Normally, a slightly raised 'fasting' glucose amid the hustle and bustle of a general medical ward is simply erroneous (or non-fasting). But what should one do about the enlarging group in the hinterland of impaired fasting glucose (IFG), with a FPG between 6.1 and 7.0 mmol/l, or IGT, with a plasma glucose level between 7.8 and 11.1 mmol/l, 2 h after a specified

5   Department of Health, Obesity among children under 11 (2005) (www.dh.gov.uk)

6   Hu et al. NEJM (2001) 345: 790–797.

7   UKPDS Group, Lancet (1998) 352: 837–854.

8   UKPDS Group, Lancet (1998) 352: 854–865.

9   4S Collaborators, Lancet (1994) 344: 1383–1389.

10 Pyorala et al. Diabetes Care (1997) 20: 614–620.

11 Joint British Societies' Guidelines, Heart (2005) 91: v1–v52.

12 NICE guidance on lipid modification (publication due January 2008) (www.nice.org.uk)

glucose load? IFG simplifies the screening of at-risk individuals circumventing the need for OGTT but IGT is a better predictor for risk of future diabetes. Both groups have 'pre-diabetes' and are high-risk populations for the development of cardiovascular disease and overt diabetes: roughly 7% of people with IFG or IGT will progress to frank diabetes every year. Although some may spontaneously revert to normal, modest weight loss, regular physical activity, some oral hypoglycaemics and other drugs have been effective in reducing progression to overt diabetes. [13,14] So, it seems sensible to recommend at least annual follow up of glycaemia and to enthusiastically promote lifestyle modification. Whether the onset of diabetes is prevented or merely deferred is an academic argument since the duration of diabetes is strongly associated with risk: lifestyle intervention is always likely to be worthwhile. Pharmacotherapy can also be useful in delaying progression to frank diabetes and now metformin, acarbose and orlistat have supporting evidence. [15] More recent trials are addressing whether other agents, such as thiazolidinediones (glitazones) and ACE inhibitors will show a sustainable reduction in the risk of developing diabetes.

TYPE 2 DIABETES

Type 2 diabetes consistently features partial beta-cell failure, and insulin resistance is almost always found. Once frank diabetes is manifest (FPG over 7.0 mmol/l), there is a continuing decline in function at a rate of about 4% a year.[16]

The acute presentation of a patient with diabetes (for whatever reason) tends to focus the mind of the admitting physician on to the prevailing random blood glucose – is it too high and do any medications need 'tweaking'? The perspective in the diabetes clinic is more one of a need to establish patients on adequate long-term therapy. Doctors need to help patients to take strategic decisions about the management of their diabetes when blood glucose is inadequately controlled by diet or oral therapy alone. General physicians may feel impotent in the management of chronic diseases when encounters are brief. However, the influence that a doctor may have at the time of an admission can be profound. Nor should the focus be on glycaemia alone – most patients will be at significant risk of cardiovascular disease in all its forms and will need statins and aspirin, and almost all will have sub-optimal blood pressure control, and may need multiple therapies to achieve systolic pressures below 135 mmHg.

....

[13] Diabetes Prevention Programme Research Group, NEJM (2002) 346: 393–403.

[14] Diabetes Prevention Programme Research Group, Diabetes Care (2002) 25: 2165–2171.

[15] Torgerson *et al.* Diabetes Care (2004) 27: 155–161.

[16] Matthews *et al.* Diabet Med (1998) 15: 297–303.

Diet

Diet and exercise regimes need to be championed before starting oral anti-diabetic agents. Dietary advice is ideally delivered by an expert dietitian who can tailor programmes to the individual. That said, the main principles are that at least 55% of the diet should be in the form of complex carbohydrate, total fat intake should be less than 30% and protein about 10–15%. However, it is difficult for the average patient to translate these naked principles into action: people need to be persuaded to eat less (since they are usually overweight), use semi-skimmed milk and low-fat cheese, to avoid fried foods, and take chicken rather than red meat. Puddings (of a traditional sort) are generally a bad idea. Those commercial 'diabetic foods' that remain on the shelves should be avoided as they are often high in fat and calories and contain bulk sweeteners that raise blood glucose levels. Moreover, they are often remarkably expensive. Exercise plays a vital role, promoting weight loss, increasing insulin sensitivity and improving cardiovascular fitness. Exercising for 4 h a week for 6 weeks has been shown to increase insulin-mediated glucose uptake by 30%.[17] Realistically however, even if lifestyle advice is successfully adhered to, the majority of patients will require pharmacotherapy to achieve or sustain near normoglycaemia. Indeed, the UKPDS demonstrated not only that drug therapy was usually required but also a need for escalating polypharmacy in the pursuit of glycaemic targets. Continuing loss of beta-cell function and the progressive hyperglycaemia that follows characterizes type 2 diabetes: this process is accelerated by further weight gain and therefore reiteration of lifestyle advice continues to be important even after pharmacotherapy has been initiated.

Starters for ten

In making initial therapeutic decisions one needs to make a 'best guess' as to where the patient lies on the continuum of insulin resistance to beta-cell failure. As a rule (although not invariably), younger patients at near-normal bodyweight are more likely to have greater insulin deficiency than obese, sedentary middle-aged patients (who will have predominant insulin resistance). It is most likely that patients will have a combination of the two and so will benefit from combined insulin sensitizer (metformin or a glitazone) and secretagogue therapy. There has been a significant expansion in the range of hypoglycaemics on the market over the last decade but the evidence base (and the clinician's experience) varies not only between classes but also between

---

[17] Dylewicz *et al.* Acta Pediatr Scand (1980) 283: 70–78.

drugs drawn from the same class. Prescribing decisions are often rather subjective, depending on a practitioner's familiarity with a particular drug (which may explain regional differences in prescribing).

Metformin should be started slowly as most people will experience some gastro-intestinal effects initially. Patients should be forewarned about this, so that they do not give up too readily: about a third will be unable to tolerate a useful dosage. Metformin is cheap and its evidence base is substantial. The UKPDS showed a 32% risk reduction in all diabetes-related endpoints ($p = 0.0023$), a 42% risk reduction in diabetes-related deaths ($p = 0.017$), a 36% risk reduction in all cause mortality ($p = 0.011$) and a 39% risk reduction in myocardial infarction ($p = 0.01$).[18] In a randomized subgroup of the UKPDS, metformin was added to sulphonylurea therapy. This group showed no difference in outcome compared to the main randomized sulphonylurea group. However, there were fewer deaths amongst those randomized to continue on sulphonylurea alone (though the same number of coronary events) than either within the main sulphonylurea group or the combined sulphonylurea and metformin group. The only rational explanation of this finding – that secondary randomization to continue on the same treatment improves outcome – is that of chance. Post-study monitoring showed no adverse effects of combined treatment.

Sulphonylureas also have a good record from the UKPDS and were used to intensify treatment in the main trial. Microvascular complications were substantially reduced, ($p < 0.015$).[19] An ongoing debate has taken place around macrovascular disease, where a 16% risk reduction ($p = 0.052$) was reported. Most accept that these data are concordant with other studies and few (if any) academics now diverge from the view that good glycaemic control yields cardiovascular benefit. Nutrient absorption modulators (such as acarbose and orlistat) may also have a role. Patients taking orlistat soon discover that a poor diet will result in immediate retribution with fatty diarrhoea and soiling!

Therapies aimed at improving beta-cell function (such as sulphonylureas and the more expensive meglitinides) are effective for the first few years of diabetes, but as beta cell function continues to decline, these agents become less efficacious.

In terms of initial monotherapy, metformin is the logical choice for overweight patients with type 2 diabetes. It is the only common hypoglycaemic therapy with which bodyweight tends to stabilize or decrease slightly. Some improvement in hyperlipidaemia can occur, particularly if weight falls. In addition,

---

[18] UKPDS Group, Lancet (1998) 352: 854–865.

[19] UKPDS Group, Lancet (1998) 352: 837–854.

there is a relatively low incidence of hypoglycaemia. The GI side effects usually subside within weeks and can be alleviated somewhat by starting with a low dose (500 mg once daily) and gradually titrating the dose up to the usual ceiling of 850 mg tds. Lactic acidosis is in reality very rare and when it occurs due to treatment with metformin, serum lactate is usually less than 2 (which is not clinically significant). More serious lactic acid accumulation occurs with superimposed shock, or in presence of conditions predisposing to metformin toxicity such as renal insufficiency, heart failure requiring pharmacotherapy or liver disease. A pragmatic rule of thumb is to stop metformin if the creatinine exceeds 150 mmol/l. In addition, when using intravenous contrast agents, metformin should be stopped 48 h prior to a procedure and restarted at least 48 h thereafter.

In the relatively rare situation where BMI is less than 25 (and so beta-cell dysfunction is likely to be particularly significant), sulphonylureas present the best initial monotherapy. In younger patients in this category, slow-onset type 1 diabetes or a rare genetic subgroup are possibilities. One should see a response in days as this class of drugs can very quickly relieve the symptoms of hyperglycaemia. Doses should be increased until fasting glucose levels are normalized. If high doses fail to do this, metformin with its complementary mode of action, should be added (or a glitazone where metformin is contraindicated or poorly tolerated).

Pulling out all the stops

If therapy with these two agents at maximum tolerated doses fails, the options are either to consider triple therapy with metformin, a sulphonylurea and a glitazone (which is licensed in the US), or to introduce insulin. With triple therapy, there may be a delay in achieving glycaemic control because the glitazones can take up to 3 months to achieve maximum effect. They act via PPAR-gamma nuclear receptors (which are most strongly expressed in adipose tissue) to increase transcription of certain insulin-sensitive genes involved in the control of lipid and glucose metabolism, hence reducing insulin resistance. This class of drug has received much interest because of their effects on various cardiovascular risk indices.

Rosiglitazone and pioglitazone are licensed for monotherapy or combined therapy (though combination with insulin is contraindicated). Pioglitazone also improves the lipid profile, increasing HDL-cholesterol and reducing triglycerides. Data were recently presented from the PROActive trial and showed some improvement in the 'principle secondary endpoint' of recorded cardiovascular events. However, the trial yielded an equivocal result when analysed for the principle outcome – an aggregate of both outcome and intervention events.[20] A sub-analysis also suggested that differential effects were not significant in those taking statins. It was reported that the pioglitazone group had an increased physician-recorded incidence of heart failure: in fact, in the absence of any echocardiographic data, this may simply have been the fluid retention – known to be a common side effect of the glitazones. These drugs are contraindicated in patients with elevated baseline liver function tests (ALT more than 2.5 times the upper limit of normal), although in clinical trials they are associated with consistent reductions in ALT. They may be used as initial monotherapy in overweight patients where metformin is contraindicated but they can cause demoralizing weight gain in a group where weight loss is so very desirable. In fact, there is thought to be a beneficial redistribution of fat, from visceral to subcutaneous, but this is unlikely to be of much consolation to the patient. In terms of triple therapy, adding a glitazone may in reality buy just a few months before insulin must be instituted but this may be helpful in those who have a great reluctance to start insulin, perhaps through fear of needles or due to real employment concerns (e.g. some professional drivers).

The other groups of oral anti-diabetic drugs, alpha glucosidase inhibitors (acarbose) and meglitinides (repaglinide and nateglinide) are potentially useful in countering post-prandial hyperglycaemia. Early in the natural history of type 2 diabetes, post-prandial glucose peaks are said to account for up to 70% of the elevation in HbA1c. Thus, when not controlled by lifestyle interventions, acarbose or meglitinides ought, theoretically, to be useful first-line management in those patients who have a combination of slightly raised basal glucose and more marked post-prandial hyperglycaemia. In practice they are not widely used. They are of potential interest in individuals who have an irregular lifestyle where meals are unpredictable, in the elderly or those with renal impairment as they have a quicker onset, shorter duration of action and non-renal excretion. They are less effective in controlling basal glycaemia. Like the other insulin secretagogues they require residual beta-cell function to be effective.

Glucagon-like peptide 1 (GLP-1) is a novel insulin secretagogue, an 'incretin' (a hormone that causes stimulation of insulin secretion). GLP-1 is secreted from the small bowel in response to glucose ingestion. A homologue of GLP-1 (exendin-4) was found in the saliva of the Gila monster (a South American lizard). It has been synthesized and is now available as exenatide. It needs to be injected, but does not cause symptomatic hypoglycaemia, and does have an additional benefit of weight loss. Native GLP-1 is rapidly inactivated by

[20] www.proactive-results.com

dipeptidyl-peptidase-4 (DPP-4) and so one way of increasing its endogenous availability is with inhibitors of DPP-4. Such inhibitors have been developed and will be available soon. They have the advantage that they can be taken by mouth, but the weight loss seen with exenatide is not reported with these agents.

Introducing insulin

Half of all patients with type 2 diabetes will need insulin within 6 years of diagnosis, as this is the only efficacious therapy once serious beta-cell failure has occurred.[21] There is no very good evidence to determine exactly when insulin therapy should be introduced and often the biggest barrier to starting is the patient's reluctance, as it can be hard to convince people solely on the basis of a high HbA1c. In practice, insulin is reserved for those who have persistently high HbA1c and do not respond to combinations of oral agents; those in whom control deteriorates despite logical and adequate drug combinations at maximum tolerated doses and patients who have either osmotic symptoms or recurrent infections. It is also called for in specific situations for safety, such as in pregnancy and in patients with severe hepatic or renal impairment. The DIGAMI trial showed that insulin improved outcomes in those with mild hyperglycaemia who had had a myocardial infarction and this is now widely implemented.[22] Insulin is doubtless underused in type 2 diabetes, due to a combination of physician inertia and patient reluctance, although with appropriate education and care in its introduction, patients tolerate it well. The incidence of problematic hypoglycaemia in type 2 diabetes is extremely low (as endogenous insulin production by remaining beta-cells is physiologically suppressed when glucose falls).

When starting insulin, sessions with a diabetes specialist nurse (including the demonstration of the much shorter and finer needles than patients expect) are invaluable to ensure a seamless transition to insulin therapy. To achieve control, patients with type 2 diabetes will require at least half a unit of insulin per kilogram and may need doses up to 2–3 units/kg where obesity and insulin resistance predominate. Insulin can usually be introduced as a simple once or twice daily basal regimen (using, for example, detemir or glargine insulin) and continuing oral therapy with metformin, which can have a significant insulin sparing effect. Less weight gain, greater reduction in HbA1c and lower insulin requirements can all be gained by continuing the metformin. Glitazone–insulin combination therapy is contraindicated because of concerns

---

[21] Matthews, Diabet Med (1998) 15: 297–303.

[22] Malmberg, BMJ (1997) 314: 1512–1515.

about precipitating cardiac failure. Insulin treatment is associated with significant weight gain which does need to be addressed proactively: patients should be told to reduce their food intake and to reduce insulin if the blood glucose becomes too low. Basal insulin should be increased until the FPG is under control. If the HbA1c deteriorates, this is the time to initiate prandial insulin, which provides a shorter acting insulin (typically aspart or lispro insulin) to cover meals. Patients may be unwilling to accept up to four daily injections and some negotiation will generally be needed.

This failure-based approach can be a long and frustrating one for both patient and doctor. First the lifestyle coaxing, then the monotherapy, followed by a number of logical combinations before the 'last resort' of insulin is called for as glycaemic control worsens. This can make clinic visits very demoralizing as the HbA1c remains stubbornly off-target. Presenting alterations in a regimen as 'optimizing therapy', as opposed to the onward and unstoppable march of the disease is a real challenge. It is useful to outline to patients early in their treatment that the condition is progressive. This removes the aspect of 'blame' as HbA1c deteriorates and therapies escalate.

Hitting the target

Although any reduction in HbA1c is to be welcomed, knowledge from the UKPDS drives current practice in which treatment is directed to the attainment of near-normoglycaemia (an HbA1c of 6.5–7.0%). This is unrealistic for many and a pragmatic approach is to aim for an HbA1c level of around 7%, but since glycaemic control is easier early in the course of the disease and complications are a function of both time and glycaemic exposure, it is sensible to strive hard early and adopt a more pragmatic approach when beta-cell failure becomes manifest. Even then, early intervention with insulin is advisable for most. Moreover, since complications are related to multiple risks, it is essential to initiate lipid lowering, excellent control of blood pressure and to vigorously discourage smoking. An HbA1c over 8.0% requires immediate pharmacotherapy. An HbA1c in excess of 9.0% a few months into treatment almost certainly means that the patient will require insulin.

To assess the response to therapy, periodic HbA1c measurement is required (every 3–6 months) and this is often accompanied by self measurement of capillary blood glucose. The price of the latter is such that cost-effectiveness in type 2 diabetes is dubious. Beware the haemaglobinopathies such as sickle cell and thalassemia, which can make HbA1c levels appear falsely low: fructosamine is a measure of shorter term glucose exposure, having a shorter half life than HbA1c, and is useful in the haemaglobinopathies and pregnancy.

The average glucose lowering effect of the major classes of oral anti-diabetic agents is broadly similar, averaging a percentage point reduction in HbA1c.

Managed care

Type 2 diabetes is so common (currently estimated as having a prevalence of around 4% in UK), that there is no possibility of all patients being routinely seen by specialist services. However, it is imperative for all to be seen by suitably trained professionals and for care to be integrated. Generally, this will involve a high level of input from primary care, with specialist nurses, dietitians and general practitioners working in teams. Some health authorities have initiated intermediate care clinics. Specialist care will be required for a minority (about 1 in 8), especially in relation to complications and complex drug regimens (including insulin). Specialist services can also support primary care through telemedicine and intranets. For Type 1 diabetes, specialist services are more important, as many teenagers default on care and reap a tragic reward of early complications as a result. Keeping in touch with these patients can be problematic but text messaging, consistency of care and flexibility all help to increase the quality of the individual's own self-management.

The wider picture

Almost all patients with type 2 diabetes should be on lipid lowering treatment. It should only be withheld from those who are at demonstrably low risk. Even the youngest patients with type 2 diabetes have a high lifetime risk of events and should be considered for statin therapy. The only important exception to this rule is around the time of pregnancy (and breastfeeding). On an intention to treat basis, the CARDS trial showed a 36% reduction in acute coronary events and a 48% reduction in stroke in type 2 diabetics treated with atorvastatin.[23,24,25] LDL-cholesterol lowering is the primary goal and the treatment target is a LDL-cholesterol of < 2 mmol/l. If hypertriglyceridaemia predominates (> 4.5 mmol/l), fibrate treatment or combination therapy may be more appropriate.

The UKPDS demonstrated that complications were related to blood pressure as well as to glycaemic control. There was no threshold of effect, and the epidemiology suggested that the lower the blood pressure, the better the outcome. For most it is reasonable to strive to keep the systolic blood pressure under 135 mmHg.

[23] Colhoun *et al*. Lancet (2004) 364: 685–696.

[24] Joint British Societies' Guidelines, Heart (2005) 91: v1–v52.

[25] NICE guidance on lipid modification (publication due January 2008) (www.nice.org.uk)

It is important to manage the diabetic patient, as all others, in the context of their overall risk. Where patients have ischaemic heart disease or albuminuria, this may influence the first choice antihypertensive agent. In the patient who remains free of such clinical manifestations, any antihypertensive is likely to reduce events and can be legitimately used as initial therapy. The ALLHAT study suggested that an ACE inhibitor is the best choice for those with poorly controlled diabetes as the fasting glucose levels dropped in this group.[26] However, where glycaemia was well controlled, thiazide diuretics were better for preventing events than ACE inhibitors and calcium channel blockers. Diabetic patients are even more likely than other groups to need a combination of several drugs. Hypertension is discussed in more detail in Chapter Six.

Usually in type 2 diabetes, one has the luxury of time: most things can be dealt with on an outpatient basis. However, emergencies do occur, most often encountered on the acute medical take as hyperosmolar non-ketotic hyperglycaemia (HONK). This condition has a phenomenally high mortality and is often diagnosed late when the comatose elderly patient in accident and emergency is noted to have a sky-high glucose (often little short of 100 mmol/l). Such a result quickly galvanizes all into a flurry of activity and unfortunately, this may lead to dangerous over-treatment with fluids. Central venous monitoring is important in these patients, where the line between euvolaemia and cardiac failure is very fine. A reasonable aim is to replace the estimated fluid deficit over 48 h, initially with 0.9% saline. There are very few situations that demand 0.45% saline, which is best avoided as it increases the risk of cerebral oedema, through overly rapid fluxes in serum sodium or osmolality.

TYPE 1 DIABETES

Type 1 diabetes was universally fatal before the discovery and purification of insulin in 1922 by Banting and Best. Before that time, some thin children survived for about a year on fat-free starvation diets – simply because in the absence of endogenous or exogenous fat, there was no ketosis.

A near-death experience

Diabetic ketoacidosis occurs in those newly diagnosed with type 1 diabetes and in those with known diabetes who stop or reduce their insulin inappropriately. The commonest reason for such a reduction is that a patient finds him/herself vomiting (perhaps due to gastroenteritis) and erroneously supposes that without

---

[26] ALLHAT Investigators, JAMA (2002) 288: 2981–2997.

any carbohydrate intake, they will become hypoglycaemic. All patients should continue their basal insulin whatever else is occurring and many will require more insulin with intercurrent illness because their insulin resistance will rise. Some teenagers and young adults manipulate their insulin with adverse consequences. Girls especially may skip insulin in order to lose weight – a highly dangerous manoeuvre. The diagnosis of DKA may be missed: the air-hunger of acidosis may be mistaken for a psychological hyperventilation or even asthma. Making the latter mistake demonstrates poor clinical observation: in DKA, rapid respiration occurs with a wide open mouth, whereas in asthma the lips are usually pursed together. The mortality of DKA remains at 2–5% and hospital audits consistently identify sub-optimal management, particularly delays in the initiation of treatment and inadequate fluid replacement (patients will generally need several litres of fluid over the first 24 h, with or without the guidance of a central venous line). Adequate monitoring during treatment is mandatory.

Persistent ketoacidosis can be detected with bedside ketone meters where available, and ketones ought to be measured hourly in the acute phase. One finger prick is enough, with a second drop of blood destined for the separate ketone-strip. Normalization of the blood glucose is not necessarily synonymous with the resolution of ketosis. Ketosis can be regarded as having resolved when ketones in the plasma are less than 1 mmol/l. The commonest causes of a failure to resolve are inadequate fluid replacement and inadequate insulin. In general, ketones should drop by about 1 mmol/l per hour when treatment is adequate. Urine and plasma ketostix are semi-quantitative alternatives where meters are not available.

DKA can present without particularly marked hyperglycaemia during pregnancy and in surgical patients, where the requirements of the foetus or vomiting result in lower than expected blood glucose levels. In such situations, patients are also prone to the development of some degree of lactic acidosis.

In addition to their use in the stabilization of the patient, sliding scales can also prove helpful as a monitoring device. Often patients are left with them running for over 72 h, which is almost never called for if the patient has begun to eat and drink. They may also be poorly managed with blocked lines, inappropriate scales and the concomitant use of dextrose (aggravating the hyperglycaemia). In general, if the blood glucose is stable in the 10–15 mmol/l range, the patient is ketone-free (< 0.5 mmol/l) and eating and drinking, then the intravenous sliding scale should be swapped over to a subcutaneous insulin regime. There is an element of guesswork here and rather than aiming to micro-manage and tighten control to levels of between 5–8 mmol/l, one should instead be satisfied with sugars in the single figures. Ideally, patients should remain in hospital for at least 24 h once on their subcutaneous regime both to ensure stability and also to provide an opportunity for consultation and education with the diabetic team. It is often useful to discharge frequent attenders with ketostix to facilitate earlier recognition of troubles at home.

Where an episode of DKA represents the first presentation, the patient should be managed by diabetes specialists. They would aim to convert the patient to a basal-bolus regime directly from the sliding scale but this does require both acceptance and willingness on the patient's part. Four injections a day, in addition to the shock of the diagnosis, may prove altogether too much and a twice-daily mixed insulin regime is a reasonable alternative. With regard to the estimation of initial dosages, there is little by way of science to it and a degree of guesswork is required. In general, one should total up the insulin requirement over 24 h from the sliding scale and then reduce this figure by 10–20%. One-third of this amount should be given as an isophane insulin at night and the rest split evenly between meals: 4–6 units of a short-acting preparation prior to meals and 6–8 units of isophane before bed would be a typical starting point. The evening isophane will often then need to be titrated up to maintain adequate fasting sugars. Where twice-daily fixed mixture regimes are used, a suitable starting regimen is a 30/70 mixture with two-thirds before breakfast and the remainder prior to the evening meal.

Hypoglycaemia

At the other end of the spectrum, hypoglycaemia will occur in most insulin-treated patients at some point, especially as diabetologists become increasingly aggressive with treatment regimes, in pursuit of optimal control. In patients with type 2 diabetes taking oral therapy but not insulin, long-acting glibenclamide is frequently the culprit when hypoglycaemia does occur, particularly if renal function is not what it should be. The autonomic symptoms of hypoglycaemia usually occur at levels below 3.6 mmol/l with neuroglycopenia (and a reduction in the level of consciousness) at values below 2.6 mmol/l. If a patient is experiencing chronic hypoglycaemia, the autonomic warning symptoms may be lost or else only apparent at more profound levels of hypoglycaemia.

Hypoglycaemia often occurs first thing in the morning (particularly where long-acting insulin is taken at night) or during the night when patients may actually wake with a hyperglycaemic response the next morning due to a surge in counter-regulatory hormones. The only symptoms to suggest such an occurrence may be morning headaches or a feeling of drunkenness. In such circumstances, a significant reduction (4 units or more) in basal insulin should be advised to bring fasting glucose levels consistently above 5 mmol/l.

Recurrent hypoglycaemia can also occur following deterioration in renal or hepatic function and this should be excluded.

Venturing on to the surgical ward

When patients with diabetes require an operation, it is ideally performed at the start of a list. Patients controlled by diet alone rarely need any specific modification, although blood glucose should be monitored. Patients on oral therapy should stop their metformin preoperatively and omit any other agents on the morning of the procedure. Blood glucose should be monitored at least 2-hourly and if it exceeds 7.0 mmol/l, a sliding scale should be instituted with dextrose. Surgical units will tend to have their own favoured scales (and woe betide any physician who suggests an alternative) but the general aim should be to keep the blood glucose in the 7–11 mmol/l range. Insulin-requiring patients undergoing a morning procedure should miss their morning insulin and start on an intravenous dextrose and insulin regimen. If on an afternoon list, half the normal morning dose of insulin should be given with breakfast and the sliding scale started at midday.

Delivering insulin

Most individuals are now treated with recombinant human insulin, and with this comes the added advantage of improved pharmacokinetics. Nonetheless, one will still encounter some patients who favour old-fashioned animal insulins (which are still available) and some also prefer traditional syringes to the more modern insulin pens. Many patients will have had many years of experience as to how best manage their diabetes: it is discourteous (and ill-advised) for any doctor to assert that he or she can manage it better after a 2-minute conversation. Insulin therapy should be adjusted only in consultation with the patient, and for sound reasons rather than for expediency.

Isophane insulin (as a basal insulin) can cause nocturnal hypoglycaemia, typically in the early hours. The newer analogues (such as detemir and glargine) may prevent this problem, having a flatter delivery profile, and providing good 20–24 h basal insulin cover. The new short-acting insulins are quicker to act than their soluble predecessors, and so match meal-induced glucose peaks more closely. Because of this, there can be greater mealtime flexibility than was previously the case – indeed one can potentially skip the occasional meal safely, adjusting the regime accordingly. The so-called 'basal bolus regimes' now more closely resemble the insulin profiles of non-diabetic individuals, although they remain far short of the physiological.

The availability of rapid-acting insulins has also contributed to the greater use of insulin pumps. Although expensive, these pumps allow for the setting of various basal rates of insulin administration and a bolus administration with each meal. Cutaneous interstitial glucose measurement and continuous automated monitoring can provide accurate real-time glucose information that is much needed in intensive insulin therapy.[27]

Much research has been devoted to non-invasive methods of insulin delivery with inhaled insulins rising to the fore. The pulmonary route is attractive as the lungs are permeable to small proteins and offer a large surface area for drug absorption. Inhaled insulin (Exubera) is quickly absorbed and so can be used at mealtimes. However, we do not yet know the long-term effects of inhaling a protein molecule with its carrier, and since insulin bioavailability is lower, NICE is sceptical as to cost effectiveness. The requisite equipment for administration is also rather bulky at present.

Although patient compliance may well be improved by non-invasive insulin delivery, exciting advances have also been made in developing possible cures for diabetes. Whole pancreas transplant is an option when a kidney is being transplanted (the combination of the two is necessary because rejection can be detected by a rising creatinine, whereas there is currently no biomarker for rejection of the pancreas itself). Islet cell transplantation is gradually increasing, and this procedure has the advantage that islets can be infused into the portal system under ultrasonic guidance as a day-case. Islets can be administered repeatedly from different donors, and although 5-year 'insulin-free' rates are disappointing, patients with severe recurrent hypoglycaemia can see their quality of life transformed. Immunosuppressive drugs are needed and the cadaveric supply of islets is limited – it is not yet a panacea.

Keeping complications at bay

Many of the current recommendations for screening and referral to appropriate specialists are now managed in primary care. However, as the general physician will often see those who slip through the net, there remains a need to be aware of care pathways.

To prevent all the complications of diabetes, optimal control of glycaemia, blood pressure and lipids (in the non-smoking patient) is the goal. To screen for nephropathy, an annual test of creatinine and microalbuminuria (such as the albumin to creatinine ratio) is required and where there is evidence of such, an ACE inhibitor or ARB should be initiated (irrespective of blood pressure).

[27] TA057 (January 2003) (www.nice.org.uk)

Where nephropathy has progressed to macroalbuminuria or the creatinine sits in the 200–250 range (in patients with average muscle bulk), the patient should be referred to a renal physician. Screening for, and treatment of, retinopathy is essential. As a minimum, patients should have initial dilated fundoscopy performed by an ophthalmologist or optometrist shortly after diagnosis and then annually thereafter (more frequently if retinopathy is progressing). Digital retinal photography is fast becoming the gold standard. During pregnancy, fundoscopy should occur at least once each trimester as some patients can develop florid retinopathy during pregnancy, the cause of which remains obscure. Prompt referral to an ophthalmologist (for laser therapy) is always required for those with macular oedema, severe non-proliferative diabetic retinopathy or proliferative retinopathy.

Ulcers

Lifting the bedclothes and removing layers of footwear, bandages and gauze is essential if diabetic foot complications are to be properly assessed. Most of those with diabetes who attend for annual review in primary care will have their feet examined with a monofilament (10 g sensitivity) and tuning fork (128 Hz). High-risk patients with active foot ulcers, or a previous history of ulcers or amputation, should be monitored by specialist diabetes podiatrists (who often run their own clinics and referral systems). A history of claudication and absent pedal pulses should prompt referral to the vascular surgeons for further assessment. In those with peripheral neuropathy, terrible problems can and commonly do occur in hospital. An immobile patient in a hospital bed can rapidly succumb to pressure sores (especially on the heels) which may go unnoticed until the smell of infection or the dampness of the bedclothes (through exudates) are seen. It is then too late and nurses, doctors and the hospital all find themselves in medico-legal territory. Infected ulcers should be deep swabbed before antibiotic therapy is instituted. Cellulitis should be vigourously treated with intravenous antibiotics combined with oral metronidazole (to cover anaerobes). Debridement must be undertaken if any dead tissue is seen, either by a competent podiatrist or a surgeon, depending upon extent. Unsurprisingly, asking for an orthopaedic opinion usually results in an orthopaedic procedure, so for foot and limb preservation the plastic surgeons (whose specialty is soft tissue) should be tried first or if the circulation is compromised, the vascular surgeons. Foul-smelling ulcers can be treated with metronidazole gel in addition to intravenous antibiotics. Maggots are extremely effective at cleaning ulcers, but some skill is needed in ushering them to the right place – they have an impressive range of speed, acceleration and direction which can prove rather disconcerting for patient and novice clinician alike. Osteomyelitis in the long bones requires specialist treatment. Osteomyelitis in the small bones of the foot can be surprisingly benign and much effort can be devoted to establishing its presence with little tangible gain in therapeutic options. Chronic indolent osteomyelitis need not be attacked surgically. The commonest cause of amputation in the UK is still diabetes. End-stage wet gangrene demands immediate surgical attention (any surgeon, orthopaedic included). Patients may need special counselling when facing the loss of limb or forefoot, but surgery is life-saving in cases where infection and dead tissue coexist. Necrotizing fasciitis is a much feared occurrence – when an infected leg seems to produce pain out of all proportion to what might be expected, beware of this catastrophic streptococcal entity. Rapid and generous debridement is the only cure.

OBESITY

More than a billion adults in the world are overweight and perhaps more alarmingly, 10% of children are obese. Obesity is by far the most important risk factor for type 2 diabetes, and unfortunately imposes a greater risk per BMI increment in those from the developing world. With our ever expanding waistlines has come a rise in associated diseases, such that obesity is set to overtake smoking as the main preventable cause of disease and premature death globally. Diabetologists, cardiologists (hypertension and coronary disease), neurologists (stoke and TIA), respiratory physicians (sleep apnoea) and orthopaedic surgeons (hip and knee replacements) will be in increasing demand. Oncologists will also be kept busy (the WHO recently estimated that overweight and inactivity account for a quarter to a third of cancers of the breast, colon, endometrium, kidney and oesophagus), along with reproductive endocrinologists (excess oestrogen causes irregular, commonly anovulatory cycles and obesity is thought to account for 6% of primary infertility). Hepatologists will have their work cut out too as obesity is set to become one of the most common causes of end-stage liver failure in more developed countries, as it progresses from the more benign fatty changes ('NASH' and 'NAFLD') to cirrhosis, portal hypertension and potentially hepatocellular carcinoma.

Despite being perhaps the easiest of all spot diagnoses to make, obesity has been much neglected in the medical arena and it is really only in the last 10 years that 'fat' has been pushed up the global agenda. Obesity can, and must, be tackled at many different levels, by many different parties. Governments have many responsibilities, including those of food labelling (through regulation) and ensuring the appropriate education of children. The food industry could and should make its profits through low calorie foods instead of fat-saturated fast food, architects must design buildings with stairs rather than lifts as their centrepiece, and the health care system needs to take obesity altogether more seriously. The experiences of the anti-smoking lobby have shown that multiple stakeholders, acting together, can bring about fundamental changes in public attitudes, achieving results despite the enormous financial interests within industry and commerce.

So what can the individual physician contribute to tackling this weighty problem? Until these big players institute real change in our culture of over eating and inactivity, it is up to the clinician to tackle the problem, one obese person at a time. With such a large proportion of our patients being overweight, there is plenty of opportunity! Perhaps the main hurdle is accepting that obesity is (or will become) a medical disorder for many patients. Rather than tip-toeing around the subject in clinic, BMI charts are useful in demonstrating to the patient that they do indeed lie in that unpleasant sounding zone of the 'morbidly obese'. Just as the representation of coronary disease with 'fat-dripping' cigarettes and graphic illustrations of the carnage of road traffic accidents have been required to make inroads into smoking and drink driving, straight talking and a degree of realism will be required to shock people off their sofas. Other than height, weight and subsequent BMI measurement, waist circumference is another potentially useful part of our assessment. However, the need to disrobe makes this an unattractive experience for many patients. Central (abdominal) obesity is now recognized as a risk factor for cardiovascular disease, dyslipidaemia, glucose intolerance and insulin resistance. There is some debate as to whether one should try to distinguish what makes up the large waist; excess subcutaneous fat versus visceral fat. Increased intra-abdominal or visceral adipose tissue creates a high flux of fatty acids to the liver through the splanchnic circulation whereas increased abdominal subcutaneous fat releases lipolysis products into the systemic circulation without direct effects on hepatic metabolism (such as glucose production and lipid synthesis). The distinction could be made with CT or MRI but for now, a tape measure suffices with the cut-offs for increased risk being 102 cm for men and 88 cm for women (measuring approximately 1 cm below the umbilicus, wherever it may hang). Of note, there are now ethnicity-specific differences in the definition of obesity recognizing the fact that certain populations are more prone to the associated diseases at a given level of adiposity.

In Asians, the WHO has redefined 'overweight' as BMI over 23, and obesity as BMI over 25. Optimum waist circumferences are also lower, at 94 cm for men and 80 cm for women.

Probably one of the reasons for our general lack of interest in obesity is that as of yet, there is no 'wonder drug'. As such, 'industry' in its widest sense currently has a vested interest in obesity and indeed the anxiety associated with it (cosmetic surgery, diet plans and gymnasia). The main challenge is to get the patient to recognize the problem and to motivate them to address it: medics are notoriously bad at achieving this and the best help really comes from specialist dietitians who can follow patients up and are better at achieving (and perhaps more importantly maintaining) weight loss. There are a number of dietary approaches including low glycaemic index diets, very low calorie diets (VLCDs) and high protein – low carbohydrate diets: it is here that the dietitian plays a key role in individualizing the approach. Behavioural psychologists are also effective but funding is scarce and if available at all, a 6 month wait is not unusual. Alongside the dietitian, a personal instructor might be expected to prove invaluable since physical activity plays a critical role in maintaining lost weight with a clear relationship between levels of activity and the degree of sustained weight loss. A new cohort of personal trainers, based in primary care, has recently been promised to patients in England. With gym sessions now available 'on prescription' from some general practitioners, clinicians may soon be exhibiting the motivational behaviours that one might expect to see on an exercise video. However, NICE has recently issued guidance on the very subject of interventions to promote weight loss: although brief opportunistic encouragement from health professionals is effective, the NICE jury is still out on the value of prescribed community-based exercise programmes, pedometers and the like.[28]

Pharmacotherapy

So what place, if any, does pharmacotherapy have? Obesity drugs have historically had a bad press, largely due to the use of dangerous concoctions of diuretics, thyroid extract and amphetamines combined with barbiturates in the 1970s and 1980s. The only drugs currently shown to be efficacious are orlistat (a pancreatic lipase inhibitor), sibutramine (a centrally acting appetite suppressant) and rimonabant (a cannabinoid-receptor antagonist). The use of drugs is limited by side effects: for example, any deviation from a low fat diet while taking orlistat results in unpleasant (and often explosive) diarrhoea. Blood pressure requires close monitoring with sibutramine as it may increase.

NICE guidance for anti-obesity medications is currently a little dated (predating the arrival of rimonabant) and a comprehensive obesity guideline is in development. At present, anti-obesity medications should be considered where the BMI is over 30 (or at a lower level where there is a persistent

---

[28] Public health intervention guidance: physical activity (March 2006) (www.nice.org.uk)

co-morbidity: over 27 for sibutramine, over 28 for orlistat). Furthermore, orlistat should be 'earned' by demonstration of a 2.5-kg weight loss in the month before a prescription is written. Continuation of the therapy requires evidence of further weight loss and is not currently recommended beyond 12 months on the basis of insufficient long-term data.[29,30] However, the Xendos study has since provided 4-year data for orlistat and similar studies are ongoing for sibutramine.[31] The impact of pharmacotherapy is limited: approximately 60% of patients treated for a year will achieve and maintain weight loss of 5% or more.

A recent addition to the appetite suppressants is rimonabant, a selective cannabinoid receptor blocker. Treatment with 20 mg daily (in addition to diet) has been shown to promote modest (mean 6.3 kg) weight loss over a 2-year period.[32]

Surgeons and staples

If all else fails, we can call upon our surgical colleagues. Laparoscopic stomach banding, Roux-en-Y (the gold standard) and other forms of gastric bypass are increasingly popular options, particularly in the US. Weight loss can be 25–30% with rapid normalization of hyperglycaemia and blood pressure in those with diabetes and hypertension. The specific intervention should be selected by the patient in conjunction with an expert. NICE has issued guidance as to the appropriate generic indications.[33] Unfortunately, the main limitation here is actually finding a local surgeon who will accept referrals for the patients who request bariatric surgery.

However, for the vast majority of those who are overweight there is no quick fix, and even with the drugs that are available, the results for weight maintenance after therapy has stopped are depressing. If we really are to alter the course of our ever-expanding waistlines, the answer lies in a concerted and profound shift in public and fiscal policy.

The deadly quartet

Along with the obesity epidemic has come the re-emergence of a syndrome first described in the 1920s as the clustering of hypertension, hyperglycaemia

29 TA031 (October 2001) (www.nice.org.uk)

30 TA022 (March 2001) (www.nice.org.uk)

31 Torgerson et al. Diabetes Care (2004) 27: 155–161.

32 Pi-Sunyer et al. JAMA (2006) 295: 761–775.

33 TA046 (July 2002) (www.nice.org.uk)

and gout. Later, central obesity and dyslipidaemia were linked to this constellation of ills that has been variably termed Reaven's syndrome, syndrome X,
the insulin resistance syndrome, the deadly quartet and more recently, the
metabolic syndrome. It has been enough of a challenge to agree what constitutes this syndrome, let alone to treat it. Most agree that the main components
are central obesity, dyslipidaemia, hyperglycaemia and hypertension. However
there is disagreement as to whether the metabolic syndrome should be defined
to mainly indicate insulin resistance, the metabolic consequences of obesity,
risk for CVD, or simply a collection of statistically related factors. How we define
the syndrome obviously impacts upon which individuals come to have it and the
favoured definition is one that is easy to use but best predicts subsequent
diabetes and cardiovascular disease. Several groups including the WHO have
attempted to construct definitions that tend to vary as to whether insulin resistance or cardiovascular risk is the main focus. The International Diabetes
Federation (IDF) proposed another definition, preferred by the authors, in 2004.

IDF definition of the metabolic syndrome

For a person to have the metabolic syndrome, they must have:

Central obesity defined as waist circumference ≥ 102 cm for Europid men and ≥ 88 cm for Europid
women (with ethnicity-specific values for other groups) plus any two of the following four factors:
* raised triglyceride level: > 1.7 mmol/l or specific treatment for this lipid abnormality
* reduced HDL-C: < 0.9 mmol/l in males and < 1.1 mmol/l in females, or specific treatment for
  this lipid abnormality
* raised BP: systolic BP ≥ 130 or diastolic BP ≥ 85 mmHg, or treatment of previously diagnosed
  hypertension
* raised FPG: ≥5.6 mmol/l, or previously diagnosed type 2 diabetes

Having settled on one of the many definitions offered, the question arises as
to what useful purpose this diagnosis serves. It is true that certain CVD risk
factors occur together more often than expected by chance but as of yet there
is no identified unifying pathophysiology: insulin resistance is present in most
who have the syndrome but this is because almost all people who have elevated
blood glucose are insulin resistant. Since there is no specific treatment for the
metabolic syndrome *per se*, one must treat the individual abnormalities
(which as they are already well-established cardiovascular risk factors, one
would hope might already be done anyway). However, importantly, the label
of metabolic syndrome can sometimes help in explaining to patients who
attend for their first appointment why they are leaving clinic with a bag full of
tablets to treat hyperglycaemia, hypertension and dyslipidaemia, in addition to
being asked to take a junior aspirin every day.

Metabolic syndrome is of course a strong predictor of future diabetes (which is hardly surprising given that the definition includes glucose intolerance). It is certainly a risk factor for CVD but is this risk above and beyond that associated with the sum risk of its individual components? Some have argued that the Framingham risk assessment algorithm is actually more predictive of future CVD events. Perhaps the most useful outcome from this clustering of risk factors is that identification of one of the risk variables in a patient should always prompt a search for others. Perhaps the only area which is likely to represent a change in clinical practice in the near future is that of pharmacological intervention for the 'pre-diabetics' and 'pre-hypertensives': pioglitazone was recently shown to reduce cardiovascular events in this group.[34] However whilst no doubt an important public health goal to treat these risk factors before progression to disease, we must be wary of labelling patients with a syndrome that may cause more anxiety, rather than have a positive impact on their health and lifestyle.

---

[34] www.proactive-results.com

Chapter 6

Peter Hill and Chris O'Callaghan

HYPERTENSION AND NEPHROLOGY

The kidney can seem something of a 'black box', with obvious inputs and outputs but mysterious and complex processes within. On the one hand, it is a delicate organ that is easy to offend with inappropriate prescribing or poor attention to fluid balance, on the other, it is an easy organ to monitor and investigate, and the only major organ for which there are proper artificial replacement therapies.

Back to basics

The kidney has three basic functions: excretory, regulatory and endocrine.

The kidney excretes toxins and unwanted products of metabolism and it removes precisely controlled amounts of water and solutes to control body fluid volume and composition. To carry out these functions, the kidney receives about 20% of cardiac output, equating to a renal blood flow of around 1200 ml/min. This enormous volume of blood drives the production of glomerular filtrate.

The glomerulus acts as a fine 'sieve'. It is composed of a ball of blood capillaries surrounded by a space into which the urine passes on its way to the renal tubules. The higher the blood pressure in the glomerular capillaries, the more filtration there will be. The pressure forces water, salts and small molecules through the filtration sieve into the urinary space. The pressure in the capillaries is determined by the afferent and efferent arterioles. Just as if one treads on a hosepipe with water running through it, the pressure will rise upstream of one's foot, but fall downstream of it, similarly, vasoconstriction of the efferent arteriole results in the pressure rising upstream in the glomerular capillaries, whereas if there is vasoconstriction of the afferent arteriole as it enters the glomerulus, the pressure downstream in the glomerular capillaries will fall. The sieve itself consists of three layers: endothelial cells lining the glomerular capillaries, the glomerular basement membrane and the epithelial cells lining the urinary space. These epithelial cells, or podocytes, have long foot-like processes, which interdigitate to produce tiny filtration slits through which filtered water and molecules pass. The size of these slits and the electrical charges around the slits determine which molecules or ions are filtered.

The kidneys produce 180 l of filtrate each day, but to drink 180 l of fluid per day would be arduous. To maintain biological homeostasis, dramatic reabsorption of water and solutes must take place. Before the filtrate is excreted it travels along the renal tubules which modify its composition and volume. Most reabsorption occurs in the proximal tubule, with fine adjustments being made in the distal tubule and collecting ducts. A series of ion channels and transporter molecules mediate these effects and a number of these molecules are now known to be the targets of commonly prescribed diuretics.

The kidney is also an important endocrine organ, producing renin, activated vitamin D, erythropoietin and prostaglandins. It is also a target for aldosterone, anti-diuretic hormone, natriuretic peptides, parathyroid hormone and once again, prostaglandins. These endocrine functions explain some of the clinical features of chronic renal failure, such as anaemia due to erythropoietin deficiency. Understanding these can influence drug therapy in renal disease, for example, prostaglandins help maintain renal vessel dilatation and hence renal perfusion. Non-steroidal anti-inflammatory agents reduce prostaglandin production and therefore reduce renal perfusion.

HYPERTENSION

Hypertension is common and the incidence is increasing as populations age and become more obese. A large chunk of health care budgets in developed countries is spent on the recognition and treatment of hypertension. Hypertension is the commonest risk factor for premature cardiovascular disease and is associated with cardiac changes including left ventricular hypertrophy. It is the most important risk factor for stroke, the incidence of which can be markedly reduced with effective anti-hypertensive therapy. The funding of General Practitioners in the UK is now directly influenced by the performance of their practices in identifying and treating hypertension.[1]

[1] Quality and Outcomes Framework (www.dh.gov.uk)

Feeling the pressure

In the general population, hypertension is broadly defined as a systolic blood pressure > 140 mmHg or a diastolic pressure > 90 mmHg.[2] In patients with diabetes mellitus or chronic kidney disease even lower blood pressures are desirable as discussed below. The diagnosis is based upon at least three properly measured readings on two or more occasions. Using an appropriately sized cuff is essential – a large arm needs a large cuff and if the cuff is too small, the pressure recorded may be erroneously high. In older patients, systolic pressure, and pulse pressure may be more powerful determinants of risk than diastolic pressure as they reflect a reduction in the compliance of the vessel walls.

White coats

White coat hypertension occurs in between a fifth and a quarter of patients and can be distinguished from other forms of hypertension using home measurements or ambulatory blood pressure monitoring. By consensus, hypertension is present when home measurements average > 135/85 mmHg or 24-h averages from ambulatory blood pressure monitoring are > 125/80 mmHg. In the clinic, the presence of hypertensive changes in the fundi, or of left ventricular hypertrophy on an electrocardiogram (ECG), can be helpful in confirming true hypertension.

Hypertension is divided into two categories; essential (with no obvious cause) in the vast majority and secondary in a small (< 5%) but important minority. Essential hypertension is characterized by an increase in peripheral vascular resistance. It can be familial and is more common in the overweight. Increased salt intake is associated with hypertension and high alcohol intake also increases blood pressure. Hypertension is more common and often more severe in the black population and may have a somewhat different pathogenesis to hypertension in the white population, as the two groups differ in their response to drugs.

Secondary considerations

Secondary hypertension is that with a discernable cause, which may be renal, endocrine or vascular. Although relatively uncommon, secondary hypertension should always be considered in the young, when hypertension is refractory to standard therapy, when it is severe (systolic BP > 180 mmHg, diastolic BP > 110 mmHg), when blood pressure suddenly becomes uncontrolled in

....

[2] Williams *et al.* BMJ (2004) 328: 634–640.

patients with essential hypertension or when severe end-organ damage is found at diagnosis.

Blockages

Renovascular disease is the most common cause of secondary hypertension. It is due to fibromuscular dysplasia in the younger, typically female patient and atheroma in the older, typically male patient. In this condition, a reduction in the delivery of blood to the kidney (on account of the stenosis) results in an increase in renin production which triggers increases in angiotensin II and aldosterone. Angiotensin II is a powerful vasoconstrictor and along with aldosterone, it also promotes sodium retention. The net effect is systemic vasoconstriction and salt and water retention. Renovascular disease can rarely present with 'flash' pulmonary oedema, due to diastolic cardiac dysfunction associated with hypertension, salt and water retention, and hyperaldosteronism. Renovascular disease should be considered if there is a history of artherosclerosis (especially peripheral vascular disease) or a significant deterioration in renal function following initiation of an ACE-inhibitor (> 20% rise in serum creatinine or > 15% fall in GFR). Renal impairment may be found on investigation, typically with hyperkalaemia, and ultrasound may show kidneys of unequal size, where a difference of 1 cm or more is considered significant. In bilateral disease, both kidneys may be symmetrically reduced. Magnetic resonance angiography is increasingly useful as an initial screening investigation, with invasive angiography being the definitive investigation. Alternatively, nuclear medicine, CT or Doppler ultrasound can be used for those who can not or will not have magnetic resonance imaging. Angioplasty and stenting are potential treatment options. The results of angioplasty alone are usually very good with fibromuscular dysplasia. With atheromatous disease, the trend is to angioplasty with stenting and lifelong antiplatelet therapy. However, small kidneys less than 8 cm in length may respond poorly to this therapy.

Atheromatous renovascular disease can lead to progressive loss of renal function in some patients and is an important cause of end stage renal disease (ESRD) in the elderly, accounting for up to 20% of patients over 50 years of age requiring renal replacement therapy. Unsurprisingly, there is an association with systemic atheroma and a 4- to 5-fold increase in myocardial infarction, congestive heart failure and stroke in patients with renal arterial disease. Reversing stenosis in the renal artery may improve renal blood flow but hypertension, hyperlipidaemia and atherosclerosis can also affect smaller vessels and contribute to the progression of renal failure in this way. Intensive medical therapy with anti-hypertensives, aspirin and statins may produce similar results.

A Cochrane review in 2003 concluded that in patients whose blood pressure could be controlled with drugs, there was no data showing an advantage to balloon angioplasty over medical therapy for blood pressure control.[3] Revascularization is not without risk; and arterial dissection, cholesterol embolism and contrast reactions are well recognized complications. The ASTRAL trial has been set up to guide revascularization decisions.[4]

Glands

Endocrine abnormalities can lead to hypertension and about half of patients with a phaeochromocytoma will have paroxysmal hypertension, with most of the remainder having what appears to be essential hypertension. Primary hyperaldosteronism should be suspected in any patient with the triad of hypertension, hypokalaemia, and metabolic alkalosis, although some patients with Conn's syndrome will have a normal plasma potassium. Diastolic hypertension is a major cause of morbidity and death in patients with Cushing's syndrome, and hypertension may also be induced by thyroid dysfunction (in either direction) and hyperparathyroidism.

Unusual suspects

Coarctation of the aorta is a rare new diagnosis in adults, although a significant cause of hypertension in children, and is characterized by decreased or lagging peripheral pulses and a vascular bruit over the back. Symptomatic sleep apnoea seems to be an independent risk factor for hypertension, although the strength of the risk is debated and the majority of patients are overweight. It is also important to remember a number of drugs are associated with increased blood pressure, particularly steroids, oestrogens and immunosuppressive agents such as ciclosporin and tacrolimus. Others culprits include amphetamines, bromocriptine and monoamine oxidase inhibitors.

Assessing the damage

Once hypertension has been established, the extent of target organ damage and the patient's overall cardiovascular risk status should be determined. A relatively limited number of investigations are needed in most cases, but it is important to be aware of the clinical clues suggesting the possible presence of secondary hypertension. Many of these disorders can be cured, leading to

----

[3] Nordmann, Cochrane Database Syst Rev (2003) Issue 3.

[4] www.astral.bham.ac.uk

partial or complete normalization of the blood pressure. The history should assess the presence of precipitating or aggravating factors, the natural course of the blood pressure, the extent of target organ damage, and the presence of other risk factors for cardiovascular disease. Hypertension can cause proteinuria and if all else is normal and the proteinuria is not in the nephrotic range (> 4 g/day), the blood pressure can be safely treated, rechecking the urine and renal function before any onward referral is made.

If secondary hypertension is suspected, appropriate investigations, other than those assessing concurrent cardiovascular risk, should be performed. The presence of primary renal disease is suggested by an elevated plasma creatinine or an abnormal urinalysis. As noted above, low grade proteinuria alone does not imply intrinsic renal disease in the context of hypertension. A phaeochromocytoma should be suspected if there are paroxysmal elevations in blood pressure, particularly if associated with headaches, palpitations and sweating. Measurement of plasma renin activity is only usually performed in patients with a possible low-renin form of hypertension, such as primary hyperaldosteronism. Measurements of plasma renin and aldosterone levels can be difficult to interpret in patients who are already on antihypertensive therapy. Otherwise, unexplained hypokalaemia is the primary clinical clue to the latter disorder for which the plasma aldosterone to plasma renin activity ratio is a reasonable screening test. Cushing's syndrome is usually suggested by the classic physical findings. Thyroid function tests and a serum calcium for hyperparathyroidism may be helpful.

Bringing the numbers down

In clinical trials, antihypertensive therapy reduces the risk of stroke by 35–40%, myocardial infarction by 20–25% and heart failure by 50%. It is estimated that bringing the blood pressure below 140/90 mmHg could prevent 19% of coronary heart disease in men and 31% in women. Optimal control to below 130/80 mmHg could prevent even more events, at 37% and 56%, respectively. Even where the impact on an individual's risk may seem modest, effects on a population basis are profound.[5]

A number of lifestyle modifications should be encouraged before pharmacological intervention. These include weight loss, regular exercise, avoidance of excess alcohol and a low-salt diet. If these measures are not effective (and they rarely will be in isolation) or the blood pressure remains elevated, drugs should be started. Increasingly, physicians will prescribe drug therapy at the

[5] Wong *et al. Am Heart J* (2003) 145: 888–895.

outset but if this is done, it is important to inform the patient of these other aspects of treatment. In the context of hypertension, smoking cessation is a priority.

Salt

Increased salt intake is associated with hypertension and may play a role in causation. There are good epidemiological data to show that when sodium intake rises above 6 g/day, essential hypertension is likely to develop, with a subsequent increase in the risk of cardiovascular events. Restricting dietary sodium to 6 g/day in hypertensive patients lowers systolic pressure by 6.3 mmHg in the over 45s, which will have an enormous impact on population morbidity and mortality. Limiting salt intake to < 6 g/day is a key goal of the Food Standards Agency in the UK.[6] This process will necessarily be a gradual one, as British palates have become accustomed to a salt intake of around double the 6 g target. Indeed, studying the effect of low-salt diets has been very challenging because it is extremely difficult to achieve one in the UK. Almost all manufactured foods, including bread, are high in salt and for patients to achieve a low-salt diet it is usually necessary for them to cook all their food from scratch. The current vogue for breadmakers is potentially helpful in this regard.

A, B, C or D?

In uncomplicated essential hypertension, low dose thiazides were seen as sensible first line drugs, in line with the results of the ALLHAT trial.[7] Thiazides also lower urinary calcium excretion, which may be beneficial in patients with hypercalciuria and recurrent calcium stones, and in those with osteoporosis. A potential drawback is that they can have an adverse impact upon glucose and lipid profiles. If low-dose thiazide monotherapy did not achieve target blood pressures in uncomplicated hypertensive patients, an ACE-inhibitor or beta-blocker has often been added, in line with the recommendations of the ABCD trial.[8] There may however be specific reasons for choosing alternative agents. For example, ACE-inhibitors improve outcomes in heart failure and also slow the progression of proteinuria and renal failure. Angiotensin receptor blockers (ARBs) have a similar impact. Beta-blockers improve survival in patients with heart failure or ischaemic heart disease. However, in the general

---

[6] www.fsa.gov.uk

[7] ALLHAT Investigators, JAMA (2002) 288: 2981–2997.

[8] ABCD Investigators, NEJM (2000) 343: 1969.

population, the combination of beta-blockers and thiazides has been associated with an increased incidence of new onset diabetes mellitus. Furthermore, in trials, beta-blockers have been less effective than other drugs at reducing major cardiovascular events, especially stroke, in the general population. Alpha-blockers, such as doxazosin, may be preferred in older men with symptoms of prostatic obstruction (although ALLHAT data suggest that they are best avoided in patients with heart failure). Calcium channel blockers are particular efficacious in black patients. If there is no specific indication for any particular drug, a recent trial (ASCOT) found that the combination of amlodipine and perindopril was able to reduce all major cardiovascular events, all-cause mortality and new-onset diabetes in hypertensives compared with atenolol and a thiazide diuretic.[9] This combination is now a good evidence-based option, particularly where a beta-blocker is poorly tolerated.

When making the choice of antihypertensive agent, ethnic background should certainly be taken into consideration. Black patients are not only more likely to be hypertensive, but they are also more prone to the associated cardiovascular complications. Based on ALLHAT data, uncomplicated hypertension responds well to dietary salt restriction and a thiazide diuretic. If thiazides are not effective or not appropriate, more black patients respond to calcium channel blockers than ACE-inhibitors or beta-blockers when given as monotherapy. Clearly if an individual has other indications for a drug, then that agent should still be prescribed.

NICE drugs

Making sense of all the trial data can be difficult. NICE has now produced useful new guidance on the treatment of hypertension in collaboration with the British Hypertension Society.[10] The guidelines suggest that young (< 55 years) non-black patients should be given an ACE-inhibitor as a first-line drug, or an angiotensin receptor blocker if they are ACE-inhibitor intolerant. Older (> 55 years) or black patients should be given a calcium channel blocker or thiazide-type diuretic as a first-line drug. If initial therapy is with a calcium channel blocker or diuretic, further therapy would be with an ACE-inhibitor. If initial therapy is with an ACE-inhibitor, a calcium channel blocker or diuretic should be added. When three drugs are required, these should be an ACE-inhibitor, a calcium channel blocker and a diuretic. A fourth drug, if

9   ASCOT Investigators, Lancet (2005) 366: 895–906.

10 CG034 (June 2006) (www.nice.org.uk)

required, may be an alpha-blocker, an additional diuretic or a beta-blocker. Black patients were defined as those of African or Caribbean descent, and not mixed-race, Asian or Chinese patients. The guidance on beta-blockers is that they are not now considered appropriate first line therapy, but may be useful in younger people who are intolerant to ACE-inhibitors and angiotensin II receptor antagonists, and in women who may become pregnant.

Hitting the target

The aim of therapy should not be to achieve only the upper limit of what is deemed allowable, but ideally to be well within the acceptable range. The goal of treatment is to maintain a blood pressure below 140/90 mmHg in the uncomplicated patient. For high-risk groups such as diabetics and patients with established renal disease, blood pressure targets are even lower. The UKPDS study of type II diabetics showed a reduced cardiovascular risk with lower blood pressures and on the basis of this study, Diabetes UK recommended a target blood pressure of < 130/80 mmHg.[11] The HOPE trial supports the same target for those with heart disease.[12] In those over 65 years of age with isolated systolic hypertension, caution is required in order to avoid inadvertently lowering the diastolic blood pressure to below 65 mmHg, since this level of diastolic pressure has been associated with an increased risk of stroke.[13]

NICE thresholds and targets

There is often confusion about the various pressures that are quoted in guidelines (see table on page 124). The threshold blood pressure is the pressure above which treatment should be started and the target blood pressure is the pressure below which the patient's blood pressure should be on treatment. Microalbuminuria (or an abnormal albumin excretion ratio) has been defined by NICE in its guidance on diabetic renal disease as an albumin: creatinine ratio > 2.5 mg/mmol in men or > 3.5 mg/mmol in women; proteinuria was defined as an albumin:creatinine ratio greater than or equal to 30 mg/mmol or albumin concentration greater than or equal to 200 mg/l. The UK CKD guidelines suggest a threshold for treatment in all forms of chronic kidney disease of > 140/90 mmHg and a treatment target of < 130/80 mmHg when the urine protein/creatinine ratio is < 100 mg/mmol. If the urine protein/creatinine ratio is > 100 mg/mmol, the

[11] UKPDS Investigators, BMJ (2000) 321: 412–419.

[12] HOPE Investigators, NEJM (2000) 342: 145–153.

[13] SHEP Investigators, Arch Intern Med (1999) 159: 2004–2009.

threshold falls to > 130/80 mmHg and the treatment target falls to < 125/75 mmHg. Where a patient has multiple conditions, such as diabetes and chronic kidney disease, the lowest relevant thresholds and targets should be applied.

Thresholds and targets in blood pressure management

Patient characteristics	Threshold BP	Target BP
General population	> 160/100	< 140/90
With 10-year CVD risk > 20% or existing CVD or target organ damage	> 140/90	< 140/90
Type 1 diabetes mellitus	> 130/85	Not defined by NICE
With abnormal albumin excretion ratio or > 2 features of metabolic syndrome	> 130/80	Not defined by NICE
Type 2 diabetes mellitus	> 160/100	< 140/80
With 10-year CVD risk > 15%	> 140/80	< 140/80
With abnormal albumin excretion ratio or proteinuria	> 140/80	< 135/75
Chronic kidney disease	> 140/90	< 130/80
With urine protein/creatinine ratio > 100 mg/mmol	> 140/90	< 125/75

About to blow

Malignant hypertension is an acute, marked and life-threatening increase in blood pressure. It is associated with high-grade retinopathy (retinal haemorrhages, exudates and/or papilloedema). There may also be renal involvement and encephalopathy due to a loss of auto-regulation of blood flow in the renal and cerebral vessels. Neurological symptoms may develop due to intracerebral or subarachnoid bleeding, lacunar infarcts, or hypertensive encephalopathy. The latter is related to cerebral oedema and is characterized by the insidious onset of headache, nausea, and vomiting, followed by non-localizing neurological symptoms such as restlessness, confusion, and (if the hypertension is not treated) seizures and coma. Magnetic resonance imaging may show oedema of the white matter of the parieto-occipital regions (termed posterior leukoencephalopathy). Direct blood vessel injury (due to high pressures) and the activation of the renin–angiotensin axis cause fibrinoid material to deposit in the lumen and thus set up a vicious cycle of worsening hypertension. Malignant hypertension is more likely to occur in patients with long-standing hypertension but it is also seen in renal artery stenosis. It can cause renal failure with the fibrinoid necrosis in blood vessels visible on renal biopsy.

Parenteral antihypertensive agents are most often used in the initial treatment of malignant hypertension. Sodium nitroprusside is an arteriolar and venous dilator, given as an intravenous infusion. Nitroprusside acts within seconds and has a duration of action of only 2–5 min. As a result, any hypotension can easily be reversed by temporarily discontinuing the infusion. However, the potential for cyanide toxicity limits its prolonged use, particularly in patients with renal insufficiency. Nicardipine is a calcium channel blocker, given as an intravenous infusion, which acts as an arteriolar dilator. Labetalol has alpha- and beta-adrenergic blocking properties and is given as an intravenous bolus or infusion: its ease of administration makes labetalol a popular choice in the emergency situation (such as prior to thrombolysis in stroke).

Oral agents can also be used. They have a slower onset of action and a lesser degree of control of blood pressure reduction. They may, however, be useful when there is no rapid access to the parenteral medications. Both sublingual nifedipine and sublingual captopril can substantially lower the blood pressure within 10–30 min in many patients. A rapid response is also seen when liquid nifedipine is swallowed. The major risk with these drugs is cerebral ischaemia, due to an excessive hypotensive response. Therefore, the use of these drugs in this manner should generally be avoided in the treatment of hypertensive crises. Indeed, sudden drops in blood pressure should be avoided in any situation.

The initial aim of treatment in a hypertensive crisis is to lower the diastolic pressure to about 100–105 mmHg over 2–6 h, with the maximum initial fall in blood pressure not exceeding 25% of the presenting value, or 10 mmHg/h. This level of control will allow gradual healing of the necrotizing vascular lesions. More aggressive therapy is unnecessary and may reduce the blood pressure below the auto-regulatory range.

Once the blood pressure is adequately controlled, the patient should be switched to oral therapy. The initial reduction to a diastolic pressure of approximately 100 mmHg is often associated with a modest deterioration in renal function; this change is typically transient and renal perfusion improves over a few months. Prognosis in malignant hypertension, even with effective treatment, is not entirely normal: most patients who have had malignant hypertension still have moderate to severe acute and chronic vascular damage and remain at risk of coronary, cerebrovascular and renal disease. When malignant hypertension results in acute renal failure, it is possible that even after 3–6 months or substantially longer, further renal recovery can be seen as the pathology heals.

KIDNEY DISEASE

The diabetic kidney

Diabetes is the cause of end stage renal disease in about a third of cases and around 40% of all diabetics will develop nephropathy. Patients with type 1 and type 2 diabetes develop nephropathy in roughly equal measure.

The pathogenesis of diabetic nephropathy is well characterized. The first step is a rise in glomerular filtration rate (GFR), probably as a result of raised pressure within the glomerular capillaries. This is followed by microalbuminuria, associated with progressive thickening of the glomerular basement membrane and mesangial cell expansion. There are also changes to the vasculature, similar to those seen in the retina, with thickening of vessel walls with glycosylated matrix. These vascular changes cause tissue ischaemia. Microalbuminuria (20–200 μg/min) is below the threshold of detection with conventional dipsticks, but can be picked up in the laboratory. Microalbuminuria can progress to overt proteinuria which is usually associated with a progressive decline in GFR. Typically it takes 15 years to develop ESRF from the onset of proteinuria, and many patients with type 2 diabetes mellitus die before this as a result of cardiovascular disease.

It is possible to slow the progression of diabetic nephropathy. In the DCCT trial, intensive insulin therapy in type 1 diabetics partially reversed glomerular hypertrophy and hyperfiltration (presumably by decreasing glycosylation and the pathological events this triggers).[14] However, this is less successful in preventing progression compared to modifying blood pressure and haemodynamic factors. In type I diabetes, giving an ACE-inhibitor to a normotensive patient with microalbuminuria decreases both albumin excretion and progression to overt nephropathy. Those with overt nephropathy also benefit from ACE-inhibitors which slow the progression of nephropathy to a greater extent than is achieved by control of blood pressure with other drugs. There is some evidence to suggest that a combination of an ACE-inhibitor with an angiotensin receptor blocker (ARB) may offer a greater reduction in protein excretion, but before combination therapy becomes standard treatment, further clinical evidence is needed.[15] In type 2 diabetes, most clinical trials have used ARBs (rather than ACE-inhibitors) to prove that modifying the renin–angiotensin system has a benefit above blood pressure control alone. It is likely the effect would be similar using ACE-inhibitors, although the financial incentive for

---

[14] DCCT Investigators, NEJM (1993) 329: 977–986.

[15] Jacobsen *et al.* Kidney Int (2003) 63: 1874–1880.

pharmaceutical companies to demonstrate this (as drugs near the end of their licences) is less. Certainly, strict blood pressure control is essential. The UKPDS study of type 2 diabetics showed that each 10 mmHg reduction in blood pressure was associated with a 12% risk reduction in diabetic complications, including cardiovascular complications and renal failure.[11]

Other factors to consider in the treatment of diabetic nephropathy are weight loss and aggressive control of hyperlipidaemia. Treatment of hyperlipidaemia with statins may benefit nephropathy by anti-oxidant or anti-inflammatory effects in addition to any anti-atherosclerotic effect.

These interventions can only slow progression of nephropathy. As the incidence of diabetes increases it is important to ensure that screening for nephropathy takes place. NICE has issued helpful guidelines on the management of renal disease in both type 1 and 2 diabetes.[16] In type 1 diabetes, annual assessment of microalbuminuria is recommended and if detected, an ACE-inhibitor or ARB should be started. Blood pressure should be maintained below 130/80 mmHg. For type 2 diabetes, the advice is similar, but the target blood pressure is 125/75 mmHg if microalbuminuria or another feature of the metabolic syndrome is present. Strict gylcaemic and lipid control is recommended. In type 2 diabetes, screening for microalbuminuria is not reliably predictive of progression to overt nephropathy. However, the presence of microalbuminuria is associated with an increased risk of developing cardiovascular disease and most patients with microalbuminuria have other reasons for therapy with an ACE-inhibitor or ARB. Once overt proteinuria is detected, aggressive blood pressure control can slow progression but the UKPDS trial demonstrated that this will require three or more drugs in many cases. NICE suggests nephrological advice when the creatinine is 150 μmol/l, but the capacity of current NHS renal services to deal with the many referrals that this advice could generate is unclear.

Proteinuria in diabetics is not always a result of diabetic nephropathy. Other glomerular diseases can also develop. Pointers to an additional superimposed renal disease include the absence of retinopathy, onset of diabetes less than 5 years ago, a rapid rate of progression in nephropathy or the presence of cellular casts in the urine.

As renal function declines, the doses of oral hypoglycaemic agents and insulin will need to be reduced because they are normally excreted by the kidney. Metformin can cause lactic acidosis and should be avoided in renal failure. Other drugs, such as tolbutamide have theoretical advantages (being largely cleared by the liver) but unfortunately lack potency. Diabetics often

---

[16] CGF (March 2002) and CG015 (July 2004) (www.nice.org.uk)

develop renal anaemia early and may need to start erythropoietin therapy sooner than non-diabetic patients. Decisions regarding the modality of renal replacement therapy should be made well in advance of the need for dialysis (as for all patients with incipient end stage renal failure). The creation of an arteriovenous fistula for dialysis access can be difficult in diabetics because their blood vessels are often small and of poor quality. Renal transplantation is performed in diabetics and improves the prognosis compared to non-transplanted diabetic patients. However, the prognosis is not as good as that of transplanted patients who are not diabetic.

The kidney in pregnancy

In pregnancy, renal blood flow increases by up to 70% following changes in vascular and interstitial fluid volumes. As a result, GFR increases by about 50% halfway through a normal pregnancy. There is a rise in plasma volume, but substantial vasodilation lowers the blood pressure (on average, systolic BP falls from 115 to 105 mmHg and the diastolic, from 70 to 60 mmHg). Haematuria is a common problem too, affecting 15–25% of pregnancies. It is usually associated with a urinary tract infection or stones. Rarely glomerulonephritis is the cause. If there is no proteinuria and provided renal function is normal, no intervention other than close observation is required.

Proteinuria before 20 weeks gestation is usually caused by renal disease, either due to a primary glomerulonephritis or a systemic disease such a lupus. In such situations, specialist advice should be sought to consider the need for a diagnostic renal biopsy to determine whether specific treatment (such as corticosteroids) is indicated. After 20 weeks, the most likely cause of proteinuria is pre-eclampsia, one of the main drivers for the establishment of routine ante-natal care. Proteinuria may precede the other signs, which are principally hypertension and oedema. In the absence of nephrotic syndrome, investigations can be limited to assessment of GFR, albumin, anti-nuclear antibodies and a renal ultrasound.

Hypertension affects 10% of all pregnancies and is defined as a BP exceeding 140/90 mmHg. Pre-eclampsia is responsible for about 30% of cases and is more common in those with pre-existing hypertension, multiple pregnancies, connective tissue disorders, obesity and black race. In pre-eclampsia, there is a fall in GFR as a result of a reduction in renal blood flow and reduced prostacyclin production, likely consequent to abnormal placental implantation and hence dysfunction. Increased renal sodium reabsorption occurs and contributes to hypertension and oedema. There is also an increase in urate reabsorption. The definitive treatment for pre-eclampsia is delivery of the placenta, with the attached baby. Bed rest may be helpful in the earlier stages and antihypertensives are usually commenced when the systolic BP exceeds 160 mmHg or the diastolic BP exceeds 90 mmHg. Methyldopa, oxprenolol, labetolol and clonidine are all suitable. Prazosin and nifedipine are sometimes used. ACE-inhibitors, ARBs and diuretics should be avoided since these drugs reduce circulating blood volumes and cause foetal hypertension. If the BP exceeds 170/110 or eclampsia develops, intravenous BP control may be needed. Hydralazine and labetolol are commonly used. After delivery, pre-eclampsia typically resolves within a few weeks with blood pressure returning to normal by 3 months. Certainly by 12 months, urinalysis should be normal and if this is not the case, an additional primary underlying renal disease should be sought.

Haematuria

Microscopic haematuria is the most common renal complaint, affecting about 13% of adults over 35 years of age. Most frequently, cystitis or urinary tract stones are to blame and in the young it is not usually a cause for major concern in the absence of other features. However, in those over 50 years of age, the risk of malignancy is significant. As dipsticks can give false positive results, the test should be repeated on a new urine sample. Transient haematuria does not need investigation except in the older patient. Myoglobinuria can cause urine dipsticks to test positive for haematuria, but microscopy is negative for blood.

In the initial evaluation of haematuria, three questions should be posed and answered: are there any clues from the history or physical examination that suggest a particular diagnosis; does the haematuria represent glomerular or extraglomerular bleeding; and is the haematuria transient or persistent? The history may point towards a specific diagnosis. For example, concurrent pyuria and dysuria are indicative of a urinary tract infection. A recent upper respiratory infection suggests either post-infectious glomerulonephritis or IgA nephropathy, depending on the time course. With IgA nephropathy, the haematuria accompanies the infection, whereas with post-infectious glomerulonephritis, the haematuria follows the infection (as the name might imply). With a positive family history of renal disease, polycystic kidney disease or Alport's syndrome (sensorineural hearing loss and nephritis) should be suspected. In the anti-coagulated, haematuria should not be put down to warfarin alone and investigation should proceed as it otherwise might. While the young may not require intensive investigation, follow up of renal function with a plasma creatinine and dipstick urinalysis is prudent to detect the infrequent case of progressive renal disease. Isolated haematuria is often associated with lower urinary tract abnormalities, and in the older patient, a urological referral is appropriate to exclude malignancy of the renal tract. However, if there are signs of glomerular bleeding with urine microscopy showing dysmorphic red cells or casts (especially red cell casts), if the dipstick is positive for protein, or if there is renal insufficiency, then patients should instead see a nephrologist for an ultrasound and consideration of renal biopsy. A biopsy is not usually performed for isolated glomerular haematuria, since the management of these patients is rarely affected by the result: the majority have IgA nephropathy. However, a biopsy should be considered (though not necessarily undertaken) if there is evidence of renal insufficiency or substantial proteinuria.

Investigations should exclude lesions in the kidney, collecting system, ureters, and bladder. Most physicians will request a plain KUB X-ray to look for stones and nephrocalcinosis, a renal ultrasound to assess the renal outline and exclude polycystic kidney disease. An iv urogram was a useful test but the spiral CT urogram has largely superseded this and provides better resolution. Urine cytology is useful in patients at increased risk of urothelial cancers, with cystoscopy in those at risk for bladder cancer (those over the age of 50 and those with specific risk factors such as heavy smoking or exposure to analine dyes).

Proteinuria

Proteinuria usually results from increased glomerular permeability, which allows the filtration of normally non-filtered macromolecules such as albumin. Proteinuria can also be caused by a reduction in tubular reabsorption of filtered proteins, for example in tubulointerstitial nephritis and from overspill proteinuria when serum levels of protein are very high, for example in myeloma. Urine electrophoresis can help identify the type of protein in the urine and this is principally used to identify immunoglobulin light chains in the urine (Bence Jones protein). Proteinuria can be transient, orthostatic or persistent. The most common type is transient proteinuria affecting about 4% of men and 7% of women, which does not need investigating as it is benign and tends to resolve spontaneously. Orthostatic proteinuria is similarly benign, primarily occurring in adolescents and characterized by increased protein excretion in the upright position, but normal protein excretion when the patient is supine. It is probably due to neurohumoral activation and altered glomerular haemodynamics. Splitting a urine collection into supine and ambulant specimens diagnoses this condition. Persistent proteinuria is more likely to reflect some underlying glomerular disease that may be primary (such as focal glomerulosclerosis or membranous nephropathy) or secondary (such as diabetic nephropathy or myeloma), or due to systemic disorder such as congestive heart failure. If obvious signs of glomerular disease are present, such as heavy proteinuria (> 4 g/day), oedema, or an active urinary sediment containing red cells (which are often dysmorphic) and red cell casts, then a nephrological referral is needed.

A 24-h urine collection is the gold standard for assessing protein excretion but it is rarely performed correctly. Patients often forget to save all their urine. A total protein to creatinine ratio, or a total albumin to creatinine ratio, on random urine specimens are useful tests to allow the trend of proteinuria to be estimated (for example when commencing an ACE-inhibitor to reduce protein excretion). They are more accurate than dipsticks, since they take into consideration the urine concentration. Quantification is important to distinguish benign proteinuric states (where proteinuria is usually below 1 g/day) from more worrying scenarios. The amount of proteinuria is also prognostic in glomerular disease. The table below compares approximate protein to creatinine ratios with true protein excretion, for a 70 kg man with normal muscle mass:

The protein to creatinine ratio

Protein excretion (g/24h)	Protein to creatinine ratio (mg/mol)
< 0.15	< 20
1	120
3.5	400
10	1200

If proteinuria persists and the history (for instance, of diabetes) is not helpful, a renal ultrasound should be performed looking for a structural lesion such as chronic pyelonephritis (scars) or polycystic kidney disease. A renal biopsy is only usually performed if there is some sign of progressive disease or if protein excretion exceeds 1 g/day, with no obvious explanation. In persistent proteinuria, annual follow-up is recommended with assessments of quantified proteinuria, renal function and blood pressure.

Nephrotic syndrome

This is a clinical syndrome of proteinuria, hypoalbuminaemia, oedema and hyperlipidaemia. Proteinuria greater than 4 g/day is often referred as 'nephrotic range proteinuria' but unless accompanied by the other clinical findings, this really constitutes only 'heavy proteinuria'. Hyperlipidaemia is likely to be a secondary phenomenon, possibly induced by endothelial changes associated with proteinuria or the loss of regulatory proteins in the urine. This syndrome has a number of causes, the likelihood of each differs according to the age of the patient. In adults, a renal biopsy is usually performed to diagnose the cause of nephrotic syndrome and determine the prognosis. Possible diagnoses include minimal change glomerulonephritis (particularly common in young people), membranous glomerulonephritis, and focal segmental glomerulosclerosis (more common in older people).

Steroid use is well documented in the treatment of minimal change disease. Treatments for the other glomerulonephritides include steroids or immunosuppressive drugs such as cyclophosphamide, ciclosporin, tacrolimus and mycophenolate, but these treatments are often less successful and the evidence for their use tends to be less compelling. Not all causes of nephrotic syndrome respond to the drugs currently available. Persistent nephrotic syndrome and proteinuria is also treated empirically: ACE-inhibitors and angiotensin receptor blockers (ARBs) reduce proteinuria, hyperlipidaemia should be treated with statins and as nephrotic syndrome is a pro-coagulative state, formal anti-coagulation may be necessary.

Rapidly progressing

Rapidly Progressive Glomerulonephritis (RPGN) is a renal disease close to the heart of most nephrologists. This is not due to the interesting pathogenesis but rather because early recognition and prompt intervention may prevent progression to end stage renal failure. As the name suggests, it is a glomerular disease (indicated by microscopic haematuria and proteinuria) associated with a progressive loss of renal function over a number of weeks if left untreated. When renal failure develops outside hospital and is associated with signs of inflammation, RPGN should be considered. The term RPGN is used to describe the clinical syndrome that on renal biopsy is often termed crescentic GN. The crescents referred to are usually inflammatory cells that infiltrate Bowman's space. When severe, the reaction can obliterate the entire glomerulus. Consider a diagnosis of RPGN when there is progressive renal impairment or systemic symptoms. Check the urine for blood, protein and red cell casts; the serum for ANCA, anti-GBM, complement, ANA, immunoglobulins and dsDNA. These tests will flag up the majority of causes of RPGN, but an early biopsy should be performed to make a tissue diagnosis and to guide specific treatment.

Anti-GBM antibody disease is a disorder in which circulating antibodies are directed against an antigen in the glomerular basement membrane (GBM) and results in an acute glomerulonephritis with crescent formation. It also goes by the name Goodpasture's syndrome when the renal lesion is associated with pulmonary haemorrhage. Early detection of this rare condition is essential since an anuric patient presenting with a creatinine over 500 μmol/l is likely to need permanent dialysis. Whereas the development of end-stage renal disease can often be prevented in less severe cases through plasma exchange (to remove the antibodies) and immunosuppression (to inhibit their ongoing formation).

Immune complex mediated RPGN are a heterogeneous group of diseases with immune complexes deposited in the glomerulus. This group includes nephritis associated with systemic disease such as Henoch–Schönlein purpura, systemic lupus erythematosus, cryoglobulinaemia, post-infectious glomerulonephritis and crescents due to primary glomerular diseases, such as IgA nephropathy and mesangiocapillary glomerulonephritis.

The most common form however, is a pauci-immune RPGN, that is a necrotizing glomerulonephritis in which no or very few immune deposits are seen deposited in the glomerulus. It is also known as renal vasculitis. The majority of patients with renal-limited vasculitis are anti-neutrophil cytoplasm antibody (ANCA) positive: cANCA (with proteinase-3 antibody) associated with Wegener's Granulomatous and the more common pANCA (with myeloperoxidase antibodies) usually in the context of microscopic polyangiitis.

Crescentic nephritis presents with hypertension, oedema and rapidly declining renal function associated with proteinuria and haematuria (usually microscopic). Red cell casts due to glomerular bleeding are frequently seen in the urine. There is often hypertension and fluid overload. There are also extra-renal features associated with these conditions. In particular, constitutional upset may occur with fever, night sweats, weight loss, malaise and arthralgia. Lung vasculitis affecting the alveolar capillaries results in pulmonary haemorrhage. This may be profound and can present as dyspnoea or haemoptysis but may equally be occult and present with diffuse alveolar shadowing on a chest X-ray or with anaemia. Lung granuloma may be seen in Wegener's, as may upper airway lesions such as sinusitis and nasal bridge collapse. In fact, any organ can be affected in these disorders. Anti-GBM disease is often associated with alveolar haemorrhage, but since ANCA-associated vasculitis is more common, vasculitis more often accounts for pulmonary haemorrhage associated with renal disease.

The treatment of RPGN can be divided into the management of renal failure, the management of the immune response and management to prevent complications of therapy. Therapy should be started at the earliest opportunity. Delaying immunosuppression until a renal biopsy has been performed is not recommended, particularly if pulmonary haemorrhage is present, anti-GBM disease is likely or the decline in GFR is precipitous. Induction therapy typically involves high dose steroids and cyclophosphamide, with plasma exchange available as adjunctive therapy. As this regimen is very aggressive, patients should be given drugs to counter the side effects of steroids and heavy immunosuppression. This should include *Pneumocystis carinii* prophylaxis with cotrimoxazole. For the maintenance phase, steroids are tapered and less aggressive immunosuppressive drugs such as azathioprine are introduced. In the future, novel immunomodulating drugs such as rituximab (an anti-CD20 monoclonal antibody) may be used if their promise is confirmed in randomized controlled trials.

SYNDROMES OF RENAL IMPAIRMENT

Acute renal failure

Acute renal failure is simply a rapid loss (usually over hours to days) of glomerular filtration and tubular function, leading to abnormal water, electrolyte and solute balance. Typically the diagnosis of acute renal failure is made by stumbling across a rise in plasma creatinine and urea rather than due to an overt or specific clinical presentation. The clinical sequelae of acute renal failure (such as pulmonary oedema or hypertension) tend to occur once renal failure is well and truly established. Studies based on laboratory findings give an incidence for acute renal failure of around 80–140 per million population.[17] In hospital-based observational studies, approximately 5% of medical and surgical admissions (elective and routine) develop acute renal failure. Despite improvements in clinical care and the available treatments, there has only been a modest change in crude mortality rates in the 50 years since dialysis began. One retrospective study of 1347 consecutive patients between 1956 and the late 1980s put the 1-year survival figure just shy of 50% – lower still in those with 'medical' renal failure. The apparent lack of improvement in survival reflects the fact that the age and co-morbidities of patients have increased dramatically over the same period. In the same series, the median age of dialysis patients increased from 41 to 62 years between the 1950s and 1980s.[18] This figure has changed little in recent years reflecting the increasingly sick patients offered dialysis.

When a case of acute renal failure presents to a physician, a rapid clinical assessment is needed to determine the aetiology. Three helpful categories can be used as a framework to clarify the underlying process: pre-renal, renal and post-renal. Pre-renal renal failure is usually due to a circulatory failure; either through loss of circulating blood volume or pressure to maintain kidney perfusion. 'Renal' renal failure is due to intrinsic renal disease resulting in a loss of glomerular filtration through glomerular, tubulointerstitial or vascular disease. Post-renal renal failure is due to obstruction of the renal tract

---

[17] Lameire *et al.* Lancet (2005) 365: 417–430.
[18] Turney *et al.* Q J Med (1990) 74: 83–104.

anywhere from the renal pelvis to the urethra. If pre-renal causes are not rapidly reversed, prolonged renal hypoperfusion leads to ischaemic damage to the kidney as acute tubular necrosis occurs. NSAIDS reduce renal blood flow and should be avoided in the context of renal dysfunction. Early ultrasound to exclude obstruction is essential in all cases and this request should not be delayed until after nephrological advice has been sought. The table gives an overview of the major causes of acute renal failure.

Causes of acute renal failure

Pre-renal	Renal	Post-renal
Hypovolaemia	Acute tubular necrosis	Intra-luminal
• Haemorrhage • Burns • Third space loss (GI obstruction or pancreatitis) • GI loss (diarrhoea or vomiting) • Renal losses following post-obstructive diuresis	• Any pre-renal cause for a sustained period • Toxins	• Stones • Papillary necrosis • Blood clot
Renal hypoperfusion	Glomerular disease	Intramural
• Renal artery thrombosis • Bilateral renal artery stenosis • Non-steroidal anti-inflammatory agents • Aortic aneurysm involving renal arteries	• Rapidly progressive glomerular nephritis	• Urethral stricture
Hypotension	Tubulointerstitial	Extraluminal
• Shock – cardiogenic, septic	• Drug-induced interstitial nephritis	• Malignancy (prostate, bladder, cervical, colorectal) • Retroperitoneal fibrosis • Bladder outflow obstruction
Oedematous states	Vascular	
• Liver cirrhosis • Congestive cardiac failure	• Haemolytic uraemic syndrome • Rhabdomyolysis	

In the majority of cases, ARF is pre-renal in origin. With prompt recognition of acute renal failure, rapid therapeutic intervention can reverse renal dysfunction and prevent ARF becoming established, requiring renal replacement therapy with the associated high mortality, morbidity and costs. In most cases, acute renal failure is associated with oliguria (< 400 ml/day) although this is not universal.

So how should a general physician initially investigate renal failure? A thorough clinical assessment is essential in the first instance. Acute renal failure should usually prompt a consultant review as the stakes are high and it often indicates that the clinical situation is grave and deteriorating. The most important steps in the management of acute renal failure are to maintain a normal fluid balance and blood pressure by making an accurate assessment of the state of the circulation, and to obtain an early ultrasound to exclude obstruction. It is important to remember that even partial obstruction, in which urine is still produced, can cause hydronephrosis and renal damage. Hypovolaemia should be rapidly addressed with prompt fluid replacement. If the patient is normo-volaemic, the circulating volume must be maintained. If the patient is fluid over-loaded with pulmonary oedema, a diuresis is usually induced with diuretics when possible and if not, renal replacement therapy is instituted to remove the fluid. Often there will have been a gradual fall in a patient's blood pressure and urine output over a number of hours to days. One must remember to stop anti-hypertensives if hypotension is a problem and all potentially nephrotoxic drugs, especially non-steroidals, should cease. NSAIDS have a particular habit of appearing on the drug charts of those in renal failure. It is often sensible to write 'no non-steroidal anti-inflammatory drugs' on the chart to prevent zealous on-call staff prescribing them in one's absence. A previous creatinine value is helpful in establishing whether the situation is chronic, or at least superimposed on a degree of chronic dysfunction, or one of acute renal impairment. ARF is usually associated with normal or large kidneys and chronic renal failure with small shrunken kidneys: an ultrasound is again essential. Time spent trying to decide whether renal failure is acute or chronic on the basis of haemoglobin, calcium or phosphate levels, is generally time better spent in the doctors' mess: this is rarely helpful and often misleading (see page 142). An intrinsic renal lesion can often be diagnosed with a good review of the medical history and a thorough clinical examination. Urine assessment by dipstick analysis, and if possible urine microscopy, can be extremely helpful too.

Reacting to results

Laboratory investigations upon an initial assessment can be divided into those that facilitate immediate management and those that may aid diagnosis. The most critical results are the plasma potassium level and pH. Hyperkalaemia and severe acidosis risk cardiac arrest and need immediate attention. The first response to hyperkalaemia if there are dangerous ECG changes is calcium (usually calcium gluconate) to provide cardioprotection. The next step is to rapidly lower the potassium level by driving potassium into cells with an infusion of

50% dextrose with insulin. Even giving glucose alone can be helpful. Salbutamol may help too. Sodium bicarbonate infusion may enhance the potassium lowering effect. Ion exchange resins, such as calcium resonium, can remove potassium from the gut but cause constipation and only work well when they reach the large bowel. Any drugs that raise potassium such as ACE-inhibitors, spironolactone and potassium supplements should of course be stopped. A severe metabolic acidosis (pH < 7.2) is concerning, particularly when associated with hyperkalaemia, since cardiac arrhythmias are even more likely to develop. Potassium and hydrogen ions must ultimately be removed from the body, either by resuscitating the kidneys if this is likely to work, or if not by dialysis or haemofiltration. Referral to the local unit sooner rather than later is better for all concerned.

Biochemical tests that help establish the cause of ARF include plasma calcium. A high calcium may indicate myeloma cast nephropathy, whereas a low calcium may point towards rhabdomyolysis or acute pancreatitis. A raised LDH is an indication of tissue necrosis and haemolysis (for example, haemolytic uraemic syndrome). Biochemical testing of the urine can be used to distinguish pre-renal from renal failure. A low fractional excretion of sodium is indicative of pre-renal failure, but this is often clinically obvious already.

A low haemoglobin is not diagnostic of chronic renal failure and is found in acute renal failure for many reasons: intravascular haemolysis from severe sepsis or thrombotic microangiopathy, haemorrhage, extra-vascular haemolysis and chronic inflammatory disease. A blood film is useful to exclude haemolysis. The white cell count and differential may be helpful. A leucopaenia may suggest severe sepsis or active SLE. A high eosinophil count hints at acute interstitial nephritis. A thrombocytopenia may indicate thrombotic microangiopathies, SLE or severe sepsis. A high platelet count is often seen in systemic vasculitis.

The urine should be examined urgently in all cases of ARF. Cells, casts, crystals and organisms can all be assessed through microscopy. Red cells should have a typical disc-like appearance. In glomerular lesions they may take on a dysmorphic appearance, but this is not a reliable change. Urinary casts come in a number of forms: red cell casts are virtually diagnostic of glomerulonephritis. They form as a result of glomerular bleeding where the red cells stack up in the tubules and then pass into the urine. Granular casts are a non-specific sign of renal injury and are formed when red cell, epithelial or white cell casts degrade.

Immunological investigations are important in the diagnosis of ARF, particularly where acute glomerulonephritis is suspected. The table below lists some key investigations. It is helpful to send these off early if there is diagnostic uncertainty, even if a renal opinion is yet to be sought, as the turn around time may be considerable.

Immunology and acute renal failure

Investigation	Results
Complement	Low C3 and low C4 in SLE, endocarditis and post-infectious GN
	Low C4, normal C3 in cryoglobulinaemia
	Low C3, normal C4 in mesangial capillary GN
ANCA	cANCA – Wegener's granulomatosis (anti-protease 3)
	pANCA – microscopic polyangiitis (anti-myeloperoxidase)
Anti-GBM	Goodpasture's disease
ANA, Anti-dsDNA	SLE
Immunoglobulins and serum electrophoresis	Myeloma associated with immune paresis and monoclonal band on electrophoresis

The majority of cases of acute renal failure are due to acute tubular necrosis following an ischaemic injury of one sort or another. In most such cases, renal biopsy is not justified unless the duration of renal failure is prolonged beyond 3–4 weeks, when a biopsy may provide useful prognostic information. Occasionally, histological examination unexpectedly identifies diseases in patients who have otherwise been asymptomatic, such as SLE, HIV or myeloma.

Intervening in acute renal failure

In ARF, the key aim is to maintain a normal circulating blood volume. Once a circulatory insult has been reversed and nephrotoxins stopped, the kidneys will often recover spontaneously. Furosemide is often given in oliguric renal failure although there is no evidence that it improves mortality or prevents the need for dialysis. It acts by inhibiting the sodium–potassium–chloride channel in the loop of Henle and, in theory, reduces tubular epithelial cell oxygen demand. There are inherent dangers with using furosemide in acute renal failure. It can only be given safely if a patient has an effective circulating volume before, during and after administration. Giving a diuretic to a dehydrated patient will make renal failure worse. Furosemide does have benefit as a diuretic in those patients with fluid overload and some residual renal function. It may, if necessary, be given as a bolus of up to 250 mg intravenously over 30 min. This may seem an excessive dose but the drug needs to be filtered by the kidney before it even reaches its target in the renal tubules. If there is precious little filtration taking place, then a higher dose will be required. If a patient remains oliguric after this bolus, there is no benefit in giving further doses – additional slugs increase the risks of ototoxicity.

Dopamine – just say no

Dopamine has theoretical benefits in the treatment of renal failure. It increases sodium excretion by diminishing its reabsorption, primarily in the proximal tubule. When infused in low dose, dopamine dilates the small renal arteries and both the afferent (pre-glomerular) and efferent (post-glomerular) arterioles. The net effect is a relatively large increase in renal blood flow with little effect on GFR. At higher concentrations (above 5 µg/kg per min), dopamine acts on alpha-adrenergic receptors to induce renal vasoconstriction. These physiological effects have led to the frequent use of low-dose, 'renal-dose' dopamine in attempts to increase the urine output and to preserve renal function in oliguric patients with ATN. However, in at least three large clinical studies of patients with oliguria and signs of shock, dopamine had no beneficial effect.[19,20] There are potential risks associated with even low-dose regimens including tachyarrhythmia, myocardial ischaemia and possibly intestinal ischaemia (due to pre-capillary vasoconstriction) which might promote bacterial translocation from the intestinal lumen into the systemic circulation. Dopamine really cannot be recommended to protect patients considered to be at risk for ATN or those with early, or indeed established, ATN.

Dopexamine has similarities to dopamine and induces a rise in renal blow flow, a natriuresis and diuresis. It activates dopamine and beta-1 adrenergic receptors but has no alpha-adrenergic effects. It has no proven clinical benefit in acute renal failure. In the future, specific dopamine A1 agonists, such as fenoldopam (which induces vasodilatation in renal vascular smooth muscle, a natriuresis and diuresis) may be of use but evidence is currently lacking.

Mannitol is an osmotic diuretic, which is filtered by the kidney but is not reabsorbed in the renal tubules. The result is an increase in the osmolality of tubular fluid, which reduces sodium and water reabsorption. Mannitol has been used in the treatment of acute renal failure for many years, but there is a paucity of evidence to support its use. Studies have shown an increase in urine output but there has been no demonstrable reduction in the need for dialysis or mortality, and its use is not recommended. The side effects of mannitol include electrolyte disturbances and an acute expansion of the extracellular

---

[19] NORASEPT II Investigators, Am J Med (1999) 107: 387–390.
[20] ANZICS Investigators, Lancet (2000) 356: 2139–2143.

volume that can precipitate pulmonary oedema. It is also directly tubulotoxic and is best avoided.

More recently, N-acetylcysteine has been used for prophylaxis of radiocontrast-induced nephropathy and following cardiac procedures. When there was pre-operative renal dysfunction (creatinine above 120 μmol/l) a trend towards a lower incidence of postoperative worsening of kidney function was seen in one randomized trial.[21] N-acetylcysteine does not have any significant side effects and is extremely cheap, so there is little to be said against its use, although its overall benefit remains unclear.

Overall, the pharmacological interventions currently available are unimpressive in the prevention of renal failure after an ischaemic insult. Close attention to the circulation and fluid balance are of much greater importance, along with assessment of biochemical parameters.

Dialysis in acute renal failure

The classic indications for immediate renal replacement therapy (RRT) are: refractory hyperkalaemia, severe metabolic acidosis (pH < 7.2), pulmonary oedema and symptomatic uraemia (especially pericarditis, encephalopathy and uraemic bleeding). Obviously, it is best that a patient is transferred between hospitals for dialysis before the situation becomes so grave. Liaison with local specialist services should start early. That way, transfer can theoretically occur in a timely fashion. Moving a patient with haemodynamic instability is a recipe for disaster. In most hospitals, intensive care units are now able to offer temporary renal replacement therapy with haemofiltration and it is best to stabilize any life threatening issues before a transfer for ongoing RRT in a regional renal unit.

In addition to these absolute indications for dialysis, patients with multiple organ failure may be commenced on RRT to treat a number of non-renal problems. In intensive care units, filtration can facilitate treatment of acute left ventricular failure, help to provide adequate volume for nutritional support and correct electrolyte and acid–base disturbances.

Until the 1960s, the development of end-stage renal disease was a death sentence. Now, there are a number of effective treatment modalities available. Not so long ago, dialysis was only offered to young patients with isolated renal failure who were otherwise well. This is not the case now and most patients are offered renal replacement therapy. Historically, acute renal failure was treated with emergency peritoneal dialysis. A physician would insert a catheter into

----

[21] Burns et al. JAMA (2005) 294: 342–350.

the peritoneal cavity and perform continuous dialysis. This is rarely performed today. Intermittent haemodialysis or haemofiltration (which can be continuous but is more often intermittent – daily) are the two most common modalities of RRT. Dialysis is a simple procedure. Blood is removed from the circulation by a simple pump, is passed quickly through a semi-permeable membrane with dialysate (dialysis fluid) on the other side to allow removal of solutes and water, before the purified blood is returned to the patient. The process lasts between 1 and 4 h. Each modality of RRT has its advantages and disadvantages and the decision on which one to use should be personalized. The most important factor to take into consideration is the haemodynamic stability of a patient with ARF. A patient with uncomplicated acute renal failure who is clinically stable should undergo intermittent haemodialysis. Where haemodynamic instability is present, a more continuous therapy should be employed (such as continuous haemofiltration). A problem with continuous therapies is the risk of bleeding as they require anti-coagulation for the duration of treatment and this may present a problem in certain clinical scenarios.

Haemodialysis and haemofiltration are different processes. In haemofiltration, blood is pumped at a slower speed and treatment takes longer. In haemodialysis, solutes usually diffuse down concentration gradients between blood and dialysate fluid, although if blood is pumped at high pressure, fluid can also be filtered out of the blood. This filtering of fluid from the blood to the dialysate is called ultra-filtration. In haemofiltration, filtration is the only process that occurs and it removes water and with it any ions and other molecules which are in solution. An appropriate volume of fluid with the desirable concentrations of ions is used to replace the fluid removed. This fluid is composed of a buffer such as bicarbonate or lactate along with physiological amounts of sodium, chloride, magnesium and calcium. Lactate is metabolized to bicarbonate in the liver, but in very sick patients, especially with liver dysfunction, lactate metabolism may be inadequate and a lactate-free buffer is required to prevent accumulation.

There are few good comparisons between haemodialysis and haemofiltration in acute renal failure and results vary. Recently, advances in membrane biocompatibility may have improved the relative performance of haemodialysis.

Distinguishing acute renal failure from chronic kidney disease

When faced with an alarming pathology report, most physicians are keen to establish whether renal dysfunction is a new and active problem, or rather part of a patient's make-up. A number of rules are often cited: sadly, many are less reliable than their advocates may think.

Is it acute or chronic?

Investigation	Acute	Chronic	Comment
Ultrasound	Normal	Small	This is the most useful distinguishing test. Small shrunken kidneys are typical of chronic renal disease.
Urea and creatinine	High	High	Not really useful, very high urea (> 50) and creatinine (> 1000) can be tolerated in chronic disease when the rate of decline is slow.
Potassium	High	High	If decline is slow, high potassium may be better tolerated.
Calcium and phosphate	Maybe normal	Often Ca^{2+} low, PO_4^{2-} high	Not a discriminating test. A normal calcium is more likely in acute renal failure, but can also be seen in chronic disease when caused by hypercalcaemia-inducing disease such as myeloma.
Haemoglobin	Low	Low	Not a discriminating test. Anaemia is common in both conditions.

Chronic kidney disease (CKD)

Chronic kidney disease (CKD) has a broad spectrum of clinical presentations, ranging from asymptomatic haematuria to symptomatic uraemia necessitating emergency dialysis. A study based upon blood samples in South East London demonstrated the presence of some degree of CKD in 5554 per million population, or 5%.[22] The gradual decline in function in patients with chronic renal failure is initially asymptomatic, but with increasing renal dysfunction, symptoms of volume overload, hyperkalaemia, metabolic acidosis, hypertension, anaemia, and bone disease develop. The onset of end-stage renal disease results in a constellation of signs and symptoms sometimes referred to as 'uraemia'. The main cause of death in chronic kidney disease is vascular disease.

Recently, an international committee devised a classification of chronic renal disease in an attempt to promote early intervention with effective treatments, as shown in the table below.[23] The Renal Association has published guidance on the management of these stages of CKD and NICE guidance on CKD is also awaited.[24] A nephrologist should generally be involved by CKD stage 3/4.

[22] John et al. Am J Kidney Dis (2004) 43: 825–835.

[23] Levey et al. Ann Intern Med (2003) 139: 137–147.

[24] www.renal.org/ckd

A classification of chronic kidney disease

Stage	Description	GFR (ml/min/1.73 m^2) by MDRD equation	Treatment
1	Kidney damage with normal or increased GFR	> 90	Observation, control of blood pressure
2	Kidney damage with mild reduction in GFR	60–89	Observation, control of blood pressure and risk factors
3	Moderate reduction in GFR	30–59	Observation, control of blood ressure and risk factors
4	Severe reduction in GFR	15–29	Planning for end stage renal failure
5	Kidney failure	< 15 or dialysis	Renal replacement therapy treatment choices

Data from the United States suggest that 5% of the population have stages 3–5 CKD, with a similar number in stages 1–2.[25] It is important to note that these guidelines are based on GFR rather than serum creatinine values. GFR is the sum of the filtration rates in all of the functioning nephrons and normal values for young people are around 120 ml/min. However, GFR declines with age and it is important to refer to the normal ranges for elderly patients to avoid unnecessary investigation in patients who are simply enjoying old age. Significant renal impairment may exist before the plasma creatinine concentration rises above the normal range. Many biochemistry laboratories now provide an estimate of GFR in addition to the absolute creatinine value and this will soon be standard. Creatinine is produced by the turnover of muscle cells, therefore, a muscular man weighing 150 kg may have a high serum creatinine of 130 µmol/l but normal renal function. However, a 45-kg elderly woman with a creatinine of 120 µmol/l has significant renal impairment. A number of equations to estimate the GFR have been developed. An easy to use formula is the Cockcroft Gault equation. It is an estimate of creatinine clearance, is most accurate when near the normal range and takes into consideration age, weight and sex.

$$CrCl \text{ (ml/min/1.73 m}^2) = \frac{(140 - age) \times \text{lean body weight (kg)}}{Cr \text{ (µmol/l)}} \times 0.85 \text{ (for females)}$$

[25] Coresh *et al.* Am J Kidney Dis (2003) 41: 1–12.

An alternative equation is the MDRD (Modification of Diet in Renal Disease – named after the study in which this formula was first used) equation, providing an estimate of the GFR. This equation is easier to use as it does not require the patient's weight, but can incorporate information about ethnicity. It is recommended by the Renal Association and UK Departments of Health in the assessment of renal disease and there is an online calculator at the Renal Association website.[26]

In CKD, the aim is to slow the rate of progression of decline in renal function, replace the non-filtration functions of the kidney, prepare a patient for End Stage Renal Failure (ESRF), and help with decisions as to the modality of renal replacement therapy (RRT), if appropriate.

Slowing the progression of renal disease has been improved with the introduction of ACE-inhibitors and better control of blood pressure. Angiotensin II may have detrimental effects that are blocked by these agents and they often improve proteinuria. Raised blood pressure in the glomerular capillaries leads to glomerular scarring (glomerulosclerosis). ACE-inhibitors or ARBs have been shown to slow the progression of renal injury in various clinical trials by reducing intraglomerular hypertension. In the COOPERATE trial, a combination of ACE-inhibitor and ARB slowed progression of renal failure in non-diabetic renal disease more than either agent alone.[27] However, problems with hypotension and hyperkalaemia are more frequently encountered with combination therapy. The greatest benefit is observed when ACE-inhibitors are started early, ideally during stage 1 of CKD. A target BP of 130/80 mmHg is currently recommended for those with low-level proteinuria, and 125/75 with high level proteinuria. In most patients, multiple drug therapy will be required starting with an ACE-inhibitor or ARB.

When commencing an ACE-inhibitor or ARB in CKD, a decline in GFR is often observed since these agents reduce GFR by their mechanism of action. The Renal Association recommends that creatinine and potassium levels are checked 14 days after starting an ACE-inhibitor and after each escalation in dose. It is acceptable for the creatinine to rise by up to 30% following the introduction of an ACE-inhibitor. Anything greater than this may indicate renal artery stenosis, in which case the drug should be stopped, the creatinine rechecked to ensure it is back to baseline, and investigations for renovascular disease considered.

As renal failure progresses, the other physiological functions of the kidneys start to fail. Disorders of fluid and electrolyte balance with oedema, hyperkalaemia, metabolic acidosis, and hyperphosphataemia occur. Anorexia, nausea,

---

[26] www.renal.org/eGFR and www.renal.org/ckd

[27] COOPERATE Investigators, Lancet (2003) 361: 117–124.

vomiting, fatigue, hypertension, anaemia, malnutrition, hyperlipidaemia, bone disease, and pericarditis develop as the patient reaches end stage. Volume overload generally responds to the combination of dietary sodium restriction and diuretic therapy, usually with a loop diuretic given daily. Hyperkalaemia is often a problem, particularly when high doses of ACE-inhibitors are used. A low-potassium diet and concurrent use of a loop diuretic, to increase urinary potassium losses, often helps. ACE-inhibitors should not be stopped unless absolutely necessary as they have the greatest proven benefit in slowing progression. Avoiding NSAIDS can help keep potassium levels normal. As renal failure develops, the kidney cannot excrete hydrogen ions and metabolic acidosis can ensue. Acidosis has detrimental metabolic effects and can promote the release of calcium and phosphate from bone. Maintaining a physiological serum bicarbonate with oral bicarbonate is ideal but the salt load can lead to oedema and hypertension.

Renal bone disease develops early in CKD. Renal impairment reduces the kidneys' capacity to remove phosphate, hyperphosphataemia occurs and this causes a fall in calcium levels, which in turn stimulates the release of parathyroid hormone (PTH). Hyperphosphataemia can be improved by giving phosphate-binding substances which bind dietary phosphate in the gut and prevent its absorption. Calcium salts such as calcium carbonate or calcium acetate are commonly used for this purpose, but can cause hypercalcaemia. More recently, non-calcium-containing binders have been developed which are not associated with this problem, but they are expensive. As the GFR falls, so too do levels of 1,25 dihydroxy-vitamin D. PTH levels can be suppressed to prevent renal bone disease using vitamin D replacement therapy with alfacalcidol. Typically alfacalcidol is introduced when the GFR falls below 40 ml/min. A problem with this drug is that again it increases serum calcium levels and may therefore accelerate vascular calcification. Calcimimetics such as cinacalcet, are able to suppress PTH levels without causing hypercalcaemia and may become first-line therapy in renal bone disease. However, they are very expensive.

With progressive renal disease, salt and water retention contributes to hypertension and high dose loop diuretics may be needed. Thiazide diuretics in conventional dosage are less effective when the glomerular filtration rate falls below 20 ml/min but can provide an additive effect when administered with a loop diuretic for refractory oedema.

Anaemia in CKD is usually normocytic and normochromic, and is due to reduced production of erythropoietin by the kidney and to reduced red cell survival. It can start to be a problem when the GFR sinks to below 60 ml/min, particularly in diabetics. Erythropoietin and iron therapy should be used to maintain haemoglobin levels, typically around 11–12 g/dl. Relevant investigations include red cell indices, reticulocyte count, B12 and folate, serum iron, transferrin and ferritin. Iron absorption is often poor in patients with renal disease and intravenous iron therapy may be required. Once iron stores have been replenished, erythropoietin should be administered in the pre-dialysis or dialysis patient to maintain haemoglobin. Darbepoetin-alpha can be given once weekly, or fortnightly.

Once the patient is in the final run-up to end-stage renal disease, signs and symptoms related to uraemia begin to occur, such as malnutrition, anorexia, nausea, vomiting, fatigue, platelet dysfunction, pericarditis, and neuropathy. Before this stage arrives, a patient should be prepared for some form of renal replacement therapy. Adequate preparation can decrease morbidity and perhaps even mortality.[28]

Early identification also enables dialysis to be initiated at the optimal time using appropriate permanent dialysis access. It may also permit the recruitment and evaluation of family members for potential organ donation. In addition, early referral allows the patient to discuss the shape of their future with a nephrologist. Excellent guidance on the management of patients with CKD and the indications for referral to a nephrologist are available on the Renal Association website.[29] Patients with CKD stage 3 should be discussed with a specialist when the estimated glomerular filtration rate is less than 60 ml/min per 1.73 m^2. Patients with low level proteinuria, and/or microscopic haematuria (with negative urological investigations) can probably be managed in primary care. Stage 4 or 5 should be referred.

RRT – the numbers[30]

Approximately 27,000 patients in England are currently in receipt of renal replacement therapy of one sort or another. Numbers are growing, with 0.40% of the population having such treatment in 1992 and 0.55% in 2001. In 2001, 91 people per million began to receive renal replacement therapy. This growth is predicted to continue at a rate of 5% per year for two decades before reaching steady state. In 2001, half of the population on renal replacement therapy were over 65 years of age, while this group represented only 11% of the dialysis population in 1984.

---

[28] Jungers *et al.* BMJ (1984) 288: 441–443.

[29] www.renal.org/ckd

[30] The National Service Framework for Renal Services. Part One: Dialysis and Transplantation, 2004 (www.dh.gov.uk)

Despite these impressive figures, other data show that there is a substantial unmet need for renal replacement in England: rates of replacement in England languish at the bottom of a table of international comparison, as shown below. In the North Thames Dialysis Study, the 1-year survival rates for patients aged 70–79 years were similar to those for all ages. Quality of life scores for these elderly patients were also similar to those of the general dialysis population suggesting that the elderly are able to cope with the demands of treatment. Older patients with chronic kidney disease should not be denied access to renal replacement therapy, however co-morbidity will need to be assessed since this may influence the response to RRT.

Comparison of international rates of renal replacement therapy in 2001 (persons per million population)

Country	Incident cases	Prevalent cases
US	336	1403
Germany	184	909
Italy	136	835
New Zealand	119	655
Wales	105	641
Scotland	101	644
Netherlands	100	639
England	91	547

Choice

Life expectancy once renal replacement therapy is initiated is modest. A 40-year-old on dialysis can expect to live for around 8 years, someone aged 60 will probably live for 5 more years.[31] However, mortality rates have fallen over the last few years.

As patients approach ESRF, they should receive counselling and consider the various treatment options available. Each therapy has its advantages and disadvantages. Some patients may opt not to have RRT and choose to have the symptoms of renal failure treated with palliative care. Otherwise, there are three forms of RRT: haemodialysis, peritoneal dialysis (continuous or inter-mittent modalities), and renal transplantation (living or cadaveric donor).

Kidney transplantation is the treatment of choice for end-stage renal disease. A successful kidney transplant improves quality of life and reduces

[31] UK Renal Registry, Seventh Annual Report, 2004 (www.uktransplant.org.uk)

mortality compared with dialysis. Pre-emptive transplantation (transplantation prior to dialysis) can improve the situation further and such patients have improved graft survival compared to those who undergo a period of dialysis before transplantation.[32] Ideally, a relative would donate a kidney before end stage disease arises. Alternatively, an unrelated person (usually a spouse) may donate. The other source of organs is the donor register: unfortunately the waiting list for kidneys far exceeds the supply, and refusal rates for organ donation have changed little in the last few years in the UK. Furthermore, fewer than 40% of dialysis patients are actually on the transplant list in the UK.[33]

The risk of death in the first year after transplantation is greater than the risk of death during a year on dialysis. If a recipient survives that first year, the survival curves cross. The early mortality is due to the surgical risk and immunosuppressive drugs. In the 1970s, immunosuppression was limited to prednisolone and azathioprine. Now patients may be given other drugs such as ciclosporin, tacrolimus, sirolimus, mycophenolate or biological agents, such as an IL-2 receptor antibody, basilizimab. One-year survival rates average 90%, but immunosuppression increases the risk of infections in the short term, and cancer in the long term.

For individuals not suitable for a transplant or those waiting for an available kidney, the choice is haemodialysis or peritoneal dialysis. Some patient, particularly the elderly and terminally ill, may decline dialysis and this can be a source of conflict between physicians, patients, and their families. Indeed, patients on a dialysis programme may choose to withdraw.

Dialysis is usually started when GFR falls below 10 ml/min/1.73 m^2 or when symptoms such as anorexia develop.

Haemodialysis

Haemodialysis requires high flow access to the bloodstream. A primary arteriovenous (AV) fistula is surgically constructed and usually takes several months to mature. An attempt at formation well ahead of the anticipated need for dialysis (often when the creatinine is around 350–400 μmol/l) is ideal. When haemodialysis is planned, venepuncture should be avoided in the arm chosen for access. Indeed, veins below the elbow should be treated with great care and not cannulated (except on the back of the hand) in renal patients in order to preserve the veins for access. Often silastic, double-lumen, cuffed and tunnelled

---

[32] Kasiske *et al.* J Am Soc Nephrol (2002) 13: 1358–1364.

[33] UK Renal Registry, Fifth Annual Report (2002) (www.uktransplant.org.uk)

catheters (Permacaths or Tesio lines) are used for vascular access. They are extremely useful in the short term but tend to become blocked and are prone to infection. Indeed, a number of interesting conclusions can be drawn from a nationwide audit of dialysis conducted by the Renal Association over 1 month in 2005.[34] The survey covered 62 main renal units and 119 satellites, a large majority of the relevant provision. Over 17,000 patients were receiving dialysis and almost 500 new patients commenced during the month. For those having haemodialysis, 69% did so with definitive arterio-venous access, although less than a third of the incident cases had functioning arterio-venous access on commencement. This is despite the fact that a majority of patients had been known to renal services for over a year prior to dialysis. These audit figures suggest that patients are even more poorly prepared than previously thought: in 2002, 67% of patients receiving haemodialysis were said to do so with definitive access, and 47% of incident cases.[35] The lack of appropriate and timely dialysis access is not simply a cause of irritation and inconvenience to patients, it is also a cause of substantial morbidity and cost. Based on the audit, it would appear that approximately 320,000 bed days are taken up by patients who need to receive their dialysis as inpatients – about a third of these due to inadequate vascular access. It is also estimated that there is an annual rate of Staphylococcal septicaemia of 13 per 100 dialysis patients and that dialysis accounts for about 10% of all MRSA bacteraemias in the UK.

Once on haemodialysis, most patients are dialysed as outpatients for 4-h spells, 3 times a week. Receiving haemodialysis 3 times a week in hospital is quite a strain for many people. Younger patients may have to work and attend dialysis, sometimes in the evening, driving themselves to and from hospital. Some are able to have home haemodialysis machines in an attempt to fit treatments around their lifestyles but the impact of renal replacement therapy on an individual and their family should not be underestimated. Dialysis also represents a significant call upon NHS resources: haemodialysis consumes between 1 and 2% of NHS monies, although patients account for only 0.05% of the population.[36]

Peritoneal dialysis

Peritoneal Dialysis (PD) is an alternative to haemodialysis. It has the advantage over haemodialysis that it can be performed at home, fluid balance is usually

[34] UK Renal Registry, Eighth Annual Report (2006) (www.uktransplant.org.uk)

[35] Pisoni *et al.* Kid Int (2002) 61: 305.

[36] TA048 (September 2002) (www.nice.org.uk)

easier to control and travel is possible since bags of solution can to taken on holiday. It needs reasonable dexterity, a high degree of motivation and attention to cleanliness whilst performing exchanges to prevent peritonitis. A catheter is placed into the abdominal cavity around 2–3 weeks before dialysis is to be started. PD fluid is then washed into the abdomen either manually or by a machine. Water and solutes move across the peritoneal membrane between the blood and the dialysis fluid. In CAPD (continuous ambulatory PD), 4 manual exchanges a day are performed. In APD (automated PD) a machine pumps PD fluid in and out overnight. For PD to be successful patients need to tolerate 2 l of fluid in their abdomen, therefore chronic lung disease and significant previous abdominal surgery tends to preclude this therapy. PD works best when patients are still passing some urine and have some residual renal function. Peritonitis is a common problem, which should be managed by the renal team, and usually responds to antibiotics.

In both haemodialysis and PD, patients are set target weights as a guide to how much fluid needs to be removed during a dialysis treatment. Dialysis patients are asked to stick to a daily restriction of around 500 ml plus their urine volume. Large weight gains (in excess of 2 kg) between dialyses result in salt and water overload. This causes hypertension, puts extra pressure on the cardiovascular system and raises mortality.

Drugs in end stage renal disease

The kidney excretes many drugs and drug metabolites, so care is required when prescribing for patients with renal disease. Drugs such as opioids can accumulate, with predictable effects, others such as NSAIDs can impair any remaining renal function. In the BNF, there is a helpful section to help guide dosing, but more comprehensive books are available on-line and in print, and they are referred to continually by the experts on renal wards. Drug interactions can be important, particularly in transplant patients. For example, erythromycin increases ciclosporin concentrations and should be avoided when possible.

Chapter 7

Christopher Kipps and Martin Lee

NEUROLOGY

ACUTE HEADACHE

'I'm very brave generally, he went on in a low voice:
only today I happen to have a headache'

Through the Looking Glass
Lewis Carroll

The lifetime prevalence of headache is around 96%, of which less than 0.5% is accounted for by serious intracranial pathology. Most general practitioners will see only 1 primary brain tumour every 10 years, and the majority of these will not present with headache alone (brain tumour is, however, a common cause of demise for leading soap opera characters). The hospital physician, on the other hand, sees a selected population, and the odds of serious pathology in patients acutely admitted to hospital or attending A&E with headache is much greater (around 15%). Patients with headache account for about 1 in 40 of all medical referrals: life is therefore rather easier for the general physician with a good working knowledge of the common causes of acute headache and the relevant management strategies. As with many branches of medicine, the take-home message when confronted by a patient with headache would be that if one only has £1 to spend, spend 95 pence on the history!

Subarachnoid haemorrhage

Subarachnoid haemorrhage (SAH) rightly retains its crown as the 'headache diagnosis not to miss'. Fatality approaches 10% immediately, 25% within the first 24 h and 50% at 3 months. These figures may be reduced by early recognition of the primary event and management of the three causes of secondary deterioration: rebleed, vasospasm and hydrocephalus.

SAH results from the passage of high-pressure arterial blood into the subarachnoid space following the rupture of a 'berry' or 'saccular' aneurysm, arising from weakening of the internal elastic lamina of the arterial wall at branch points along the circle of Willis. Risk factors for the development of aneurysms include the usual vices of smoking and alcohol, together with hypertension, a strong family history, polycystic kidney disease and other congenital abnormalities of connective tissue (such as Ehlers–Danlos syndrome). These are not very useful diagnostic associations. Rupture is usually spontaneous but may also be hastened by use of recreational sympathetomimetic drugs, particularly cocaine.

Fortunately, not all aneurysms rupture. Pathological studies have shown cerebral aneurysms in 2–5% of the population, yet the population incidence of SAH is only 1 in 10,000, with peak age incidence around 50. Unfortunately, there is often no prior warning in those that do, although 'sentinel' headaches, associated with a minor leak, do probably occur in some. The frequency of warning headaches is disputed, ranging from 10 to 43%. In general, it is foolhardy to dismiss any new, unusual, sudden-onset severe headache, especially if associated with nausea, neck stiffness or failure to settle rapidly. Rupture may also be preceded by aneurysmal enlargement causing local compression, as in the classical case of a painful, pupil-involving, third nerve palsy due to a posterior communicating or basilar artery aneurysm.

Most SAH presents with sudden-onset severe 'thunderclap' headache, vomiting, meningeal signs and retained consciousness. Days after the event, patients may report lower-back pain if asked, signalling a lumbar arachnoiditis secondary to dependant lumbar CSF blood. Some patients deteriorate rapidly into deep coma when neck stiffness may be absent, and SAH should always be considered in the differential of coma. Seizures and localizing signs occur early in a minority of patients with SAH and the sudden rise in intracranial pressure may cause retinal subhyloid or vitreous haemorrhages resulting in blindness with an absent red reflex (Terson's syndrome).

Unfortunately, SAH is well camouflaged diagnostically among benign thunderclap headaches that outnumber it by 10 to 1. Vomiting occurs in both but neck flexion stiffness signals SAH. More than two episodes of severe-onset headache makes SAH unlikely, avoiding unnecessary investigation in patients with repeated episodes of coital or exertional headache. However, the distinction may not be clear for a first attack.

Grading in SAH is useful for guiding prognosis and management (Glasgow coma scale score and the World Federation of Neurological Surgeons, or WFNS, grading scale) as well as appeasing neurosurgical registrars on the phone.

A head CT scan is 95% sensitive for subarachnoid blood within the first 24 h after SAH. This falls to 75% by day 3 and to only 30% in 2 weeks. The figures are

WFNS grading system

Grade	GCS	Motor deficit
Grade I	15	Absent
Grade II	13–14	Absent
Grade III	13–14	Present
Grade IV	7–12	Absent or present
Grade V	3–6	Absent or present

probably better with newer fifth-generation CT scanners. Lumbar puncture (LP) for the detection of haemoglobin breakdown products in the CSF at least 12 h after headache onset remains the gold standard and is almost 100% sensitive for up to 2 weeks, but the sensitivity has fallen to less than 40% at 1 month. Xanthochromia refers only to the colour on visual inspection of CSF contaminated by haemoglobin breakdown products. Guidelines have recently been published regarding CSF analysis in SAH.[1] The guidelines assert that spectrophotometry of CSF involving bilirubin quantification is the recommended method of analysis and that this should be done on the final bottle of CSF to be collected. An increased CSF bilirubin is the key finding that supports the need for further investigation (although bilirubin will usually be accompanied by oxyhaemaglobin). The occurrence of oxyhaemaglobin alone is most often artefactual.

False positives may occur in other conditions where blood products reach the subarachnoid space such as herpes encephalitis and sagittal sinus thrombosis, and this may mislead if time has not been spent on the clinical history. Traumatic CSF taps occur with an agitated patient but are of little consequence if the CSF is spun down immediately for bilirubin measurement. In addition, a traumatic tap rather than SAH is suggested by a clear reduction in the number of CSF red cells between the first and third collected bottles. A traumatic tap does, however, contaminate the CSF for any subsequent analysis, emphasizing the importance of performing the correct analysis first time. Occasionally, the CSF may show a moderate lymphocytosis, a mild increase in protein and a reduction in glucose secondary to a chemical meningitis following SAH.

Confirmed SAH is usually followed by transfer to a regional centre after liaison with neurosurgical and anaesthetic colleagues. Intra-arterial angiography

[1] Van der Wee, Ann Clin Biochem (2003) 40: 481–488.

is usually diagnostic though possibly falsely negative in the presence of significant vasospasm, requiring a repeat study at a later date in rare cases. A peri-mesencephalic pattern of haemorrhage on CT, characterized by blood confined to the cisterns around the midbrain, occurs in 10% of SAH. This has a benign prognosis, and no evidence of an arterial aneurysm tends to be found: venous thrombosis may play a role in these bleeds. Other causes of subarachnoid blood include arterial dissection, venous sinus thrombosis, dural arteriovenous malformation and pituitary apoplexy, which may need to be considered when the history or angiogram does not suggest an underlying aneurysm.

A recent Cochrane review and meta-analysis reconfirms that nimodipine reduces poor outcome and CT evidence of secondary ischemia after SAH, particularly when given orally.[2] Patients should be hydrated with intravenous isotonic fluids (at least 1 l normal saline every 8 h) and placed on bed rest. Treating acute hypertension is avoided unless mean arterial blood pressure is above 130 mmHg (diastolic plus a third of the pulse pressure). Risk of rebleed is 25% within the first 2 weeks and is highest from day one, whereas the risk of vasospasm peaks on days 4–6. Both factors suggest that early intervention may be preferable in patients who are well enough, though there are no randomized data to support this.

Management of confirmed SAH has benefited from the rapidly developing specialty of interventional neuroradiology that offers an alternative treatment option to surgery. Treatment for defined aneurysm is dependant upon location and accessibility, but the International Subarachnoid Aneurysm Trial (ISAT) showed that in patients eligible for either surgery or endovascular coiling, coiling was associated with a 22% relative risk reduction of death or severe disability at 1 year, increasing to 27% at 2 years.[3] It is important to note that patients were entered into the trial on an uncertainty principle, and the study involved patients in whom surgery was not 'clearly the best option'.

The widespread use of MRI has created an additional dilemma: the management of identified asymptomatic intracranial aneurysms that occur in up to 4% of the general population. Scanning the brain of patients with dizziness, paraesthesia or chronic headache may lead to the conversation 'the good news is there is no serious cause for your symptoms, the bad news is you have a small aneurysm', which causes more anxiety in the patient and physician than was there prior to scanning. There is now some data to guide further management

[2] Rinkel *et al.* Cochrane Database Syst Rev (2005) CD000277.

[3] Molyneux *et al.* Lancet (2002) 360: 1267–1274.

in these cases. The retrospective and prospective international study of unruptured intracranial aneurysms (ISUIA) has suggested that asymptomatic aneurysms less than 10 mm within the anterior circulation have a low risk of rupture of no greater than 0.05% per year, and treatment of these is not usually undertaken.[4,5] The annual rupture rate for larger aneurysms or those in the posterior circulation approaches 1% per year or more, and intervention may be appropriate after taking into account various factors including the risks of treatment, patient age and aneurysm location. Guidelines also suggest that screening for patients in whom there is a family history is advised only if there are two or more first-degree relatives with a ruptured intracranial aneurysm.

Arterial dissection and venous sinus thrombosis

At least as frequent (but generally less commonly recognized) causes of acute- or subacute-onset headache include arterial dissection and venous sinus thrombosis. They are more commonly associated with focal neurological signs than SAH. Arterial dissection may occur spontaneously or in response to relatively minor trauma and, with the advent of MRI, is an increasingly recognized cause of stroke in young people. Dissection is commonly extracranial, affecting either the vertebral or carotid vessels and can be bilateral. Downstream cerebral pathology may occur as a result of blood tracking between the intima and media of the lumen wall and causing occlusion, or more commonly from an embolus arising from the intimal tear. Neck, face or periorbital pain and Horner's syndrome (20%) are the hallmarks of carotid dissection. Cases linking cervical arterial dissection and stroke during activities involving prolonged neck extension such as 'hair salon stroke' have been reported but remain anecdotal. Most focal neurological sequelae due to distal emboli occur within 24 h, although events have been reported up to 2 months after documented dissection. Vertebral dissection causes posterior neck pain and occipital headache and focal neurological symptoms related to the posterior circulation. Full anticoagulation for 3 months followed by a further 9 months of aspirin is conventionally used, although the evidence base is weak. The Warfarin versus Aspirin for Secondary Stroke Prevention (WARSS) trial suggested that anticoagulants may be no more effective than antiplatelet agents in preventing recurrent arterial thromboemboli.[6] A formal trial of aspirin versus anticoagulation in arterial dissection is needed.

---

[4] ISUIA Investigators, N Engl J Med (1998) 339: 1725–1733.

[5] Wiebers *et al*. Lancet (2003) 362: 103–110.

[6] Mohr *et al*. N Engl J Med (2001) 345: 1444–1451.

Cerebral venous sinus thrombosis is always worth remembering when the brain scan and CSF are initially unhelpful but the patient is unwell. Venous blood exits the brain via superficial and deep cerebral veins that drain into the peripherally located dural venous sinuses. The superior and lateral sinuses are most commonly affected by thrombosis that may be precipitated by a wide range of local, systemic and haematological prothrombotic states. Common precipitants include pregnancy, dehydration, infection and the oral contraceptive pill. Prothrombotic tendencies, including factor V Leiden, protein C and S and antithrombin III deficiencies, malignancy and antiphospholipid antibodies, may also be worth excluding.

Blockage of the outflow pipe due to cerebral venous thrombosis causes two primary problems: raised intracranial pressure resulting in headache and papilloedema, and cortical irritation with subsequent seizures and limb weakness. CT scanning may show multifocal infarction or haemorrhage and subtle high signal in the sinus to those looking for it, or an 'empty delta sign' if contrast is given. MRI and MRV are better. Lumbar puncture (LP) may help exclude alternative diagnoses such as meningitis, and SAH and will confirm raised pressure. Treatment is based on limited evidence, but full heparinization appears to improve outcome as does early diagnosis. There has been only one randomized trial, and that was stopped early after only 10 patients had been randomized to each arm, when it was found 8 patients had recovered in the heparin arm compared with one in the placebo arm.[7] Reassuringly, retrospective studies do not appear to show an increased risk of haemorrhage with heparin therapy, even in the presence of venous haemorrhage. The difficulties surrounding dose titration mean that low-molecular-weight heparin is now often used in cases of cerebral sinus thrombosis and the anecdotal outcomes appear similar. Raised intracranial pressure may respond acutely to osmotic agents, acetazolamide or shunting but these do not rectify the underlying cause of the raised pressure. Selective endovascular thrombolysis may be considered in patients who continue to deteriorate despite adequate heparinization, although only good outcomes tend to be reported, as case reports, in the literature. Pulmonary embolus from a dural sinus thrombosis is described and carries a poor prognosis.

Intracranial haemorrhage

Although severe headache, early impaired consciousness and progression are touted as markers of primary intracerebral haemorrhage, there are no clinical features to reliably distinguish ischemic stroke from primary intracerebral

---

[7] Einhaupl *et al.* Lancet (1991) 338: 597–600.

haemorrhage, highlighting the importance of early imaging in stroke patients. Deep cerebral haemorrhage affecting territories supplied by perforating arterioles is commonly hypertensive in aetiology in those with appropriate vascular risk factors over the age of 40 years. Vascular anomalies and other alternative causes should be excluded in more peripheral lobar cortical haemorrhage, usually by angiography or follow-up MRI. A drug history and toxicology screen should always be considered in the young. Patients with intracerebral haemorrhage who develop an above-knee deep-vein thrombosis or pulmonary embolus in hospital often require placement of an IVC filter. Longer-term anticoagulation may be considered, but the risk of recurrent peripheral thrombosis must be weighed against an increase in the baseline risk of primary intracerebral haemorrhage recurrence (0.5–2%) with anticoagulation, for which data are not available.

Raised intracranial pressure headache

The physician should be alert to the possibility of the headache of raised intracranial pressure in the context of any novel progressive headache syndrome with associated features. The brain has developed within a tight bony box for protection from trauma with the only decent sized exit being the foramen magnum. This has some drawbacks as any increase in intracranial volume rapidly results in increasing pressure, which ultimately leads to either obstruction of arterial inflow or herniation through the foramen magnum – both devastating events. There is some initial facility to compensate for an expanding intracranial volume as both the cerebral venous and CSF volumes (about 80 ml each) may be compressed and excluded from the cranial vault without serious sequelae but after this, deterioration is often rapid. In addition, if the primary problem relates to the venous or CSF system (such as in hydrocephalus), this buffer is removed. The possibility of raised intracranial pressure should be considered in any subacute progressive headache syndrome in which an alternative positive diagnosis cannot be made, particularly if features such as headache on waking from sleep, nausea and vomiting are present or exacerbation occurs with bending or driving over bumps in the road! Cognitive decline, ataxia and drowsiness are late warning signs.

Low-intracranial-pressure headache

Low intracranial pressure also causes headache, and here the history is diagnostic. Headache is exacerbated by standing and relieved by lying, the significance of which may be missed. This rarely occurs if the patient has recently had an LP or spinal surgery but CSF leak may also arise from a dural tear associated with degenerative disc disease, overenthusiastic shunting or even after trauma. CSF hypotension and hypovolaemia is associated with subdural collections and increased meningeal enhancement on MRI scanning. CSF pressure at supine LP is usually less than 5 cm H_2O, and aspiration may even be required to extract a CSF sample. Dural repair or blood patching may be required if symptoms persist.

Neuromythology has often dictated that strict bed rest for several hours after LP is required to reduce post-LP headache, but several studies have shown that this is not the case. Patients may generally mobilize immediately afterwards. Bed rest, fluids and caffeine may speed resolution of any post-LP headache that does occur, the majority of which resolve within 3–5 days. Refractory post-LP low-pressure headache is effectively treated by a dural blood patch in 90% of the rest.

Other secondary causes of headache in hospital

Systemic infection or illness is a common cause for isolated headache in hospital patients. Catches include meningitis in the elderly or comatose (that may occur without meningism), glaucoma and giant cell arteritis in those over 55 years of age. Medication is often forgotten, but is also a frequent cause of headache.

Primary headaches

The general physician might quite reasonably feel that their job is done once a serious secondary cause for headache has been excluded. However, this has not provided the patient with a diagnosis or management strategy, and a positive early diagnosis of a primary headache syndrome may remove the need for extensive investigation in all patients. Primary headache can usefully be divided into migraine, tension-type headache, trigeminal autonomic cephalgias and a rag bag of others including cough, coital and hypnic headaches.

Migraine

Migraine is common and a frequent cause of acute medical admission, often raising concerns about meningitis, SAH and encephalopathy. The old adage that 'when in doubt, wait it out' remains pertinent with migraine, as spontaneous improvement is usually seen within 24 h. Migraine is usually asymmetric, gradual in onset (usually over more than 30 min) and is associated with nausea and sensitivity to light and noise. A previous history, family history and the age of the patient are helpful additional features.

Distinguishing migraine aura from stroke is a common puzzle, and the history again usually trumps investigations unless there is ready access to diffusion-weighted imaging. Associated migraine aura is distinguished by its chronicity.

Functional imaging studies illustrate a slow-spreading cortical depression (at the rate of a few millimetres per minute) that precedes migraine headache and mirrors the associated clinical aura. Hence, visual and sensory migraine aura progress and develop over minutes, unlike a stroke or seizure. Aura are also typically positive phenomena if visual (scintillating scotomata or teichopsia) or sensory (paraesthesia rather than sensory loss). Despite what is often found in the textbooks, it is common for patients to report persistent altered hemisensory perception for hours or sometimes days after a migraine attack that occurs in the absence of clinical signs or imaging changes.

Occasionally, known migraine sufferers present with 'status migranosis' to the emergency department. Treatment options include the subcutaneous triptans, intravenous prochlorperazine combined with dihydroergotamine, sodium valproate, neuroleptics (such as chlorpromazine) or steroids, in addition to regular analgesia. As outpatients, acute migraine treatment usually involves the use of 5HT1 agonists such as sumatriptan, but efficacy in terms of numbers needed-to-treat is not dramatically better than that for high-dose (900 mg) dispersible aspirin. The benefits of acute migraine treatment are improved by treating early and are dependant upon the route of administration. Oral wafers, nasal spray and subcutaneous injectable formulations are useful where nausea is prominent. 5HT1 agonists may be combined with nonsteroidal and codeine-based analgesics but should be used with caution in patients with cardiovascular disease. β-blockers, tricyclic antidepressants and antiepileptics are all used as prophylactic therapy in troublesome migraine.

Migraine in pregnancy is a misery. Luckily, most migraines will occur in the first trimester and not much beyond. This is an evidence-poor zone for obvious reasons, and, to date, little is regarded as safe other than paracetamol. Widespread use of metoclopromide in pregnancy for other indications is reassuring, and it may help reduce nausea and vomiting, if present, with migraine, and perhaps even the headache itself. True migraine occurring for the first time during pregnancy, particularly if there are focal signs, needs to be taken seriously, and many neurologists would offer the patient an MRI scan to ensure that there is no rare but sinister cause, such as an arteriovenous malformation or meningioma, which might cause problems during the remainder of pregnancy or delivery. For many migraine sufferers, pregnancy will actually reduce their headache frequency.

Cluster headache deserves mention as the presentation is characteristic, the pain excruciating and the condition treatable. One of the so-called 'trigeminal autonomic cephalgias', it is characterized by severe unilateral head and periorbital pain, autonomic features of lacrimation, conjunctival injection and rhinorrhoea. Unlike migraine, it is short lived (usually less than 1 h), and the patient (more commonly male) invariably moves around with the pain rather than lying still. Also known as an 'alarm clock headache', it often occurs at the same time each day, more often the early hours of the morning, and the pain is so bad that the patient may bash his head on the wall in an attempt to gain some form of relief! High-flow oxygen in hospital eases the pain acutely though is usually impractical at home. Subcutaneous sumatriptan is sometimes effective, and the cluster of attacks may be aborted by prescribing a short tapering course of prednisolone 60 mg together with verapamil, which may be continued if episodes fail to settle within a few days. Headache syndromes with shorter or continuous unilateral stabbing head pains often prompt a normal CT head scan if they result in acute hospital admission. These patients should be tried on an NSAID, which helps a significant proportion.

When to take pictures

The setting and clinical suspicion strongly influences this decision. In the primary care setting, the chances of demonstrating significant intracranial pathology in nonacute (present for greater than 4 weeks) headache with no neurological signs or features of raised intracranial pressure approaches that of asymptomatic patients (< 0.5%). Scanning should be performed when underlying pathology is suspected or the diagnosis remains unclear. Associated focal neurological signs, meningism, altered sensorium, personality change, seizures or syncope, age over 65 and predisposing medical conditions (such as immunosuppression or warfarin therapy) are reasonable grounds for investigating further with imaging. For other cases, a period of observation may be appropriate.

THE DIZZY PATIENT

> *"There can be few physicians so dedicated to their art that they do not experience a slight decline in spirits when they learn that their patient's complaint is giddiness"*
> W. B. Matthews
> Practical Neurology. Oxford, Blackwell, 1963

Few physicians are rarefied enough to avoid all contact with the dizzy patient, and a logical and simple approach, guided by a few principles, helps demystify the syndrome. Two features are key: are the episodes paroxysmal and are they truly vertiginous? The addition of a Hallpike and head impulse test completes the necessary armoury.

The differential diagnosis of paroxysmal symptoms usually includes syncope, seizure, hypoglycaemia and hyperventilation, as well as a peripheral vestibulopathy. The first three are associated with altered consciousness rather than imbalance, although, unfortunately, it is surprising how many patients are unable to distinguish between these. If uncertainty remains, patients with potential cardiac disease should have further cardiological evaluation, although the pick-up rate from 24-h ECGs is depressingly low. Complex partial seizures may be associated with gastric, gustatory, olfactory or psychic aura or prolonged recovery, and a witness account may highlight cyanosis, motor automatisms and verbal arrest. Hypoglycaemia usually occurs in the context of treated diabetes, although it is important to remember that blood sugar via a finger-prick glucometer after an episode may be normal and falsely reassuring. Nocturnal events in diabetics require regular blood sugar monitoring before this diagnosis can be excluded.

True vertigo is the sensation of movement or rotation of either the person or environment and is caused by asymmetric vestibular input, a result of dysfunction of the semicircular canals, vestibular nerve or nuclei. It is always made worse by head movement, and the absence of this feature in the patient with persistent dizziness suggests that true vertigo is unlikely.

Panic attacks, especially with hyperventilation, commonly cause a sense of dizziness that is not truly vertiginous. The symptoms usually occur in specific places or situations, and are associated with a distressing sense of anxiety. Associated features such as limb and peri-oral paraesthesia with hyperventilation are helpful, and patients are best helped by a clear nonjudgemental explanation. Reproducing the patient's symptoms by asking them to overbreathe for 1–2 min (this can be tested by threading a paper towel along a tendon hammer and asking the patient to keep blowing to keep the towel horizontal) can be very helpful, both diagnostically and therapeutically.

The most common (and treatable) cause of recurrent or paroxysmal vertigo is benign paroxysmal positional vertigo (BPPV). The history is virtually diagnostic, with symptoms occurring when rolling over in bed at night, hanging out the washing or turning the head to reverse the car. Paroxysmal symptoms on neck extension are usually BPPV and not 'vertebrobasilar insufficiency'. The natural history is of an acute bout of recurrent movement-induced attacks (a clear history of vertigo is not even necessary) with gradual reduction in frequency and severity of episodes. Recurrence of symptoms at a future date is quite common. BPPV is caused by the movement of stray otoconial particles within the duct of a (usually posterior) semicircular canal. It is an important diagnosis to make as not only can the patient be reassured, but it is also possible to remove these particles through repositioning manoeuvres and effect an instant cure. A Hallpike manoeuvre is all that is required to confirm the diagnosis; the general neurological examination should be normal between episodes. From a seated position, the patient's head is turned to one side and the patient is pitched backwards (in the plane of the posterior semicircular canal). There is usually a lag of 10–15 s before the onset of rotatory nystagmus and vertigo, which subsequently settles. Persistent symptoms or nonrotatory nystagmus suggests that a structural brain lesion should be excluded. An Epley manoeuvre may be performed from this position if the test is positive and will relieve symptoms in 4 out of 5 patients. This is performed by slowly rolling the patient's head through 180 from the most provocative position towards the normal side.[8] If this provokes a further paroxysm of vertigo, success is more likely. BPPV is common after head injury and unusual in the very young. Atypical or long-standing cases may require exclusion of intracranial pathology with imaging and referral to a vestibular testing lab.

Recurrent episodes of non-movement-sensitive, prolonged vertigo usually have either migraine or Menière's disease as the cause. The presumed pathophysiological basis of Menière's disease is episodic endolymphatic hypertension, which produces devastating attacks of spontaneous vertigo with nausea and vomiting, together with a low-frequency hearing loss, and a sense of fullness or blockage in the affected ear. The usual key feature is the association with tinnitus although this may develop later. The vertigo usually lasts for a few hours, but the tinnitus and hearing loss might continue for days. An audiogram and ENT referral are usually appropriate. Vertigo attacks in migraine often respond to medications used to treat migraine headaches such as a triptan, or even dispersible aspirin, and in some patients the vertigo attacks can be prevented by regular treatment with a β-blocker, verapamil, sodium valproate or acetazolamide.

A slightly different problem faces the doctor assessing a patient with their first ever episode of intense spontaneous persistent vertigo, nausea and vomiting, where the diagnosis usually lies between cerebellar stroke and labyrinthitis. It is often assumed, usually correctly, that the patient has labyrinthitis, although middle-ear infection may be diagnosed and a prescription written for an antibiotic, as well as prochlorperazine by mouth. Acute otitis media does not cause vertigo unless there is a suppurative labyrinthitis. In labyrinthitis (or probably, more correctly, acute vestibulopathy), nystagmus is always unidirectional. Bidirectional-gaze-evoked nystagmus excludes the diagnosis and is often due to drugs. Vestibular nystagmus is, to some extent, also suppressed by visual fixation and may be induced by bringing the back of the hand to within about 5 cm of the eyes so that focussing and fixation cannot occur. Several clinical tests help distinguish acute labyrinthitis (of presumed viral, postinfectious or vascular origin) from an acute central cerebellar lesion (usually a stroke), but the head impulse test is probably the most useful.[9] This is done by rapidly

[8] McClure *et al.* Baillieres Clin Neurol (1994) 3: 537–545.

turning the head (5–10°) in the direction of the vestibulopathy, with the eyes fixed on a distant stable midline object (often the examiner's nose). With a peripheral vestibular lesion, the vestibulo-ocular reflex fails and the eyes move from the midline before correcting with a 'catch up' saccade. On the intact side, the eyes remain in the middle position. A normal head impulse test in the setting of acute vertigo and an inability to stand with the eyes open are features that suggest a central lesion.

There are many reasons for a patient to be off balance while standing or walking, a symptom that many patients will insist on calling 'dizziness' but this is not true vertigo. Whereas it is true that the older the patient the less likely that a single diagnosis can be made to account for the problem, aminoglycoside toxicity merits consideration. This causes bilateral loss of vestibular function, ataxia and oscillopsia (sensation of movement of the external environment when the head is moved), but not vertigo. In the absence of any significant and relevant hearing loss, it can cause some diagnostic difficulties because an aural cause might not be considered in the differential diagnosis of imbalance. The patient will be able to walk perfectly well heel-to-toe but will be unsteady with their eyes closed. Systemic gentamicin is rarely cochleotoxic in humans, but the vestibular system is highly susceptible, and gentamicin vestibulotoxicity should be considered in any patient who notices imbalance after a hospital admission (during which they received gentamicin).

BRAIN SURGERY FOR THE GENERAL PHYSICIAN

Raised intracranial pressure

Whether the nearest neurosurgical opinion is three wards or 100 miles away, the first port of call for most patients requiring neurosurgical management is the general physician. Raised intracranial pressure causes more than its fair share of anxiety but diagnosing the problem and initial management are aided by a few general principles.

A variety of lesions may occupy space and provide a catch for the unprepared, including intracranial haemorrhage, vasogenic (tumour) and cytotoxic (stroke) oedema and hydrocephalus. In all cases, the patient may appear well until the compressible volumes (venous blood and CSF) are exhausted, when a sudden linear increase in pressure is experienced — the so called 'Monro-Kellie doctrine'. The patient who talks and walks after head injury but then deteriorates is a classic example.

....

9 Bronstein, J Neurol Neurosurg Psychiatry (2003) 74: 289–293.

Warning symptoms of raised intracranial pressure include headache that is exacerbated by coughing, bending and lying but these features are neither sensitive nor specific, and any new progressive headache should be taken seriously. Papilloedema should be sought but may be absent (particularly in the elderly). Vomiting, cranial nerve palsy and impairment of consciousness signal significant raised intracranial pressure and incipient deterioration, which may be accompanied by relative bradycardia and hypertension, the 'Cushing response'. Temporising measures to reduce intracranial pressure may include sitting the patient up, ensuring adequate oxygenation, using 20% mannitol and giving a diuretic. Intravenous dexamethasone may also help in cases of vasogenic oedema. Urgent neurosurgical advice should be sought. These measures may buy a short period of time (4–6 h), but are usually futile unless definitive surgical decompression is an option.

The evidence to guide the indications for surgical evacuation in focal brain haemorrhage or craniotomy for cerebral swelling after trauma or large hemispheric stroke is lacking, although trials are planned or underway. Cases should be discussed on a case-by-case basis with the local neurosurgical team.

Changes in the management of primary malignant intracranial tumours over the last 30 years do not appear to have dramatically impacted on survival rates. Debulking and radiotherapy after histological diagnosis may confer some small benefit over radiotherapy alone but, in general, malignant glioma is a microscopically disseminated disease at diagnosis, and surgery is rarely curative. Better 5-year survival rates may be achieved with less common tumour subtypes, such as oligodendrogliomas, and a histological diagnosis should nearly always be sought to guide therapeutic options, inform prognosis and exclude alternative diagnoses.

Shunts

Shunts can be life saving in hydrocephalus. Hydrocephalus may be due to reduced resorption of CSF across the convexity of the meninges into the venous circulation via the arachnoid granulations (communicating hydrocephalus) or due to mechanical obstruction of drainage at some point earlier in the outflow tract from lateral to third and fourth ventricles before entering the basal cisterns (noncommunicating hydrocephalus). The diagnosis is usually confirmed by brain CT scan, although MRI with flow-sensitive sequences may be required to exclude aqueductal stenosis. However, dilated ventricles on CT do not in themselves confirm high pressure and should be interpreted in the context of the history and associated features such as generalized atrophy. Most unsteady octogenarians with dilated ventricles do not have hydrocephalus and are unlikely to improve with shunting! Shunts for hydrocephalus are usually ventriculoperitoneal, but may be ventriculoatrial or ventriculopleural.

Patients with shunts may re-present with complications of shunt insertion, often to the nearest general hospital. Within the first few weeks, this is usually infection related, although it may also be due to early shunt failure. Shunt infection may not play fair and present as a typical meningitis but instead the patient may be nonspecifically unwell with raised inflammatory markers alone, or may present with abdominal pain or peritonism, and little in the way of headache or meningism. Diagnosis may be made by isolating the organism from the blood or the CSF via a shunt tap (after neurosurgical discussion) or, once a noncommunicating hydrocephalus is excluded by imaging, by LP. Shunt blockage presents with features of recurrent hydrocephalus and raised intracranial pressure including headache, vomiting and cognitive decline. Imaging may show ventricular dilatation but a previous comparison film is not always available. X-rays of the shunt itself may show breakage or kinks. An easily compressible reservoir suggests distal shunt patency, but is not 100% sensitive. A blockage in the shunt proximal to the reservoir prevents reservoir refilling or aspiration. Ultimately, if the problem is subacute, referral for CSF pressure studies and shunt revision may be required.

Spinal cord compression

If you consider it, you need to exclude it! Spinal cord compression needs to be considered in any patient presenting with acutely weak legs (even in the presence of absent reflexes). A sensory level and early bladder involvement help differentiate from early Guillain-Barré syndrome, but it is difficult to criticize the physician who excludes a treatable cord lesion with imaging in ambiguous cases. The timing of imaging, the use of steroids and acute surgery in spinal cord injury (SCI) and compression remains controversial. The National Acute Spinal Cord Injury Studies (NASCIS) I and II suggested improvement in motor function and sensation in patients with complete or incomplete SCIs who were treated with high doses of methylprednisolone within 8 h of injury. However, there are concerns about the statistical analysis, randomization and clinical endpoints used in this study, and a number of professional organizations have revised their recommendations. The Canadian Association of Emergency Physicians is no longer recommending high-dose methylprednisolone as the standard of care. The Congress of Neurological Surgeons has stated that steroid therapy 'should only be undertaken with the knowledge that the evidence suggesting harmful side effects is more consistent than any suggestion of clinical benefit'. Early imaging (within 6 h) in cases of acute compressive myelopathy may allow decisions about early surgical intervention, but there are no studies to confirm an additional therapeutic benefit from early intervention although, as always, absence of evidence is not necessarily evidence of absence.

INFLAMMATORY CNS DISEASE

Multiple sclerosis

Although present for many hundreds of years, it is perhaps a marker of the clinical heterogeneity of multiple sclerosis (MS) that it was not until just before the turn of the twentieth century that the French neurologist J. M. Charcot, best known for his work on hysteria, first drew together a clear description of the clinical and histological features of MS. Such was the phenotypic variability of MS and the fashion for diagnosing hysteria in women at that time that it was initially believed to be a rare condition, more common in men. Such is the awareness of the condition today that the pendulum has perhaps swung too far the other way, and MS is now the first thought in any young adult with sensory symptoms. What is known is that multiple sclerosis is one of the commonest neurologically disabling conditions to affect young adults and may be found in 1 in 800 people in the UK, a similar frequency to type 1 diabetes. It is, therefore, high on the differential in young adults presenting with *de novo* neurological symptoms, patients who often present, at least initially, to the general physician.

The disease is an autoimmune condition characterized by patches of inflammation, demyelination and axonal damage within the central nervous system. It occurs predominantly between the ages of 20 and 50 and is a touch more prevalent in women (roughly three to two). It is difficult to think of an aetiological theory that has not been suggested to explain multiple sclerosis, but currently a combination of exposure to one or several, as yet undefined, environmental agents in association with a genetic susceptibility appears the best guess. Family and twin studies suggest a polygenic influence; particularly the HLA-related gene complex region, and it is clear that certain ethnic populations (including the Inuit and Romany gypsies) are not susceptible to MS. An environmental influence might explain the increasing risk with latitude and the reported clustering of cases but to date there is no convincing data for any single agent.[10] The usual suspect infectious agents have all appeared in the dock at various times but on each occasion the evidence has not stood up to scrutiny, and there have been trials of nearly every antibiotic and antiviral agent in patients with multiple sclerosis. A 'slow virus' also appears unlikely.[11] Patients can at

[10] Kurtzke, Neurol Sci (2000) 21: 383–403.

[11] Prusiner, N Engl J Med (2001) 344: 1516–1526.

least be reassured that the condition is not contagious and, on current knowledge, not something they could have taken action to avoid.

Most patients with MS (85%) initially present with attacks and remission of neurological symptoms, interspersed with periods of clinical stability, the so-called relapsing and remitting form of the disease. As time goes by, relapses become less frequent and, by 10 years, half will have developed the secondary progressive form of the disease. A small proportion of patients present with progressive disease without relapses from the outset, which may present more of a diagnostic challenge. Common initial symptoms include: an asymmetric partial transverse myelitis, hemiparesis and hemisensory disturbance, dysarthria with ataxia, and optic neuritis. Gradual onset, positive sensory phenomena and a lack of constitutional symptoms in an appropriately aged patient are the clues. Other symptoms such as Lhermitte's (lightning-like limb pains with neck flexion) and Uhthoff's phenomena (reproducible exercise and heat-induced neurological symptoms) and stereotyped short-lived but multiple paroxysmal tonic limb spasms also suggest inflammatory CNS lesions. However, not all that tingles is MS and significant anxiety is often induced by raising the possibility of MS prematurely in a patient with isolated sensory symptoms. Reassuring patients with a normal neurological examination and appropriate negative imaging is an important therapeutic intervention.

> 'By the method of exclusion, I had arrived at this result,
> for no other hypothesis would meet the facts.'
>
> A Study in Scarlet
> Sherlock Holmes[12]

This preceding adage applies well in MS, which remains a diagnosis of exclusion. Atypical symptoms that should prompt exclusion of an alternative diagnosis include seizures, confusion, headache, fever and a progressive neurological syndrome in the young. A confirmed diagnosis of MS requires evidence of separation of lesions in time and space within the CNS (usually two spontaneously resolving clinical episodes) and no better explanation. New MS diagnostic criteria now allow diagnosis after a single attack if there is follow-up MRI evidence of new brain lesions at 3 months.[13] A first attack may be difficult to distinguish from acute disseminated encephalomyelitis (ADEM), although this occurs more commonly in children and is associated with headache, drowsiness, meningeal signs and CSF pleocytosis, all of which would be

---

[12] Conan Doyle, A Study in Scarlet, OUP, Oxford, 1999.

[13] McDonald *et al.* Ann Neurol (2001) 50: 121–127.

unusual in multiple sclerosis. Brain MRI may be indistinguishable from MS but new lesions are not seen on follow-up in ADEM.

The brain MRI scan is abnormal in 90–95% of patients with clinically established MS. This figure is less in those with early disease or in primary progressive patients in whom (it is assumed) pathology is predominantly in the spinal cord. In MS, lesions are typically located within the corpus callosum (unusual in ischemia and perpendicularly orientated in MS) and cerebellar peduncles in addition to classically located periventricular white matter lesions. In addition, lesions within the spinal cord are not commonly seen in vascular disease. A normal scan should prompt the search for an alternative cause or supplemental support for a diagnosis of MS. Spinal cord imaging will detect lesions in a significant proportion of patients with MS and is a useful additional investigation in these situations. Additional support for the diagnosis with unpaired oligoclonal bands in the CSF and asymmetrically delayed visual-evoked potentials may also be helpful. A matched serum sample for oligoclonal bands should always be sent.

Patients with optic neuritis are often aware of the association with MS. A history of pain on eye movement and gradual onset monocular visual loss with a relative afferent papillary defect in a young adult suggests the diagnosis, and approximately 40% will subsequently have developed MS in 10 years. Atypical features including painless loss, poor recovery or established optic atrophy at presentation require imaging to rule out a compressive lesion. Brain MRI may also help prognosticate in patients with clinically isolated syndromes consistent with a first demyelinating episode, such as optic neuritis.[14] The presence of an abnormal brain MRI at presentation predicts an approximate 80% risk of conversion to clinically definite MS at 10 years compared with a negative scan (10% conversion risk), although a larger percentage have developed abnormal MRI scans. This information may not always be helpful to patients and needs to be assessed on a case-by-case basis.

Treatment in MS can be divided into treatment of acute demyelinating episodes, disease modifying therapy and symptomatic treatment. The first and last of these are most likely to involve the general physician. Relapses in MS may be associated with systemic infection, which should always be treated or excluded first. NICE guidelines suggest that a 5-day course of very-high-dose steroids may be given orally for acute relapse (such as Solu-Medrone in orange juice), a route that may avoid admission for intravenous steroids. Serum levels appear similar, irrespective of the route of administration. Patients can be told that evidence suggests that steroids speed the rate of recovery but do not

[14] O'Riordan *et al.* Brain (1998) 121: 495–503.

appear to affect the extent of recovery or disease course in the long term. Symptomatic treatments include management of neuropathic pain, often with a combination of antiepileptic and tricyclic medication. Spasticity responds to physiotherapy, removal of exacerbating factors such as pain, constipation and urinary retention and the judicious use of antispasmodics. Some spasticity may be helpful if the patient remains mobile. Urinary urgency can be treated with anticholinergic medication, with residual volumes under 100 ml. Unfortunately, disabling symptoms such as fatigue, cognitive impairment and tremor are more difficult to treat.

Four products are now licensed in the UK for disease modification, three types of interferon-beta and a separate product, co-polymer 1. All reduce relapses by an average of a third, are expensive, are given by subcutaneous or intramuscular injection and require the patient to be ambulatory and to have had at least 2 relapses in the last 2 years. Effects on long-term disability are less clear. Unfortunately, there is no licensed therapy for progressive disease. The Internet has become a source of unregulated information for patients on many different putative therapies. A sensitive and open discussion regarding the paucity of unbiased evidence for these treatments in peer-reviewed scientific journals is often helpful to patients who present with sometimes confusing and conflicting information.

MS mimics

Fortunately, in many cases, the diagnosis of MS is straightforward, but a wide range of other inflammatory conditions may enter the diagnostic ring in patients presenting with disabling neurological symptoms. Many systemic immunologically mediated conditions have neurological sequelae and present with subacute and relapsing neurological dysfunction that may mimic MS.

Chance favours the prepared. An elicited history of migraine may prompt further enquiry into evidence of seizures, recurrent miscarriage, livedo reticularis and peripheral venous thrombosis in the antiphospholipid syndrome. Serum testing may show thrombocytopenia and a raised APTT. Antiphospholipid antibodies should be checked but may occur following acute infection and should be confirmed by repeat testing. The venous and arterial thrombosis and small-vessel vasculopathy associated with this condition are usually treated with anticoagulation. Migraine is also a feature in CADASIL (cerebral autosomal dominant arteriopathy with subcortical infarcts and leucoencephalopathy) due to mutations in the Notch3 gene on chromosome 19, which presents in the young adult with cognitive decline and stroke-like episodes. Brain MRI shows confluent deep white matter lesions that may be characteristic. Gene testing is available, and skin biopsy shows granular osmophilic material ('GOM') found on electron microscopy in vessel walls.

Mitochondrial disorders also present with multifocal neurological symptoms and stroke-like episodes, usually in the context of short stature, diabetes and deafness. MRI abnormalities (subcortical and non-large-vessel-distributed lesions) are unlikely to be confused with MS. An increased lactate/pyruvate ratio in serum and CSF, genetic testing and a muscle biopsy help confirm a mitochondrial abnormality.

Connective tissue disease may present with a relapsing or progressive spinal cord, optic nerve or neuropsychiatric syndrome mimicking MS. Constitutional symptoms, arthralgia and rash suggest systemic lupus; keratoconjunctivitis sicca and xerostomia suggest Sjögren's syndrome. An ESR and autoantibody screen are useful in patients in whom the diagnosis is possible. Cerebral vasculitis enters the differential in patients with a subacute history with headache, meningism, encephalopathy, seizures and progressive neurological deficits in the absence of a known systemic vasculitis or connective tissue disorder. Serological markers are often absent, MRI may show supra- and infra-tentorial white matter lesions, and CSF analysis typically shows a raised protein and lymphocytosis. Angiography may show nonspecific areas of focal spasm or may be normal. Definitive diagnosis may elude even brain biopsy, but this is often undertaken to exclude alternative causes before starting long-term combination immunosuppressive therapy.

Behcet's disease is concentrated in the Mediterranean basin and Japan. Diagnosis is made by highlighting a history of recurrent oral ulceration (greater than three episodes per year) in association with a combination of genital ulceration, skin lesions (typically papulopustular lesions, pseudofolliculitis or erythema nodosum) and uveitis. Pathergy may also be present but is less common in Caucasians. Neurological involvement occurs in around 5% of patients and presents either as cerebral venous thrombosis or a relapsing brainstem syndrome. Optic neuritis and progressive transverse myelitis have also been described. Relapses may be associated with fever, headache and a raised ESR, all of which should prompt the search for a systemic disorder. MRI scanning usually shows characteristic brainstem and basal ganglia involvement, and the CSF is usually pleocytic with a slightly raised protein level. Immunosuppressive therapy is required for relapsing disease.

It is perhaps worth mentioning neurosarcoidosis at this point, if only to place it into perspective. Often the diagnosis of the intellectually destitute when presented with an unusual neurological case at the Grand Round, isolated neurosarcoid is rare. Neurological involvement does occur in about 5% of patients with systemic sarcoid. In these patients, a steroid-responsive relapsing optic neuritis, brain stem, spinal cord or nerve root disease may mimic MS. Sarcoid is typically a meningeal disease unlike MS, providing diagnostic clues such as meningeal enhancement on MRI and CSF leucocytosis. Hilar lymphadenopathy may be demonstrated with a chest x-ray and, if possible, with high-resolution CT. Abnormal respiratory function tests are found in most cases of systemic sarcoidosis. Gallium-67 SPECT scanning may show characteristic tracer uptake in salivary and lacrimal glands, chest and spleen. Ophthalmologic examination for evidence of uveitis can be useful. Definitive diagnosis requires histological confirmation of noncaseating epithelioid cell granulomas. Serum and CSF angiotensin converting enzyme levels do not appear sensitive or specific. Response to treatment can be disappointing.

Other clinical conditions that may present with a meningoradicular syndrome and a marked CSF leucocytosis (> 50 lymphocytes) include Lyme (*Borrelia burgdorferi*) disease, crypotococcal infection and HIV. Lyme disease occurs in temperate forested regions of Europe and Asia and in the northeastern and upper midwestern areas of the US. Significant regional variation occurs in the UK. A history of tick bite, characteristic rash (erythema chronicum migrans) and constitutional symptoms in association with a painful polyradiculopathy, facial palsy or meningoencephalitis are typical (but rare). Confirmation is by detection of intrathecal IgM against *Borrelia*. Neurosyphilis still occurs, more commonly in the HIV population. Diagnosis is considered when headache and seizures are associated with pupillary abnormalities and an active CSF. The diagnosis is highly unlikely in the presence of a negative serum *Treponema pallidum* haemaglutination (TPHA) assay. A positive CSF VDRL confirms the diagnosis in the presence of a positive serum.

In summary, it is always worth considering an inflammatory CNS condition in the patient with subacute-onset fluctuating neurological symptoms. The brain is an exquisitely sensitive organ dependant on a rich immunologically packed vascular supply and responds poorly to unsolicited inflammation.

Progressive weakness

Here, the first step is usually to determine whether weakness is upper motor neurone or 'neuromuscular' (pathology distal to the anterior horn cell in the spinal cord: peripheral nerve, neuromuscular junction and muscle) in pattern. Upper motor neurone lesions usually present with hemiparesis or paraparesis and pathologically brisk reflexes. Neuromuscular causes usually affect all four limbs and are not associated with exaggerated reflexes. Areflexia, wasting, distal limb weakness and sensory symptoms suggest a neuropathy. Myopathies affect proximal limb function: patients complain of being unable to rise from a chair, and have difficulty getting out of the bath and climbing stairs. Difficulty with washing hair in the shower or hanging out the washing quickly distinguishes proximal arm weakness from distal weakness causing difficulty with jar tops, turning keys in locks and fastening bras. Myopathies are associated with retained reflexes, an absence of sensory symptoms and signs and no evidence of early wasting. Neuromuscular junction disorders such as myasthenia gravis appear similar to myopathies but more commonly have ocular and facial involvement, and a fatigable ptosis in this setting is virtually pathognomonic. A diagnosis of motor neuron disease requires the presence of both lower and upper motor neuron signs and is usually suggested by the presence of progressive wasting, weakness and fasciculations in the context of pathologically brisk reflexes and an absence of sensory features. It is primarily a clinical diagnosis. Neurophysiology may be extremely helpful in confirming or distinguishing between neuropathies, myopathies and neuromuscular junction disorders but is time consuming, operator dependant and most effective when a particular clinical question is being asked.

Neuromuscular Respiratory failure

Bulbar and respiratory assessments are essential in patients with neuromuscular weakness. Neuromuscular respiratory failure is a disorder of ventilation and inadequate tidal volume. Diaphragmatic and respiratory intercostal muscles work along a very narrow tension–length relationship, and failure is often precipitous outside of this. Pulse oximetry is usually normal in early neuromuscular respiratory failure. By the time the oxygen saturation drops, the decline may be catastrophic. Arterial gases are similarly insensitive, and peak flows do not sensitively reflect falling lung ventilatory volumes. The most sensitive test is measurement of lung volume or forced vital capacity. A vital capacity approaching 15 ml/kg or a rapidly declining vital capacity requires intensive care assessment and usually intubation, as assisted ventilation and not the provision of supplemental oxygen (which can be dangerous) is required. A count of 20 in a single breath equates approximately to a vital capacity of 2 l. Patients counting to less than 10 are approaching imminent respiratory failure.

Bulbar function

Early recognition and assessment of bulbar involvement is important in patients presenting with evolving weakness, especially as there may also be respiratory compromise. Aspiration and acute respiratory deterioration may be abrupt if precautions are not taken early. Neurogenic dysphagia affects liquids more than solids. Nasal regurgitation occurs with palatal weakness and occurs early in myasthenia gravis and Guillain-Barré syndrome. Swallow is best assessed empirically rather than by using a surrogate such as the gag reflex. Swallow should be tested with water looking for double swallow, choking and signs of a 'wet' or 'croaky' count to ten. If the patient is felt to be at risk, a nasogastric tube should be placed.

Flaccid paresis

Flaccid paresis implies areflexia and is usually neuropathic. Guillain-Barré syndrome is the most common acute (less than 4 weeks) progressive neuropathy, with an average-sized hospital expecting to see 5–10 cases per year. The diagnosis may be missed early on when the patient presents with limb paraesthesia and vague complaints about reduced mobility and poor balance. An acute neuropathy may also occur with vasculitis, diphtheria (pharyngeal exudates and absent pupillary accommodation reflex), porphyria (associated hyponatraemia and urinary porphobilinogens), arsenic (deliberate self-harm or poisoning), hexacarbon toxicity (history of glue sniffing), botulism (dilated pupils and ptosis) and infective causes of meningoradiculopathy, particularly HIV infection. Tick paralysis should be considered in travellers from the US or Australia.

Guillain-Barré usually presents with distal ascending weakness and paraesthesia. A sensory ataxic gait and foot drop may occur early. However, unlike toxic neuropathies, the inflammatory demyelinating neuropathies may also be patchy and proximal, and the patient may present with facial or asymmetric limb weakness. Reflexes may be preserved early in the clinical presentation. Sensory symptoms point away from a myopathic or neuromuscular disorder. A history of preceding respiratory (cytomegalovirus) or gastrointestinal (campylobacter) infection, vaccination or surgery may be elicited. Lower-back pain with a positive Kernig's sign or impaired straight leg raise is a useful diagnostic clue reflecting nerve root inflammation. Autonomic instability occurs in about 60%, and nonmobile patients should be on a cardiac monitor. Investigations include those required to exclude alternative causes, occasionally with cervical cord imaging. CSF analysis typically shows a raised protein without significant pleocytosis. Nerve conduction studies may be nondiagnostic in the early stages, but typically show marked conduction slowing. Axonal variants (seen more commonly in association with campylobacter infection) have marked early motor involvement and a poorer prognosis and may be diagnosed electrophysiologically. Glycolipid antibodies may be associated with particular syndromes (GQ1B – Miller-Fischer variant with ataxia and ophthalmoparesis, MG1 – motor variants) but do not currently influence early management.

Trials have shown that plasma exchange improves outcome, reducing the average time to regaining the ability to walk by about a month. Fortunately, intravenous immunoglobulin appears to be equally effective and does not have the logistical and haemodynamic implications for the patient.[15] There is no published evidence that demonstrates a clear benefit with combined or repeated therapy, although there is a theoretical basis to suggest that patients who continue to deteriorate despite immunoglobulin might also benefit from plasma exchange to remove persistent pathogenic antibodies. Good general medical and nursing care is also paramount with bulbar, respiratory and haemodynamic monitoring and venous thrombosis prophylaxis. Neuropathic pain may be severe, and often requires combination therapy for good symptomatic relief. The psychological impact of being 'locked-in' should not be forgotten, and visiting and counselling services offered by past patients through the Guillain-Barré syndrome support group can be extremely helpful in the UK.[16]

Paresis with retained reflexes

Myopathies and neuromuscular junction disorders present with proximal weakness, retained reflexes and the absence of sensory symptoms. Patients complain of difficulty in climbing stairs, washing their hair, lifting their arms or raising their head from the pillow in the mornings. Myasthenia gravis, caused by antibodies to the nicotinic acetylcholine receptor on the postsynaptic neuromuscular junction, is characterized by fatigability, early ocular and bulbar features and always needs to be considered when there is ptosis. The diagnosis is almost certain if greater than 50% ptosis develops on sustained upgaze. Ophthalmoparesis is not seen in inflammatory myopathies or motor neurone disease. Signs of paradoxical breathing and a vital capacity should be checked in all these patients. The diagnosis is increasingly recognized in the elderly who may declare neck weakness by surreptitiously supporting their head by placing their chin on their hand like Auguste Rodin's *The Thinker*. Exacerbations may be triggered by infection, drugs or as part of the natural history. Oral pyridostigmine may improve symptoms transiently but will not prevent progressive decline, the need for a nasogastric tube or ITU admission. Diagnosis is confirmed by a positive antibody test (80% sensitivity in generalized MG, 50% in ocular MG) and nerve conduction studies showing decrement with repetitive stimulation. Antibody-positive patients should be screened for thymoma. Thymectomy in younger patients doubles the chance of drug-free remission. A Tensilon test

[15] Van der Meche *et al.* N Engl J Med (1992) 326: 1123–1129.

[16] Guillain-Barré Support Group, Lincolnshire County Council Offices, Eastgate, LINCS NG34 7EB.

carries risk and may be equivocal although, on occasion, it can be useful in the acute setting. Intravenous immunoglobulin or plasma exchange may improve the weakness over days, steroids over weeks and azathioprine over months. Deterioration may also be caused by cholinergic crisis due to pyridostigmine overuse, suggested by the history and presence of salivation, lacrimation, urinary symptoms, diarrhoea, gastric upset and emesis (the SLUDGE syndrome).

Acetylcholine receptor antibody negative cases occur with antibodies to separate sites on the post-synaptic membrane. Antibody testing for anti-muscle-specific tyrosine kinase antibodies is now available. The Lambert-Eaton myasthenic syndrome is characterized by relative ocular and bulbar sparing, attenuated reflexes that augment with activity and an association with small cell lung carcinoma. The neurophysiology is distinctive, and circulating antibodies to the presynaptic voltage-gated calcium channel can be measured.

Treatable inflammatory myopathies present over weeks or months, although admission may be precipitated by abrupt decline. Bulbar, neck and proximal limb weakness predominates, reflexes are preserved and there may be stigmata of an associated connective tissue disease or underlying malignancy. Dermatomyositis may have cutaneous features including a heliotrope rash on the eyelids, a V-shaped 'shawl sign' of photosensitive skin rash around the neck and Gottron's patches on the hands. Electromyography confirms the clinical suspicion of a myopathy, but muscle biopsy is usually required before immunosuppressive therapy. Prednisolone is used in the chronic setting, but intravenous immunoglobulin may also help acutely.

Drug-induced myopathy should be considered. Steroids and statins are the primary offenders. The risk with statins may be increased when given with cytochrome P450 enzyme inhibitors (such as macrolide antibiotics), and new-onset myalgias, exertional cramping or a marked rise in the creatine kinase (CK) should prompt a change to an alternative medication. Hyperthyroidism may be associated with muscle pain and stiffness, a raised CK and muscle hypertrophy. Polymyalgia does not cause muscle weakness or an elevation of CK.

Not unsurprisingly, critically ill patients often develop limb and respiratory weakness following their stay in the intensive care unit. This may be related to a pre-existing undiagnosed condition (myasthenia gravis, myotonic dystrophy, Guillain-Barré syndrome) or, more commonly, secondary to an ITU-related acquired neuropathy or myopathy. Often, the two coexist with a predominantly distal sensory and motor neuropathy and proximal myosin-loss myopathy. Difficulty in weaning from the ventilator may be the first clue. Both disorders arise in the context of a systemic inflammatory response syndrome (SIRS), although myosin-loss myopathy appears associated with the use of nondepolarizing neuromuscular junction blockers, particularly in the presence of steroids.

Nerve conduction studies may aid diagnosis. Recovery may occur but is prolonged, and there is no specific therapy.

Seizures, status epilepticus and 'funny turns'

Seizures can be simply divided into two groups: partial, with focal onset, and generalized (formerly grand mal) where all parts of the cortex are involved simultaneously, with loss of consciousness at the onset. Adding the words 'simple' or 'complex', implying retained or altered awareness, respectively, allows the generation of a hierarchy of descriptive terms, much loved by neurologists. An accurate description of a seizure remains the single most useful clinical tool, and optimal treatment can depend on the correct seizure classification. For generalized epilepsies, sodium valproate and lamotrigine are the drugs of choice, with the latter being preferred in women of childbearing age. Lamotrigine can cause a particularly nasty rash of the Stevens-Johnson variety, and should be instituted slowly and with care. For focal epilepsies, particularly in those where there is a defined central lesion, carbamazepine remains the workhorse and phenytoin remains loved by neurosurgeons. Both are relatively easy to initiate. However, phenytoin is subject to first-order kinetics in the lower part of the notional therapeutic range, before metabolism is quickly saturated and zero-order kinetics prevail. Elimination does not increase as the dosage increases, and the potential for toxicity is therefore nonlinear. Dosages should be increased cautiously when approaching the therapeutic range. With the exception of phenytoin, there is seldom much call for anticonvulsant levels, which tend to merely reflect compliance rather than efficacy. When measuring phenytoin levels, one must make sure that this is done at least 6 h post dose, or at a trough. The nystagmus, ataxia and confusion of phenytoin toxicity are well-known, and are similar to the symptoms when carbamazepine is the offender. Both lamotrigine and valproate occasionally cause encephalopathy. In the elderly, the least toxic anticonvulsant is probably gabapentin, although it may exacerbate peripheral oedema. Epilepsy surgery now offers the hope of cure in some, particularly in those with temporal lobe seizures secondary to mesial temporal sclerosis.

Status epilepticus is a state of recurrent seizure activity with little or no return of consciousness between episodes. Although the World Health Organization has defined this period as lasting for 30 min or more, there is ample evidence to suggest that even 4 min of seizure activity can cause distress to neurones, and that any period of seizure activity lasting more than 2 min should be considered a medical emergency.[17] For immediate treatment of the episode, give

---

[17] Gastaut, Dictionary of Epilepsy. World Health Organization, Geneva (1973).

oxygen, 2–4 mg intravenous lorazepam, followed by a similar dose (if needed) after 10 min, and subsequent intravenous phenytoin loading. Intravenous valproate is also efficacious in status epilepticus. In the unlikely event that these measures are unsuccessful, transfer to the intensive care unit for induction of therapeutic coma with propofol or thiopentone is warranted, initially for a period of 24 h.

Women with epilepsy who are of childbearing age have additional issues to deal with. The risk of neural tube defects with valproate is approximately double that of the other antiepileptic drugs, despite the addition of 5 mg folate, which every epileptic woman should be taking prior to conception. Lamotrigine or carbamazepine are currently favoured, and should be established well in advance of pregnancy if possible. There is a balance between the adverse effects of seizures on the foetus and those of anticonvulsant drugs, which raise the background teratogenic risk to 2–4%. The principle of the lowest dose of the single most efficacious drug in the individual patient should be maintained and any changes minimized once conception has occurred.

Contraception is influenced by the use of agents that induce hepatic metabolism (carbamazepine, oxcarbazepine, phenobarbitone, phenytoin, topiramate and, after new evidence, lamotrigine), and at least 50–60 mcg of oestrogen is needed in an oral contraceptive preparation when used in combination with these drugs. The progesterone-only 'mini-pill' is ineffective in this situation, and the dose of the morning-after pill needs to be increased by 50%. Following menopause, consideration should be given to protection against the accelerated bone mineral loss caused by many common anticonvulsants.

A normal EEG can never confidently exclude epilepsy, something that is far better achieved by a careful history from the patient, and preferably an observer. The combination of a standard EEG and a sleep-deprived EEG, when there is appropriate clinical concern, will usually provide as much diagnostic certainty as the test is ever likely to give. The reflex request for an EEG when faced with a complaint of collapse, without taking an adequate history is pure folly, generating unnecessary false-positive reports. An MRI scan is indicated when a focal epilepsy syndrome is suspected, but likely to be of less use in the case of idiopathic generalized epilepsy. It remains the case that at least 50% of blackouts are cardiovascular, and, of the remaining 50% that are initially undiagnosed, half will also have a cardiovascular cause.[18] Relatively few cases of undiagnosed collapse will turn out to be neurological. Pseudoseizures cause more than their fair share of misery for patients and physicians alike; however, it is wise to

[18] Kapoor, New Eng J Med (2000) 343: 1856–1862.

remember that even the most prolific pseudo-fitter can have the occasional genuine seizure thrown in for good measure. Hard and fast rules for determining which seizure is not genuine are difficult to come by, but the patient who retains consciousness with bilateral limb shaking is not having a generalized seizure. The usual seizure markers of tongue biting, incontinence, muscle soreness, injury, retrograde amnesia, post-ictal confusion and sometimes headache are usually absent. Forced eye closure, pelvic thrusting and post-ictal tearfulness might raise an eyebrow in the right circumstances. Be careful not to dismiss the patient with nonconvulsive or complex partial status epilepticus who may present bizarrely, but often have automatisms such as lip smacking, or subtle facial twitching and grimacing (see page 181). A normal prolactin level does not exclude an epileptic seizure and is a useless investigation in this context.

Lastly, sudden unexplained death in epilepsy (SUDEP) has received attention recently, and accounts for around 500 deaths annually in the UK. These cases are unassociated with trauma or drowning and are believed to be related to seizure activity. Young adults are at most risk, and the greater the number of seizures, the greater the risk. When discussing the benefits of treatment with epileptics, it is important to mention these issues, especially in those with frequent seizures or poor drug compliance.

Parkinsonian syndromes

When the regimented nature of hospital drug rounds collides with the individual patient who has Parkinson's disease (PD), a great deal of frustration and unnecessary anguish is often the result, particularly if the patient is 'playing away from home' on a surgical ward. Most patients with PD are extremely adept at manipulating their drug regimens, and should be allowed to do so as far as is possible. Anti-Parkinsonian drugs come in a variety of forms, and understanding a few principles of drug therapy makes it easier to make rational changes.

Replacing missing dopamine with L-Dopa is good at relieving bradykinesia and rigidity, but not particularly good at helping tremor. Formulations of L-Dopa are combined with a dopa decarboxylase inhibitor, which prevents peripheral conversion of the drug. There remains debate about the timing of L-Dopa initiation, with some evidence to suggest that earlier treatment results in earlier emergence of complications such as dyskinesia. This is not, however, a reason for delaying therapy in the presence of treatable symptoms that impact on the quality of life. It is probably preferable in younger patients to use a dopamine agonist initially, delaying L-Dopa introduction until later. The issue is different with older patients where this is less of a concern, and the aim should be to control the symptoms with the minimum dose: an initial starting dose of 50–100 mg of L-Dopa, before a meal, increasing to t.d.s. dosing as and where needed is often appropriate. If a trial of 200 mg L-Dopa t.d.s. does not improve symptoms, the diagnosis is extremely unlikely to be PD, and one of the atypical variants should be considered.

Commonly, motor fluctuations develop with unpredictable end-of-dose off effects, or dyskinesias (excess movement), particularly at peak blood levels of L-Dopa. These are particularly common in younger-onset patients. In general, most patients far prefer to be a little dyskinetic and mobile, than to be 'off' and rigid. L-Dopa, is relatively short-acting, with an effect lasting 2–3 h – over time, this means that t.d.s. dosing may need to increase to 4 or 5 times daily. The duration of action of L-Dopa can be prolonged to about 3–4 h with the addition of catechol-O-methyl transferase (COMT) inhibitors. Quicker absorption and, thus, onset of effect is possible by using liquid or dispersible formulations, which can be used as 'rescue doses' when needed. Controlled release formulations of L-Dopa are available, and may be of use overnight, or in patients with unpredictable 'off' effects; absorption is often erratic, making this unsuitable for many.

Dopamine agonists are an alternative to L-Dopa initially, but the use of L-Dopa is almost inevitable at some stage in the disease, and combination therapy is common. Although efficacious, the older agonists have the potential complication of vomiting (especially pergolide), peripheral oedema (cabergoline) and retroperitoneal, pulmonary or valvular fibrosis. Annual auscultation, chest X-ray and ESR should accompany the use of these ergot agonists, although it is acknowledged that this may not be the most effective means of screening. Newer nonergot agonists (such as ropinirole and pramipexole) may not cause this problem. All patients taking agonists should be warned about excessive somnolence, which in some cases has been abrupt, and has the potential to impact adversely on driving (sudden-onset sleep syndrome). Parkinsonian patients with cognitive impairment are particularly susceptible to confusion and even psychosis on the longer-acting agents. Apomorphine infusion may be useful for patients with motor fluctuations and dyskinesias. In recent years, deep brain stimulation has emerged as an alternative for some patients with medically refractory PD.

Surgical procedures cause particular difficulty for many patients. Whenever possible, drugs should be continued at their standard doses, down the nasogastric tube if necessary, and they should be recommenced immediately postoperatively: Sinemet can be crushed and given via the nasogastric tube in a small amount of water. Prompt reinstitution hastens recovery and reduces complications of immobility, intestinal ileus and aspiration. Abrupt discontinuation of dopaminergic agents can be dangerous and induce a neuroleptic malignant-like syndrome, with death occurring in some cases.

The failure to respond to Parkinsonian medications suggests an atypical variant of Parkinson's disease, such as progressive supranuclear palsy (PSP), corticobasal degeneration (CBD) or multisystem atrophy (MSA). Both PSP and CBD can present with either a movement or cognitive disorder. PSP is notable for marked axial (rather than appendicular) rigidity, early falls, vertical gaze palsy and a frontal dementia characterized by extreme slowness of thinking and frontal release signs (grasp, pout, palmomental reflexes). The presence of an alien limb (i.e. one that is not under full control of the patient) suggests CBD, and may be accompanied by apraxia (inability to use a limb despite normal power and sensation) and dystonia (co-contraction of antagonist muscles). In CBD, cognitive impairment often manifests as visuospatial dysfunction. MSA can present as pure autonomic impairment or cerebellar dysfunction, but more commonly with variable degrees of Parkinsonism. It is often transiently responsive to L-Dopa, and these patients tend to have less in the way of cognitive impairment. The postural hypotension can be particularly disabling for these patients, but it may respond to compression stockings, fludrocortisone or midodrine — of course, it is made worse by L-Dopa.

Confusion and hallucinations are particularly common in diffuse Lewy body disease, where there is a marked sensitivity to neuroleptics, and use of these agents can induce profound rigidity or even neuroleptic malignant syndrome at relatively low doses, and the use of an atypical neuroleptic is recommended. The cholinesterase inhibitor drugs, used more commonly in Alzheimer's disease, are useful for treating hallucinations. Any acutely confused patient with Parkinson's disease should be considered as having a medical cause (until excluded), with urinary and chest infections being particularly common.

Dementia, delirium and coma

The delirious or acutely confused patient is well-known to most junior doctors, particularly at 2 AM, and the presentation is usually of an agitated, disoriented and easily distractible patient who may be hallucinating. While the common causes of confusion are found in most general medical textbooks, things sometimes get a bit tricky when one has checked the glucose and found that there is no drug that seems to be causing the problem, the patient is not constipated, does not have a urinary tract or chest infection and that the blood tests are all distinctly unexciting, including the blood gas, sodium and ammonia levels! CT scan of the brain and CSF examination can help; herpes simplex encephalitis is sometimes the cause, as is a stroke in 'silent' brain areas, particularly the right hemisphere or thalamus. CNS lymphoma and diffuse brain metastases (particularly breast) are also potential, more chronic, causes and may be more easily detected by MRI scanning (although the patient and radiographer may not relish this experience). Typically, most metabolic causes of delirium spare pupillary reactions and ocular movements – Wernicke's encephalopathy is a notable exception to this rule, and the opportunity to treat it immediately with thiamine should never be wasted.

A rare, but completely treatable form of acute confusion is nonconvulsive status epilepticus, which presents with a variable change in consciousness, confusion and slow thinking. There may be automatisms such as stereotypic hand or lip movements, and it may also be associated with marked anxiety, fear or irritability. Episodes can be almost continuous, but may also have ictal and interictal phases. Those who are unaware of this diagnosis may misinterpret these seizures as psychogenic, and it can be difficult to distinguish the two. An EEG during an episode should be diagnostic – likewise, a dose of intravenous lorazepam (2–4 mg) may abolish the seizure activity.

The power of infection to render an elderly patient drowsy, even to the point of coma, is always worth remembering. Before this, paratonia (*gegenhalten*), a resistance to limb movement that disappears when the limb is moved slowly, is often seen. When coma happens suddenly, it is worth paying special attention to the eyes. Posterior circulation strokes, particularly those blocking the basilar artery ('top of the basilar syndrome') present with altered consciousness and a variety of gaze palsies. Visual-field defects and pupillary abnormalities reflect the involvement of the occipital cortex, the thalamus and midbrain. Once anaesthetized with propofol and intubated for airway protection, usually immediately after admission, all eye signs are unreliable, so the first look is quite important. Treatment with thrombolysis (which is addressed in Chapter Eight) may have a role in these cases.

Prolonged coma after a stay in the intensive care unit is not uncommon. Although establishing and treating the initial cause of coma where possible is important, later, the use of sedating agents, depolarizing drugs and the consequence of severe illness may cause the patient to take far longer than expected to wake up. Midazolam infusions cause particular difficulty, as the drug can accumulate in severe illness, prolonging its effect, particularly in those with organ failure. The elderly are particularly susceptible, and one has to allow enough time for adequate drug clearance before making a decision to withdraw treatment. When a significant brain injury has occurred, such as with prolonged or out-of-hospital cardiac arrest, the absence of any motor activity (M1 on the Glasgow Coma Scale) on day 3 has a particularly bad prognosis, especially if there has been generalized myoclonic status epilepticus. Although there is much media attention about individuals who wake up many years after coma, the reality is much less dramatic. One should be aware and wary of eye-opening as a sign of reemerging consciousness, as this inevitably happens after about a week of coma, and has no bearing on the ultimate prognosis.

The one-third of those reading this chapter who will ultimately develop Alzheimer's disease will hopefully have more treatment options at their disposal than at present. While education might be felt to be protective, no doubt it is really the insensitivity of measuring instruments that is the real explanation for this. A number of cholinesterase inhibitor drugs are currently available. The benefit is very modest, entirely symptomatic and individual. NICE has recommended that they be only used in patients with moderately severe Alzheimer-type dementia.[19] Many carers feel that the drugs make patients easier to manage, and they do indeed seem to increase alertness. The difference between them essentially relates to the side-effect profile.

Not all dementia is Alzheimer's disease, particularly if the onset occurs under the age of 65. Surprising persistence is sometimes needed to uncover the autosomal dominant family history in Huntington's disease, both a movement disorder and a dementia. Often, suicide, homicide, alcoholism or abandonment obscure this aspect of the history. Frontotemporal dementia is a prevalent form of early-onset dementing disorder and typically presents either as a progressive behavioural disturbance or as one of two language syndromes where the meaning of words is lost and objects are no longer recognized, or as a nonfluent syndrome with agrammatism. Sadly, there are few therapeutic options available. Screening for reversible causes of dementia should always be performed. Although the yield is low, the consequences of missing a treatable condition are profound. A CT scan will exclude the rare unsuspected frontal meningioma, and thyroid function tests, B12 and folate and an ESR are recommended. An antinuclear antibody titre and syphilis serology often give troublesome results, and opinion is divided as to their worth in a screening panel. In younger patients, a much more extensive set of investigations and specialist referral is warranted.

INFECTION

Prion disease

No account of neurology in the UK can fail to mention the issue of CJD, variant or otherwise. vCJD occurs in younger age groups, and the initial features are usually psychiatric, with anxiety and depression being common. This is frequently accompanied by sensory disturbance such as limb paraesthesia

---

[19] TAO19 (2001) & Press Release (January 2006) (www.nice.org.uk)

or discomfort. Cognitive decline follows and may be associated with rapid progression, ataxia and myoclonus (brief shock-like jerks). EEG changes, typical of sporadic CJD, are absent, but there may be hyperintensity of the pulvinar on MRI, and tonsillar biopsy may help establish the diagnosis. The prognosis is grim, and death inevitable in little more than a year following onset. The number of new vCJD infections, however, appears to be declining, in contrast to sporadic and familial CJD, where the prevalence remains constant. In the UK, 17 blood donors are known to have later developed vCJD, and of the 50 recipients of their blood products, two have become infected. One has died with clinical vCJD, but the other died of unrelated causes.

Bell's palsy

A single episode of Bell's palsy can usually be regarded as unlucky; a second is distinctly suspicious and suggests consideration of sarcoid, Lyme disease, Guillain-Barré and its variants or diabetes, all of which need further investigation. Most Bell's palsies have a degree of subjective sensory disturbance, and peri-auricular pain is common. It is important to confirm the involvement of the ipsilateral frontalis muscle by asking the patient to raise the eyebrows. This can sometimes be quite subtle. Rarely, a focal brainstem lesion can mimic seventh-nerve palsy, but, as fibres of the abducens nerve wind their way around the nucleus of the facial nerve, these are inevitably affected, causing loss of abduction (lateral rectus) on that side.

Herpes simplex virus (type 1) is thought to play a role in the aetiology of Bell's palsy, and has been recovered from surgical specimens of the facial nerve. For this reason, acyclovir (or its derivatives) at treatment dose may be of benefit early in the course, and should be continued for about 5 days, although the evidence for benefit is far from conclusive. The additional use of prednisolone (60 mg tapering course) is thought to reduce swelling and consequent local infarction of the nerve in the facial canal. However, a recent Cochrane meta-analysis showed no benefit from studies in 176 patients.[20,21] The most neglected feature of this problem is local eye care, and, if there is any doubt about the ability of the patient to maintain complete eye closure, early ophthalmologic review should be sought. The eye should be patched and lubricating ointment applied several times a day to prevent corneal desiccation. Treatment is otherwise expectant in the majority: only around 10–15% will fail to recover and need specialist follow-up.

....

[20] Grogan *et al.* Neurology (2001) 56: 830–836.

[21] Salinas *et al.* Cochrane Database Syst Rev (2004) CD001942.

Acute zoster and postherpetic neuralgia

Postherpetic neuralgia occurs in 10–15% of people following an acute herpes zoster rash, although occasionally the neuralgia occurs without the rash. Since about half of those who develop the pain will not respond to any treatment, the early use of antiviral agents is recommended. Anticonvulsants or tricyclic antidepressants are the most effective treatments for neuropathic pain. Many do indeed get better with time.[22,23]

[22] Kost *et al.* N Engl J Med (1996) 335: 32–42.

[23] Dubinsky *et al.* Neurology (2004) 63: 959–965.

Chapter 8

Matthew Giles and Andrew Coull

STROKE MEDICINE

Stroke is unusual in that despite its 'specialty feel', the vast majority of stroke patients are managed by general physicians in the acute phase. The concept of the stroke physician has been slow to emerge in the UK. The condition's broad spectrum of manifestations and the wide range of skills required in its management (from hyper-acute interventions to long-term rehabilitation, and from close liaison with surgeons to multidisciplinary team working) mean that stroke medicine is not fully at home under the umbrella of any one branch of medicine. This is despite stroke being the most important cause of adult disability and the number three cause of death in the UK. Happily, in recent years, stroke has moved up the political agenda with burgeoning research interest and the expansion of dedicated stroke services. Despite this, the National Audit Office published a report, critical of the Government's stroke services, in late 2005. Ministers responded by committing to inject significant energy into the area over the next decade.[1] Stroke is now set to become a fast-moving medical field and one with which general physicians will need to keep abreast.

A mixed bag

The definition of stroke is troublesomely broad, housing a wide range of diverse conditions (including cerebral vasculitis, amaurosis fugax and primary intracerebral haemorrhage). The diagnosis of ischaemic stroke (IS) should not be made lightly as it demands a lifetime of secondary prevention

---

[1] Reducing brain damage: faster access to better stroke care, National Audit Office, November 2005 (www.nao.org.uk)

(with anticoagulation where appropriate). The general physician should avoid the temptation to diagnose stroke in the many patients seen on the general take with 'funny turns', dizziness, falls, slurred speech, confusion, non-specific visual disturbance, pre-syncope or syncope, unless there are further focal features which support the diagnosis. In the absence of focal neurological symptoms or a sudden onset, the diagnosis of stroke is often wrong.

Fiddling with physiology

Once the patient with IS has passed through the front door and onto the ward, further pitfalls await the general physician. The thorny subject of acute blood pressure control following IS has long vexed doctors and although some guidelines have been published, answers in the stroke literature are hard to come by (perhaps a sign that none exist). The rationale for acute blood pressure intervention post-stroke can be argued both ways – either that a high blood pressure is required to maintain cerebral blood flow in the face of disrupted cerebral autoregulation, or that a high blood pressure could cause cerebral oedema or haemorrhagic transformation in the recently infarcted brain. A pragmatic approach used in many centres is to recommend the continuation of previously prescribed anti-hypertensives, sometimes parenterally if necessary, and acute intervention only when there is evidence of end organ damage or accelerated hypertension. Aggressive blood pressure control is of course recommended 1–2 weeks down the line for secondary prevention. Guidance is rather more specific in the context of thrombolysis.

Other physiological manipulations in the acute phase post-IS are frequently discussed on the stroke unit. Post-stroke fever is a common finding. There are several possible causes to consider and top of the list would be sepsis, next comes venous thrombosis and then drugs. However, stroke itself can cause fever, either through direct cerebral damage to thermoregulatory mechanisms or as an inflammatory response to infarcted brain. Fever carries poor prognostic implications post-stroke and the concept of reducing cerebral infarction by cooling is an attractive one as this is effective in animal models, as well as following neurosurgery, cardiac surgery and cardiac arrest. However, although clinical trials have shown that inducing hypothermia is feasible, there is no trial evidence to show that it is clinically beneficial. A pragmatic approach adopted in many centres is the aggressive treatment of any identified cause of fever as well as the fever itself with paracetamol and cooling.

A very similar account could be written for post-stroke hyperglycaemia. This, again, is a frequent finding (even in the non-diabetic) and is a consequence of the stress response mediated through cortisol and adrenaline release.

In vitro work shows that hyperglycaemia worsens neuronal damage and this is born out in studies in which hyperglycaemia is associated with a worse clinical outcome, haemorrhagic transformation of an infarct and reduced recanalization with thrombolysis. At the same time, glycaemic control with insulin infusion has been shown to be beneficial in other parts of the hospital – CCU and ITU – and the rationale for its benefit post-stroke is persuasive. However, as for temperature control, studies have shown that although glucose control is feasible post-stroke, there is no evidence for a better clinical outcome. Again, a pragmatic approach adopted in many centres is to establish glycaemic control in diabetics with an insulin infusion and to treat blood glucose over 12 mmol/l in others.

A fistful of tablets

The question of which anti-platelet agents (and when) is one that is hotly debated on wards and in stroke clinics up and down the land. The role of aspirin is well established following the CAST and IST trials, which together randomized over 40,000 patients with major IS to either aspirin or placebo.[2,3] Meta-analysis of these trials showed that aspirin significantly reduced the risk of recurrent IS (1.6% aspirin group versus 2.3% controls), death (5.0% versus 5.4%) and recurrent stroke (of any sort) or death (8.2% versus 9.1%) over the study period, at the cost of a small and non-significant excess in symptomatic intracranial haemorrhage. It is worth pointing out, however, that although benefits are significant, they are small in terms of absolute risk reduction. Another interesting point to arise from CAST and IST is that there was no excess in haemorrhagic stroke among the 9000 patients randomized before their CT scan and among the 800 who were inadvertently randomized after haemorrhagic stroke, there was no net harm. The implication from these observations is that aspirin can be started prior to a CT scan establishing whether or not a stroke is ischaemic. However, this should not be used as an excuse by radiology departments to delay cerebral imaging in stroke patients; this should always be performed as soon as practically possible – particularly as the UK enters the thrombolysis era.

Although the place of aspirin in acute IS is widely accepted, the role of other anti-platelet agents and combinations is more controversial. Clopidogrel has,

2 CAST Steering Committee, Lancet (1997) 349: 1641–1649.
3 IST Steering Committee, Lancet (1997) 349: 1569–1581.

until recently, been aggressively marketed by the pharmaceutical industry. The CAPRIE trial showed it to be no worse than aspirin alone in preventing a combined endpoint of IS, myocardial infarction (MI) or vascular death in patients with IS and so its use as an aspirin alternative in patients who are truly aspirin intolerant is accepted.[4] What is more divisive (and is probably now unacceptable except in a few specialist settings) is the use of the combination of aspirin and clopidogrel. The oddly designed MATCH trial found that this combination was no better than clopidogrel alone in preventing a primary endpoint of IS, MI, vascular death or hospitalization for ischaemia in 7599 patients with either IS or TIA and another vascular risk factor.[5] Furthermore, there was a significant increase in major or life-threatening bleeding. Although a direct comparison with aspirin alone does not exist, these findings have put combination aspirin and clopidogrel out of favour for long-term secondary prevention following IS. The combination, however, has found some favour in the hyper-acute phase post minor stroke or TIA in which the rates of recurrent stroke are higher and the dangers of haemorrhagic transformation of an IS lower, thus improving the overall risk–benefit ratio.

Just like clopidogrel, the star of dipyridamole has waxed and waned, although in the UK (at the time of writing), it is currently in favour. Its chequered past arises first from a number of early, small trials reporting conflicting results regarding its benefit in IS, second from the largest and most positive trial of its use in IS being heavily criticized for its conduct and, third for its frequent adverse effect of headache. However, the most recent meta-analysis of its use in combination with aspirin compared to aspirin alone in IS, found that it was superior in reducing both recurrent stroke and a combined endpoint of non-fatal stroke, non-fatal MI and vascular death.[6] At the same time, its role has recently been rubber stamped by the National Institute for Health and Clinical Excellence (NICE) in the enticingly entitled 'technology appraisal number 90', recommending the use of a combination of aspirin and dipyridamole for 2 years post TIA or IS.

Time is brain

There are few topics that exercise UK stroke physicians more than thrombolysis. Everyone has their own entrenched view, ranging from it being 'the best

[4] CAPRIE Steering Committee, Lancet (1996) 348: 1329–1339.

[5] Diener et al. Lancet (2004) 364: 331–337.

[6] Leonardi-Bee et al. Stroke (2005) 36(1): 62–68.

thing since sliced bread' to it being 'quite impossible in the NHS' (probably the commonest). A very few seem to regard it as the Devil's work. The answer, doubtless, lies somewhere in between. The rationale is simple and elegant – that perfusion of an ischaemic brain can be re-established by lysing an occlusive thrombus – but the drawback lies in the possible haemorrhagic consequences. A host of RCTs have gone about studying this issue using different agents, doses and time intervals after IS. Summarizing a fierce two-decade debate is challenging. However, the proponents argue that RCTs conclusively show that thrombolysis with intravenous tPA given within 3 h of IS onset significantly and substantially increases the odds of a favourable outcome (measured by Rankin score) at 3 months, compared to placebo, and benefit in longer time windows after stroke onset may be possible.[7] The opponents argue that benefit is outweighed by an excess of symptomatic intracranial haemorrhage and maybe death caused by thrombolysis. Those perching on the fence point out that a thrombolysis service requires rapid presentation of a patient to a hospital which has 24-h immediate CT scanning, a stroke unit and a physician with specialist training. Even then, the vast majority of stroke patients would not be eligible for such a service because they fall outside the time window for treatment. A Canadian study reported in 2005, demonstrating the effectiveness of thrombolysis in the 'real world'. Of 1135 enrolled patients, 37% experienced significant clinical improvement. Symptomatic haemorrhage occurred in around 5% of patients, the majority of whom died.[8] Ultimately, all of these arguments have some validity and one's stance on thrombolysis may boil down to the temperament of clinician and patient rather than evidence-based decision-making!

Pragmatically, however, the arguments are becoming stale as, realistically, there will be no further RCTs within this particular realm of thrombolysis because tPA treatment within 3 h is now 'standard' treatment in North America and some parts of Europe. Currently, in the European Union, thrombolysis with tPA given within 3 h of IS is licensed, as long as patients are recorded in an international stroke registry (SITS-MOST). The routine use of thrombolysis in IS in the UK may depend on the findings of SITS-MOST but the Canadian effectiveness study certainly represents a significant line in the sand. There are many reasons to manage stroke with a sense of urgency, almost irrespective of thrombolysis. Obtaining imaging and introducing patient and

---

[7] Hacke *et al.* Lancet (2004) 363: 768–774.

[8] Hill *et al.* CMAJ (2005) 172: 1307–1312.

expert to one another at the earliest opportunity gives the initial part of the stroke care pathway much greater impetus. Additionally, a recent trial giving activated factor seven to patients with primary intracranial haemorrhage (again within a 3-h time window) suggests that this therapy is highly promising.[9] A confirmatory study is eagerly awaited.

The TIA emergency

The early risk of recurrent stroke after TIA or minor ischaemic stroke (MIS) has recently been shown to be approximately 10% within the first week and 15% at 1 month, much higher than previously estimated.[10] It has long been noted in specialist TIA clinics that non-attenders are common: referred patients had subsequently been admitted to hospital with a major stroke, ahead of their clinic appointment. However, previous studies of the prognosis of MIS and TIA failed to demonstrate this risk for a simple methodological reason; prognosis was often estimated from clinical trial data in which patients were recruited some time after their initial 'event'. Thus, the high-risk patients, who went on to have a major stroke after their TIA or minor stroke were never included in the studies as they became 'major stroke patients' and therefore fell outside the inclusion criteria. This high early stroke risk has been shown in population- and clinic-based studies in the UK and US as well as in patients attending emergency departments in the US and Canada. The early risk of recurrent stroke is similarly high in both groups.[11] Much research is currently directed into calculating the early stroke risk of individual patients and it seems that the presence of motor or speech disturbance, longer duration of symptoms, increasing age, diabetes and higher blood pressure at presentation all carry a poor prognosis, as does the presence of carotid stenosis and, when available, diffusion/perfusion mismatch on diffusion weighted MRI.[12] How specialist TIA services should be organized in the UK to deal with this risk is yet to be seen.

Back to basics

One of the greatest but least glamorous steps forward in inpatient stroke medicine in the last decade has been the emergence of the dedicated stroke unit. The story of this rise is interesting in that it centres on the effectiveness of

---

[9] Mayer *et al.* NEJM (2005) 352: 777–785.

[10] Coull *et al.* BMJ (2004) 328: 326–328.

[11] Giles *et al.* Expert Rev Neurother (2005) 2: 203–210.

[12] Rothwell *et al.* Lancet (2005) 366: 29–36.

good, basic clinical care rather than any pharmacological intervention or new technology. Organized inpatient stroke care improves outcome. Stroke unit care encompasses several different models including a geographically defined ward or a mobile stroke team providing care in a number of different settings. Regardless of the model studied, stroke unit care has been shown to reduce mortality (both related and unrelated to stroke), dependency and institutionalization at discharge and up to 5 years after.[13] Benefit has been shown regardless of stroke severity on admission, age and sex. Because stroke unit care is heterogeneous, comprising many different components, it is difficult to postulate which single aspect, if any, is key. There is no room for complacency as the existence of a stroke unit does not guarantee access for those who need it, as highlighted by the Royal College of Physicians' Sentinel national stroke audit.

A surgeon on the stroke unit?

Of obvious interest within the stroke world is the aetiology of stroke. A recent meta-analysis studying the risk of recurrent stroke according to aetiology found that patients with large artery disease (generally carotid stenosis) had a significantly higher risk of recurrent stroke than other groups.[14] By pooling patients from all population-based studies reporting early risk of recurrent stroke according to subtype, it can be shown that in patients with large artery disease, the risks of recurrent stroke at 7 days, 1 month and 3 months are 4.0, 12.6 and 19.2%, respectively. The corresponding risks for those with cardioembolic stroke and small vessel stroke are shown in the table below. Thus, although patients with large artery atherosclerosis comprised only 14% of the 1709 initial strokes studied, they represented 37% of the recurrences at 7 days and 31% of the recurrences at 3 months.

Percentage risk of stroke recurrence over time

	Time		
Type of stroke	7 days	1 month	3 months
Large artery disease	4.0	12.6	19.2
Cardioembolic	2.5	4.6	11.9
Small vessel disease	0.0	2.0	3.4

[13] Stroke Unit Trialists' Collaboration, Cochrane Database Syst Rev (2001) Issue 3.

[14] Lovett et al. Neurology (2004) 62: 569–574.

This observation is particularly important when considering the role of carotid endarterectomy. The procedure has been shown to be highly effective in reducing the risk of recurrent stroke in patients with symptomatic carotid stenosis of ≥ 70% without near-occlusion. What has been less clear is the timing of surgery as previous studies have shown that this can be harmful in patients with large infarcts or evolving symptoms. A recent analysis of data from NASCET (North American Symptomatic Carotid Endarterectomy Trial) and ECST (European Carotid Surgery Trial) showed that benefit from surgery was highly dependent on the time from the last symptomatic event to randomization and fell rapidly with increasing delay.[15] It concluded that in TIA and MIS patients with symptomatic stenosis ≥ 70% who are neurologically stable, carotid endarterectomy should be performed within 2 weeks for maximum benefit. Another finding of interest to the general physician was that greatest benefit was observed in those over 75 years old. Again, the implications for TIA services in the UK, where delays before endarterectomy can be of the order of 3–6 months are considerable. A national audit began in 2006 to examine the experiences of those undergoing carotid endarterectomy in the UK.

While the evidence for carotid endarterectomy for symptomatic stenosis is clear and compelling, asymptomatic disease is a rather different question. The most recent study is the UK-based ACST (Asymptomatic Carotid Surgery Trial) which randomized 3120 patients with asymptomatic carotid stenosis (of over 60%) to either immediate carotid surgery or 'indefinite deferral'.[16] It found that the risk of all fatal or disabling stroke at 5 years was reduced by surgery from 6.1 to 3.5% and the risk of all strokes (including peri-operative events) fell from 11.8 to 6.4%. It is yet to be seen whether this benefit would either be observed in routine clinical practice or be favourable enough to persuade patients to chose surgery in an asymptomatic condition.

As with the rest of vascular surgery, radiologists are now muscling in on carotids. It seems likely that stenting may replace the open procedure in the not too distant future. A carotid duplex may one day be added to the aortic ultrasound, faecal occult blood and battery of other screening tests offered to people to occupy their time in early retirement!

---

[15] Rothwell *et al.* Lancet (2004) 363: 915–924.

[16] Halliday *et al.* Lancet (2004) 363: 1491–1502.

Chapter 9

John Frater and Nicola Jones

INFECTIOUS DISEASES

HIV AND AIDS

The number of HIV infections continues to rise on a global basis as well as within the UK. The epidemiology of the disease in the UK is changing from predominantly gay, white males to include a greater proportion of black African heterosexuals. By the end of 2005, the Health Protection Agency (HPA) estimated that there were 58,300 individuals infected with HIV in the UK.[1] Of these, approximately a third were unaware of their status. Men who have sex with men (MSM) remain the highest risk group for acquisition within the UK and, according to the HPA, the incidence of new infections remains roughly unchanged year-on-year at around 1700 cases. Heterosexual spread of HIV within the UK is less common but on the increase. Since 1999 there have been more new diagnoses of heterosexually acquired infection identified within the UK than new infections in MSM. This is thought to be predominantly the result of infection being imported mostly (70%) from Africa rather than contracted within the UK.

As far as the origin of HIV is concerned, there is increasing evidence that the retrovirus crossed from primates into man through blood spilt at the time of hunting. For example, one study in Cameroon tested blood from 930 bush hunters who were regularly exposed to fresh primate blood. The study revealed that 11 hunters had been infected with 6 different primate-derived viruses of which two were novel retroviruses, designated HTLV-3 and HTLV-4. Evidence such as this supports the popular 'cut hunter' explanation for HIV and opposes the well popularized explanation that HIV was the result of infected polio vaccinations, as described in Ed Hooper's book, '*The River*'.

---

[1] www.hpa.org.uk

Management of HIV-infected patients has become a sub-specialty in itself but nevertheless; all physicians need to be aware of the general principles. The British HIV Association (BHIVA) has recently updated its guidelines and its website is a valuable resource.[2]

Testing for HIV has always been an emotive area. Some physicians feel that HIV tests and results should be as freely available as other investigations. The current policy is that HIV testing can and should be carried out by any physician without the need for any 'specialist' counselling. However, the physician should be aware of the updated regulations of the Association of British Insurers which used to allow insurers to know whether a client had ever been tested or even counselled for an HIV test.[3] These guidelines have now been amended to suggesting the following question: 'Have you tested positive for HIV/AIDS or are you awaiting the result of such a test?' There may be some circumstances, especially if there is a high pre-test probability of a positive result, when it may be more appropriate for the test to be deferred and carried out by a GUM or HIV clinic where access to post-test counselling and guidance is more readily available.

Once a positive diagnosis has been reached, the physician needs to define the state of disease progression (based on clinical findings, AIDS-defining illness and surrogate markers such as plasma viral load and CD4 cell count) and to determine whether the patient requires antiretroviral therapy. Highly active antiretroviral therapy (HAART) is having a dramatic impact on HIV-related morbidity and mortality both in the industrialized world and now also in sub-Saharan Africa. However, it is well recognized that HAART cannot eradicate HIV from an infected person and is not a cure. The aim of therapy is to suppress viral replication and thereby to prolong and improve quality of life for as long as is possible.

There are three groups of patients in whom therapy might be considered. Those who are symptomatic, those who are asymptomatic but have low CD4 cell counts and those with primary infection (or 'seroconverters'). The former are straightforward and should all be considered for treatment, but the latter two groups are more complicated. The seroconverter is a particularly thorny area as biological data suggests that viral suppression in early infection might allow some preservation of the immune response. However, as yet, there has been no substantive clinical trial to support this. At the time of writing,

---

[2] www.bhiva.org

[3] www.abi.org.uk

the SPARTAC trial is recruiting recently infected patients in what is likely to be the last realistic opportunity to answer this question. Accordingly, BHIVA guidance is that any newly infected HIV positive individual should be offered entry to a clinical trial designed to assess the role of HAART at this stage of the illness. From a public health perspective, treatment of seroconversion may be particularly important in reducing the incidence of new infections, as it is possible that it is predominantly seroconverters who are responsible, in turn, for causing the majority of new transmission events.

In chronically infected asymptomatic patients, the aim is to treat when CD4 cell counts are less than 350 cells/µl with the intention of preventing further decline to less than 200 cells/µl. Of note, 40% of newly diagnosed cases of HIV infection in the UK have a CD4 cell count of less than 350 cells/µl, and are therefore immediately eligible for therapy. More recent data has suggested a benefit in commencing therapy even earlier (e.g. in terms of a lower incidence of non-Hodgkin's lymphoma), however the evidence is not robust enough to support this change and one needs to consider that HAART is intended to be life-long and an asymptomatic patient may have 10 years of potentially toxic therapy in front of them.

The decision regarding which therapy to start is based on many clinical trials, none of which is particularly definitive. Three basic classes of drug are available: the reverse transcriptase enzyme inhibitors (the 'nucleoside' class – NRTI – and the 'non-nucleoside' class – NNRTI) and the protease enzyme inhibitors (PI). Standard therapy should include three drugs based around a backbone of 2 NRTIs and a PI or an NNRTI. The major change in PI prescribing is based on the realization that ritonavir – one of the earlier PIs – is an extremely potent cytochrome P450 inhibitor. Accordingly, most PIs are now prescribed as part of a 'boosted' formulation which includes a low 100 mg dose of ritonavir which has minimal antiviral effect but which results in much greater plasma levels of the therapeutic drug. Other drugs are available and – unlike antibiotics – new drugs are around the corner. The NRTIs have been pharmacologically manipulated to make them more active, resulting in the nucleotide reverse transcriptase inhibitors, such as tenofovir. The advantage of these agents is a broader antiviral spectrum, including against Hepatitis C. The 'entry-inhibitor' class of drugs (e.g. T20 – enfurvitide) are peptides which must be injected and inhibit viral replication by inhibiting the Gp41 protein, which is key to virus cell-entry. Other agents include the CCR5 and CXCR4 antagonists some of which are in clinical trials and offer a novel therapeutic approach. One therapy that is not available within the anti-HIV armoury and which does not figure on the horizon is a vaccine – whether protective or therapeutic. The ability of the virus to mutate and 'escape' from immune responses has resulted in most candidate vaccines being ineffective. At least one professor working in the field has announced the sale of all his vaccine company shares.

There are two main metabolic complications of HAART that should be recognized by the general physician: lipodystrophy and mitochondrial toxicity. Lipodystrophy syndrome results in stigmatization and is often responsible for a reduction in drug adherence. The main components of the syndrome are raised plasma cholesterol and triglycerides, insulin resistance, fat accumulation in viscera and breast tissue, and subcutaneous fat loss (lipoatrophy). Although data from prospective studies are not adequate to be conclusive, PIs appear to have an increased risk and the NRTI stavudine (particularly in conjunction with didanosine) has also been implicated. There are data to suggest that switching patients off these drugs can result in improvement of symptoms. Accordingly, a number of physicians try and avoid PIs as first-line antiretroviral medication and drugs such as abacavir and tenofovir may be favoured. Metformin may help with associated glucose intolerance and if a statin is required to treat hypercholesterolaemia, pravastatin has the fewest interactions with HAART. The majority of interventions for lipodystrophy are not successful and therefore new options include injectable skin 'fillers' such as polylactic acid (New-fill), which are now being offered, with reported success, at a number of HIV centres.

The nucleoside analogue class of antiretrovirals was first found to be associated with mitochondrial damage over 15 years ago. The NRTIs inhibit DNA polymerase gamma, required for mitochondrial DNA replication. Although the mechanism is unclear, the downstream impact of this is lactic acidosis. The risk of developing lactic acidosis on HAART may be as high as 2% per patient per year, and asymptomatic hyperlactataemia may be present in over 16% of patients on HAART. The management of affected patients is to withdraw HAART and look for other precipitating causes. The reintroduction of therapy remains uncharted territory. Agents which augment mitochondrial metabolism (such as thiamine, riboflavin and co-enzyme Q) have all been tried with varying degrees of success.

HIV drug resistance has major implications for antiretroviral prescribing and is increasingly being monitored in the clinic through viral RNA sequencing both prior to starting therapy and at the point of drug failure. One consolation has been that resistant viruses are possibly disabled by their mutations and are less virulent. However, there has been recent concern regarding the rise of drug-resistant strains that maintain a high degree of virulence. In March 2005, the Aaron Diamond AIDS Research Center in New York reported on such a strain. The patient was a gay male who tested positive for HIV in

December 2004 with a CD4+ cell count which was less than 200 cells/µl.[4] The infecting virus was resistant to all three major classes of antiretroviral drug. Tests suggested that infection had been recent implying that this virus was unusually virulent. Whether this is an isolated case or a marker of a more widespread trend is not yet clear.

EMERGING INFECTIOUS DISEASES

The potential threat of an emerging infectious disease can be illustrated in terms of the deaths associated with the 1918 influenza epidemic or the current AIDS crisis. Despite numerous earlier predictions that technology would eradicate infection from the medical problem list, the number of deaths worldwide due to infection is second only to those caused by cardiovascular disease. New infections emerge (SARS) and old ones return (human monkey pox or West Nile fever). We are able to speculate on the arrival of new epidemics. As this book goes to press, concerns over avian influenza and its potential to mutate to allow person-to-person spread of infection continue to make headline news, causing a degree of anxiety amongst public health physicians and policy makers.

Influenza

Influenza remains a major cause of mortality worldwide, being responsible for up to half a million deaths in around 5 million infected people each year. However, current concerns are focused on the outbreak of influenza in chickens and other birds in Southeast Asia and Eastern Europe. In 1997, the Hong Kong Health Department reported an outbreak of H5N1 influenza A in chickens and humans – the first documented transmission of the 'avian' influenza virus from birds to humans. Eighteen patients were hospitalized, and 6 died. Those particularly at risk were laboratory workers and others who were directly exposed to poultry. There was no evidence of human–human transmission. In 1997, the entire poultry population of Hong Kong (estimated at about 1.5 million birds) was destroyed and this may have prevented an epidemic in the short term. Nevertheless, in 2003, two further human cases were reported in China. The H5N1 strain continues to spread across Asia, in particular Vietnam, South Korea, and Japan. By Autumn 2006, bird-to-human transmission had resulted in well over 100 deaths.[5] The WHO website is regularly

---

[4] Markowitz *et al*. Lancet (2005) 365: 1031–1038.

[5] www.who.int/csr/disease/avian_influenza

updated to give a running total of the number of reported infections and attributable deaths worldwide. The Chief Medical Officer for England predicted a potential 50,000 excess deaths, as the result of an H5N1 pandemic in the UK. An enormous amount of research is being carried out to identify the mutations and viral transformations that may be required to allow avian influenza to trigger a human pandemic. The H5N1 strain is most commonly mentioned, however a second strain – H9N2 – is also infecting birds, has infected humans and has the potential to transform into an epidemic-driving virus. The significance of such mutations is placed in context by the influenza outbreak of 1918 which is speculated to have killed up to 50 million people – more than the First World War, and in significantly less time. When – or even whether – the H5N1 strain will mutate is unknown. After all, the virus has been endemic in Asia for many years without mutating. Nevertheless, responsible governments must prepare for such an eventuality. By 2006, the drug oseltamivir ('Tamiflu') was being stockpiled by government agencies but had also been the subject of panic-buying by the public over the Internet. As a reminder that nature is usually one step ahead of the pharmaceutical industry, a report in Nature in October 2005 described an oseltamivir-resistant H5N1 variant circulating in birds in Vietnam.[6]

West Nile virus

Since 1999, the United States of America has had to cope with the influx of an infection previously only seen in Africa, Asia, the Middle East and some regions of Europe. West Nile virus was first identified in 1937 in Uganda. Infection is caused by a flavivirus (belonging to the same family as Yellow Fever virus – relevant because vaccines to Yellow Fever may be adapted to protect against West Nile Virus). The primary viral hosts are migratory bird populations, but the Culicine mosquito vector incidentally infects both horses and man, with no on-going transmission. Infections in the United States are seasonal, peaking in August and September. The strain currently travelling westwards across the United States and infecting increasing numbers of individuals each year is similar to an isolate from Israel and is particularly lethal to crows. During 2005, 3000 human cases were reported to the CDC in 44 US states with 119 deaths.[7] West Nile virus may result in an asymptomatic

----

[6] Le *et al.* Nature (2005) 437: 1108.

[7] www.cdc.gov/ncidod/dvbid/westnile/

infection in man or disease ranging from a mild febrile illness through to aseptic meningitis and encephalitis. At the time of writing there have been no cases in the UK, although surveillance via the HPA continues.[8]

SARS

SARS (severe acute respiratory syndrome) is caused by a coronavirus (SARS CoV). SARS most probably had its origins in Guangdong Province in China, where the first human cases were identified in November 2002. In March 2003, the WHO issued a warning regarding the new epidemic. By 5 July, 2003, worldwide spread had been contained and the infecting pathogen characterized. The 2003 outbreak, involving more than 300 cases in Hong Kong, may have initially been due to contaminated sewage in a hotel bathroom. The infection was subsequently disseminated by a physician from Guangdong Province who stayed for one day at the hotel on 21 March, 2003 and transmitted the virus to other hotel guests, before travelling to Vietnam, Singapore, and Toronto. In 5 months, the WHO reports that SARS infected 8400 people in 32 countries. During the epidemic, there were four probable cases in the UK, all of whom recovered. Between July 2003 and May 2004, four more small outbreaks of SARS were reported worldwide. Of these, three appeared to stem from poor laboratory practice. The origin of the fourth outbreak is not clear. All four outbreaks were rapidly contained. These events are a warning that SARS re-emergence is highly likely and surveillance programs are key in all at-risk regions. The speed with which SARS, and the coronavirus that causes it, were identified and characterized, and the subsequent containment of the infection is a success story and a tribute to excellent public health and infection control procedures.

It is believed that the SARS coronavirus originated from animals – markets that traded in live game animals were the potential source of interspecies transmission. The average number of secondary cases was between 2 and 4, but some patients were 'super spreaders'. The incubation period is 2–10 days, but may be as long as 20 days. Asymptomatic and mild cases are documented but uncommon; they do not appear to be important in transmission, and viral isolation has not been successful in these patients. Transmission is primarily in healthcare settings, usually at least 5 days after the onset of illness and primarily from those who are most seriously ill. The major mechanism of transmission is from respiratory droplets to mucous

---

[8] www.hpa.org.uk

membranes in the eyes, nose or mouth; aerosol-generating procedures such as intubation or bronchoscopy also amplify transmission.

The initial features of clinical illness are fever, myalgia, malaise and cough.[9] Features that distinguish this from other common respiratory infections are watery diarrhoea and the lack of upper respiratory symptoms. The initial chest X-ray is abnormal in 60–100% of patients, depending on the time interval from onset of fever to hospitalization. About one-third improve; the rest have progressive disease with persistent fever, dyspnoea and oxygen desaturation. In these patients, chest X-ray findings reveal multiple areas of consolidation, and occasionally, pneumomediastinum – a characteristic sign of SARS. About 20–30% require care in the ICU, primarily for mechanical ventilation. For patients over 65 years of age, the mortality rate exceeds 50%. There is no treatment with documented benefit. In vitro tests suggest potential viral inhibition by interferon beta, glycyrrhizin, and, to a lesser extent, interferon alfa. There is also anecdotal evidence that steroids are helpful.

Prion diseases – vCJD

Part of the family of Transmissible Spongiform Encephalopathies (TSEs), Creutzfeldt–Jakob disease (CJD) is a progressive and fatal degenerative diseases of the brain which is caused by an accumulation of mutant prion proteins. The original version of CJD was described over 80 years ago, but more recently a new form – variant or vCJD – has resulted in human fatalities and is now widely accepted to be the result of contaminated beef from animals suffering with 'Mad Cow Disease' or Bovine Spongiform Encephalopathy (BSE). The initial report of deaths was 3 in 1995; this subsequently increased to a peak of 28 in 2000 and decreased to 18 in 2003. Despite earlier apocalyptic predictions, as of September 2006, HPA data reveal a total of 156 UK deaths from definite or probable vCJD and 6 people living with the diagnosis.

Although steps have been taken to eradicate infected meat from the human food chain, current concerns revolve around human-to-human transmission from blood transfusions, blood products and contaminated surgical equipment. These are real risks. 2003 saw the first death of a recipient of an infected blood transfusion. The blood donor had died in 2000 but had been well at the time of donation in 1996. A second likely case was reported in 2004. Accordingly, the UK government in conjunction with the Spongiform Encephalopathy Advisory Committee (SEAC) ruled that as of April 2004,

---

[9] Levy et al. Am J Respir Crit Care Med (2005) 171: 518–526.

anyone who had received a blood transfusion after 1980 was not eligible to donate blood. Those who have received an 'at risk' transfusion are required to be traced to determine the potential on-going risk in terms of contamination of surgical equipment and those who donated blood to patients who subsequently develop vCJD also need to be contacted to assess their risks of disease. As a precautionary measure, leucodepletion of all blood components was implemented by the UK government in 1999, but the true efficacy of this process is unknown as vCJD is also present in plasma and non-white blood cell components.[10,11]

The impact of vCJD on surgical procedures has resulted in infection control guidelines to reduce the potential for cross-infection should an infected or 'at-risk' patient undergo surgery. Essentially the risks can be stratified according to the material being operated on (tonsillar and brain tissue being at high risk) and the exposure risk of the patient. The major impact has been in the adoption of single use instruments in many surgical procedures. Implications and the financial impact of guidelines can be far-reaching. For example, once a £30,000 endoscope has been used on a patient with haemophilia who has previously received blood products, it must be quarantined and not used on any other patient.

THE RETURNING TRAVELLER

The natural habitats of certain pathogens are restricted to tropical regions, often as a result of the distribution of the transmitting vectors. However, the rise in international travel and the increasing availability of low-cost flights means that 'fever in the returning traveller' is now a common presentation on the acute medical take as well as to the infectious diseases out-patient clinic. The presentation is frequently non-specific with no localizing symptoms. The timing of the onset of the fever may be helpful as shorter incubations (less than 3 weeks) might favour dengue, typhoid, leptospirosis, malaria or yellow fever, whereas a longer incubation period is more commonly found with acute HIV infection, brucellosis, leishmaniasis, melioidosis, schistosomiasis and tuberculosis. A thorough history should look for exposure to pathogens. For example, mosquito bites might suggest malaria, dengue, filariasis or yellow fever; fresh-water exposure might suggest leptospirosis or schistosomiasis; animal contact might indicate a risk of brucellosis, Q fever, rabies or tularaemia.

---

[10] Turner, Br J Haem (2000) 110: 745.

[11] Sivakumaran, Br J Haem (2000) 110: 234.

A detailed and unremitting sexual history is essential – a significant proportion of travellers have new sexual encounters and admit to unprotected sex. Do not be afraid to ask the well-dressed businessman with a wife and two kids in the Cotswolds about recent homosexual experiences.

Malaria

Of those consultations that identify a pathogen in the returning traveller, malaria is the most common diagnosis and should be considered in anyone evaluated for fever travelling from an endemic region. In particular, patients from areas where malaria is endemic, who having been living abroad for a protracted period, may lose protective immunity to malaria. Unaware of this, when they return for a visit home, many such patients do not take malaria prophylaxis assuming they are protected, and accordingly, become infected. Malaria is transmitted from person to person through the intermediary of a female Anopheles mosquito. Malaria is found throughout the tropical and sub-tropical regions of the world and causes more than 300 million acute illnesses and at least 1 million deaths annually. About 90% of deaths due to malaria occur in sub-Saharan Africa mostly amongst young children. Most will recall that there are four types of human malaria: *Plasmodium vivax*, *P. malariae*, *P. ovale* and *P. falciparum*. However, a fifth strain, *P. knowlesi* has also been discovered which infects both man and chimpanzees. *Plasmodium vivax* and *P. falciparum* are the most common, and *P. falciparum*, the most deadly. Malaria can kill by destroying red blood cells and by clogging the capillaries that carry blood to the brain (cerebral malaria) or other vital organs, causing renal failure, jaundice, coagulopathy or pulmonary oedema and ARDS. Most patients will have fever, headache and myalgia, although gastrointestinal symptoms such as diarrhoea and vomiting are common and may be misleading. In those who take chemoprophylaxis the presentation may be more benign. The 'gold standard' of diagnosis remains the thick and thin blood films to identify intraerythrocytic parasites. Many diagnostic laboratories also provide rapid antigen testing facilities. These are based on ELISAs for malaria proteins such as HRP-2 or parasite LDH. They are in the form of dipstick or cassette-type tests and generally produce a result in less than 20 min. Compared with microscopy which can detect 50 parasites/μl (0.001% parasitaemia), rapid tests can detect above 100 parasites/μl (0.002% parasitaemia). Although sensitive for *falciparum*, rapid tests – especially those based on HRP-2 – are less good at detecting non-*falciparum* species. Some investigators feel that the tests can also be used as a crude monitor of parasitaemia during treatment. This is based on the principle that parasites seen following therapy may be non-viable and therefore do not produce LDH. In contrast, HRP-2 persists for longer following clearance of parasites and therefore is less useful as a guide for treatment. A thorough review article on rapid tests for malaria is referenced below.[12] Patients with a marked systemic inflammatory response, severe anaemia, renal failure or a parasitaemia greater than 3%, can be characterized as severe and should be considered for intravenous therapy. To exclude the diagnosis of malaria, three negative films are required as, although one negative film is sensitive, diurnal variation of the parasite life cycle and sequestration means that peripheral blood parasitaemia may not always be reflective of total parasite burden.

Falciparum malaria should be considered to be chloroquine-resistant unless one has good evidence to believe otherwise. Accordingly, in the UK, quinine and artemether derivatives are the treatments of choice. If the parasitaemia is greater than 5–15% an exchange-transfusion may be beneficial, although this is controversial. Major complications of falciparum malaria are hypoglycaemia (both due to increased metabolism of infected red blood cells and hyperinsulinaemia associated with quinine therapy) and bacterial sepsis. Steroids, anticoagulation and immune serum offer no benefit in the management of malaria. If the parasitaemia has not fallen within 48 h of commencing oral therapy, one needs to consider whether the patient has a resistant infection and whether intravenous therapy is warranted. Daily blood films are required until three consecutive films are negative.

There is now widespread global resistance of *P. falciparum* to conventional antimalarial drugs, such as chloroquine and sulfadoxine-pyrimethamine. However, in China the 'wormwood' plant has been harvested for its antimalarial herbal medicine, qinghao, for many centuries. Indeed, the herb is referred to in writings from a 2000-year-old Chinese tomb. This has now led to the introduction of a new group of antimalarials, the artemisinin compounds (artesunate, artemether and dihydroartemisinin). Artemesinins are active against multidrug-resistant *P. falciparum* malaria, produce a very rapid therapeutic response, are well tolerated by patients and reduce transmission of malaria through activity against gametocytes.[13] After a series of very encouraging studies of artemesinin in Thailand, the WHO has recommended that all countries experiencing resistance to conventional monotherapies should use combination therapies containing artemisinin

---

12 Moody, Clin Microbiol Rev (2002) Jan: 66–78.

13 Ashley *et al.* Curr Opin Infect Dis (2005) 18: 531–536.

derivatives with lumefantrine, mefloquine, or sulfadoxine/pyrimethamine for the treatment of falciparum malaria. In the UK, Riamet, a combination of artemether and lumefantrine, is now licensed for the treatment of all but severe malaria, in which case intravenous quinine is currently the recommendation. With increasing data from large clinical trials, it might be expected that Riamet – for which an intravenous formulation is available but unlicensed – may soon become first-line therapy for all cases of falciparum malaria.

Dengue

Dengue fever and dengue haemorrhagic fever are present in urban areas in the Americas, Southeast Asia, the Eastern Mediterranean and rural areas in Africa. Dengue fever causes a severe, flu-like illness that affects infants, young children and adults, but seldom causes death. The incidence of dengue is on the increase and approximately 2.5 billion people are at risk in over 100 endemic countries. Up to 50 million infections occur annually with 500,000 cases of dengue haemorrhagic fever and 22,000 deaths, mainly amongst children. There is a spectrum of disease ranging from a mild febrile syndrome to the classic incapacitating disease with abrupt onset of high fever, severe headache, pain behind the eyes, muscle and joint pains and rash. Dengue haemorrhagic fever and dengue shock syndrome are potentially deadly complications that are characterized by high fever, haemorrhage and circulatory collapse. Potentially fatal gastro-intestinal, cerebral and pulmonary haemorrhage are associated with derangement of coagulation and thrombocytopaenia. The condition may progress to shock with circulatory failure. Without treatment, death follows in 12–24 h in 20% of cases, but with intensive supportive therapy mortality can be as low as 1%.

Aedes aegytpi and *A. albopictus* mosquitos transmit four distinct, but closely related, viruses that cause dengue. Person-to-person spread of infection does not occur. Recovery from infection provides lifelong immunity against that serotype but confers only partial and transient protection against subsequent infection by the other three types. There is good evidence that sequential infection increases the risk of more serious disease resulting in haemorrhagic fever. In recent years, *A. albopictus* has become established in the United States, Latin America, the Caribbean and in parts of Europe. The fear is that dengue fever may then follow. Often blamed for this are the rubber tyres exported from Asia: small collections of water in the tyres may support the larvae of the mosquitos and facilitate their worldwide dissemination.

Viral haemorrhagic fevers

Viral haemorrhagic fevers (VHF) include Lassa, Ebola, Marburg and Congo–Crimean haemorrhagic fevers. Cases rapidly grab the headlines due to the fear they evoke. The epidemiology of Ebola and Marburg fever is unknown, but Lassa is acquired from contact with mouse urine in West Africa, and Congo–Crimean haemorrhagic fever from tick bites in Asia and Southern Africa. These diseases have a high mortality, from approximately 5% for Lassa to over 80% for Ebola. They are associated with fever, massive bleeding and multi-organ failure. Transmission to other patients and healthcare workers occurs, especially in resource-poor settings, and isolation and strict barrier nursing should be commenced. Where available, admission of the patient to 'dangerous pathogen isolation facilities' is advocated and public health services should be informed of a patient with a suspected VHF.

Lassa fever is an acute illness caused by Lassa virus, an arenavirus. The disease was first identified in a missionary nurse in Lassa, Nigeria in 1969 and subsequently was found in other areas of West Africa. It is acquired from the multimammate rat and is endemic in Nigeria, Sierra Leone, Liberia, Guinea and the Central African Republic. Person–person spread can also occur through contact with bodily fluids including semen. Disease symptoms may initially be non-specific (fever, headache, sore throat, vomiting, chest and abdominal pain) but may progress to hypotension, haemorrhage, encephalopathy and mucosal bleeding. The overall mortality is around 5% with an estimated 5000 deaths per year globally. Treatment is limited, although ribavirin may be effective if given within a week after the start of symptoms.[14] To date there have been six 'imported' cases of Lassa to the UK and all have been contained.[15]

Ebola haemorrhagic fever was originally recognized in 1976 and has a much higher associated mortality than Lassa fever. Infection is with the Ebola virus (after the Ebola River in the Democratic Republic of the Congo), one of the *filoviridae*. Of the four known strains of Ebola, three are pathogenic in man: Ebola-Zaire, Ebola-Sudan and Ebola-Ivory Coast. Ebola is thought to be zoonotic, and, after much searching, the animal reservoir is now thought to be various species of fruit bat.[16] Although cases of Ebola generally occur in western Africa, a case in the UK has been reported following a needle-stick injury. It is thought that epidemics start with zoonotic spread to an index case and then person-to-person spread follows as a result of exposure to bodily fluids, including aerosols, particularly within healthcare settings. Symptoms are of

[14] Bossi *et al.* Euro Surveill (2004) 9: E11–E12.

[15] Crowcroft *et al.* J Infect (2004) 48: 221–228.

[16] Leroy *et al.* Nature (2005) 438: 575–576.

rapid onset and, like Lassa, are initially non-specific. They may include fever, headache and myalgia. This may be followed by gastrointestinal upset and, eventually, internal and external bleeding. Diagnosis is via ELISA and PCR, although treatment is supportive. As the host is unknown, infection control procedures must focus on strict isolation of infected individuals once an epidemic has commenced.

HOSPITAL-ACQUIRED INFECTIONS

An increasingly common arena in which the general physician is likely to be involved is hospital-acquired, or 'nosocomial', infection. The increasing number of medical interventions promotes infection. Hospital-acquired pneumonia, antibiotic-associated *Clostridium difficile* diarrhoea and catheter-associated urinary tract infections are prevalent on the general medical wards. In more specialized units, infections of venous access lines, implanted cardiac defibrillators, temporary pacing wires or intracranial shunts all require well-designed antibiotic-treatment plans and regular review and advice from infectious disease physicians and microbiologists.

Intravascular cannulae

In the United States alone, over 1000 million intravascular devices are used each year, 15 million of these being central venous access catheters. The potential healthcare burden that line infections represent is significant. A number of units are now using 'peripherally-inserted central catheters' (PICC lines) which are inserted via the antecubital fossa and are deemed to be more acceptable than standard central lines, with fewer complications. Where long-term intravenous access is required, tunneled lines – either partially (Hickman or Groshon lines) or totally implanted (Portacath) – are favoured. Infections of central lines have a significant morbidity and mortality (some report up to 20% for line-associated bacteraemia) and invoke costs due to extended patient admissions.

Line infections can be thought of as being either localized or systemic. The features of a localized infection may be as obvious as pus or erythema around the line exit site, with a positive Gram stain confirming the presentation to be infection rather than mechanical irritation. The subcutaneous course of a tunnelled line may also become infected and may not be associated with exit site inflammation. The more serious complications are systemic and may result in bacteraemia with metastatic spread of infection. For example, any patient with a line-associated *Staphylococcus aureus* bacteraemia must be investigated to exclude endocarditis, septic thrombosis, septic arthritis and discitis.

Diagnosis of a venous line infection is not always straightforward. Paired peripheral and line-derived blood cultures may be of help when the culture from the line 'flags' at least 2 h before the peripheral set. Microbiology can also be helpful if the same bacterium with the same drug-sensitivity 'antibiogram' is repeatedly isolated from blood cultures, especially in the presence of on-going therapy. This is a particularly useful method for identifying infections caused by low-grade pathogens such as coagulase-negative *Staphylococci* and *Enterococci*.

A common laboratory method in the UK for the diagnosis of line-related infection is the semi-quantitative method in which the line tip is rolled across the surface of an agar plate. The test has a sensitivity of 60% for diagnosing line infection if more than 15 colony-forming units are counted on the plate after incubation. Line removal remains the simplest route to a diagnosis. In simple infections, defervescence may rapidly follow, and low-grade pathogens may only require minimal antibiotic therapy. If the patient remains unwell despite the removal of the catheter, an ultrasound of the cannulated vein may reveal infected thrombus – or thrombophlebitis – which may not respond to antibiotics alone and may even require surgical intervention.

Clostridium difficile diarrhoea

Clostridium difficile is a spore-forming bacterium, initially identified in the stools of babies in the 1930s. Since the 1970s it has been implicated in antibiotic-associated diarrhoea. *C. difficile* is present as part of the normal intestinal flora in approximately 3% of healthy individuals. However, following the administration of broad-spectrum antibiotics, such as cephalosporins, ampicillin and clindamycin, infection with *C. difficile* may result in symptoms ranging from diarrhoea to pseudomembranous colitis and toxic mega-colon. Approximately 1–3% of patients with *C. difficile* colitis develop severe signs and symptoms of disease, requiring admission to an intensive care unit. Two toxins cause the diarrhea: toxin A – which has enterotoxic and cytotoxic activity – and toxin B, which is only cytotoxic. Toxins are internalized by colonic luminal cells, which then die resulting in ulceration and diarrhoea.

It is possible that in mild cases, cessation of the antibiotic will result in cure. However the majority of patients are now treated with either oral metronidazole or oral vancomycin. In the first instance, keeping the patient off antibiotics is the key intervention. However, if antimicrobial therapy is a requirement certain antibiotics – such as aminoglycosides, macrolides and tetracyclines – have a lower tendency for *C. difficile* infection. In all patients, fluid resuscitation and avoidance of anti-diarrhoeal agents such as loperamide is important.

Infection control policies are critical in preventing spread, as the majority of cases are likely to be transmitted nosocomially rather than resulting from an overgrowth of the host's own flora. Handwashing is critical. Alcohol hand gels, which have replaced soap and water in many hospitals for non-soiled skin, do not kill *C. difficile* spores, although whether this impacts on disease prevalence has not been formally evaluated. The duration of therapy ranges from 10 to 14 days, although it is acceptable to continue treatment for the same duration as a concurrent course of antibiotic therapy. Other therapies have been evaluated to varying degrees. Other agents such as fusidic acid and teicoplanin (given in tea) have shown clinical responses in patients with *C. difficile* diarrhoea, however metronidazole remains the drug of choice.[17]

Most patients fully recover, however approximately 20–30% relapse. This may be a result of initial failure to cure, or re-infection with the same or different strains. In the event of relapse, management is initially the same as for the first episode, although it is sensible to exclude other causes of diarrhoea and in more severe cases to undergo sigmoidoscopy and biopsy. In the event of multiple relapses, further interventions such as intravenous immune globulin, anion-binding resins such as cholestyramine and even administration of bacteria (either through rectal infusions of laboratory cultures, oral bacterial yoghurts or faecal enemas from healthy relatives) have shown some effect in small clinical studies. Of note, cholestyramine binds vancomycin and therefore there should be a reasonable interval between the administration of these two agents. A number of trials have looked at the yeast *Saccharomyces boulardii*, suggesting that in certain patients, co-administration with antibiotics reduces the incidence of *C. difficile* diarrhoea. This is not yet an accepted practice and the best way to avoid antibiotic-associated diarrhoea is through rigid adherence to antibiotic guidelines policies and effective infection control.

Urinary catheter-associated infection

Urinary tract infection (UTI) is one of the more commonly diagnosed infections, particularly in the elderly. A 'positive' urine dipstick is frequently used to explain a number of acute presentations of elderly patients to the Medical Assessment Unit referred as 'confused' or 'off legs'. The appropriateness of this assertion is not always apparent. The indwelling urinary catheter (IUC) is, however, a risk for urinary sepsis and bacteraemia. The catheter surface – like much prosthetic material – is a potential site for microbial adherence and retention.

---

[17] Aslam *et al.* Lancet Infect Dis (2005) 5: 549–557.

This can result in a biofilm that minimizes elimination by host defences and reduces antimicrobial penetrance. Once an IUC has been inserted, it becomes colonized with bacteria at a rate of approximately 5% per day – every patient with a long-term urinary catheter will have evidence of bacteriuria, mostly asymptomatic.

As with uncomplicated UTI, *Escherichia coli* is frequently a causative pathogen. However other organisms, often with more resistant antibiotic profiles, are frequently to blame. In particular, these include Gram-negative organisms such as Enterobacter species and *Pseudomonas aeruginosa*, as well as Gram-positive organisms, particularly MRSA and Candida species. Polymicrobial bacteriuria is also common and in chronically catheterized patients, the flora may change twice or three times per month.

The clinical presentation of UTI associated with IUC can be varied, from asymptomatic bacteriuria to frank sepsis. The infection can be located within the bladder only (cystitis) or may spread to involve the kidneys (pyelonephritis) and prostate gland (prostatitis). Perinephric or prostatic abscess formation should be considered, especially in the presence of systemic features of sepsis or positive blood cultures.

Definitive diagnosis of UTI in catheterized patients is difficult. Urine can be collected for microbiological examination by aseptic aspiration from the urinary catheter port. As biofilms are frequently present in such catheters, urine samples are frequently abnormal and often contain bacteria. The significance of positive cultures is thus difficult to determine. The standard benchmark for diagnosing uncomplicated UTI of more than 100,000 colony forming units per ml of urine has a specificity of around 90%, but is only 37% specific in catheterized patients.

Antibiotic prophylaxis for long-term catheterization is unlikely to be helpful, although there have been some more favourable reports with fluoroquinolones. In asymptomatic patients, the treatment of bacteriuria is not warranted if the catheter is to be retained. The Infectious Diseases Society of America (IDSA) guidelines, however suggest that following removal of a catheter, persistent bacteriuria for greater than 48 h warrants treatment, even if asymptomatic. If the patient is symptomatic and urine culture is negative, a second or third generation cephalosporin or fluoroquinolone is likely to be effective. *P. aeruginosa* can be treated with a carbapenem or extended-spectrum penicillin (e.g. Tazocin – piperacillin-tazobactam). Enterococcal infection will respond to either amoxicillin or vancomycin and MRSA will be vancomycin sensitive. Fungal growth – usually with Candida species – is common in catheterized patients. This usually represents colonization and a very low proportion of patients progress to fungal sepsis and candidaemia.

Duration of therapy should be kept to 5–7 days in uncomplicated cases of IUC-associated UTI, but should be continued for 14 days if pyelonephritis is suspected. Removal of the IUC is normally only required if it is blocked or malfunctioning. The need for further imaging of the urinary tract should be considered if structural abnormality is suspected.

The rise of drug resistance

The impact of increasing resistance of bacteria and viruses to antimicrobial agents needs to be regarded as a significant threat to public health. Although well publicized in the media, methicillin-resistant *Staphylococcus aureus* (MRSA) represents only a part of the problem. Increasing evidence suggests that many Gram-negative organisms and viruses are developing drug resistance. This includes the enterobacteriaceae and pseudomonads, the bacillae responsible for the majority of significant Gram-negative sepsis. In addition, resistant strains of HIV are becoming more frequent and, at least anecdotally, there appears to be a concurrent rise in the burden of HIV-associated disease.

MRSA

According to figures from the HPA, the proportion of *Staphylococcus aureus* bacteraemias due to MRSA has risen from 2% in 1990 to 40% in 2004. Although this may reflect an increase in reporting, there is clearly a growing problem. Methicillin resistance is defined as a minimum inhibitory concentration (MIC) greater than 4 μg/ml. Resistant isolates were identified within a year of the drug's introduction in 1959. The significance of methicillin-resistance is that it is a marker of resistance to all beta-lactam agents including cephalosporins, and may suggest resistance to quinolones. Resistance is mediated by the mecA gene, which encodes for the PBP2a protein. This permits cell-wall synthesis in the presence of β-lactam antibiotics. The mecA gene is on a mobile genetic cassette that can transfer horizontally to methicillin-sensitive staphylococci rendering them drug-resistant. This is thought to have been a major method by which resistance became widespread.

Although initially a hospital-acquired infection, there is increasing evidence for community acquisition of MRSA – the so-called community-associated MRSA. Interestingly, the community-associated MRSA appears to carry a version of the mecA gene (SCC mecIV) which differs from hospital-acquired MRSA and encodes less resistance. Community-associated MRSA is frequently sensitive to ciprofloxacin as well as to trimethoprim-sulfamethoxazole and clindamycin. One recent observational study in the United States of patients presenting with skin and soft tissue infections revealed that 76% of MRSA cases were community-associated. However, a study from the UK suggests that a significant proportion of patients presenting to hospital with MRSA may have acquired it, not in the community, but on previous exposure to healthcare facilities.[18]

Hospital-acquired MRSA is generally transmitted to the patient from healthcare workers, other patients or environmental contamination. Patients are likely to represent the greatest reservoir of infection and this is associated with the duration of in-patient stay, antibiotic therapy with broad-spectrum agents, admission to ITU and surgical site infection. The role of transmission from the environment is not clear but a small American study from 1997 suggested that the rooms of patients who have MRSA in their wounds or urine are disproportionately contaminated, as are the uniforms of the healthcare workers looking after them.[19] Colonization of healthcare workers is frequently transient, even for less than 24 h. However carriage may last for longer periods – possibly for years – particularly in individuals with dermatological conditions, such as dermatitis. The nose is the most frequently colonized site and transmission may be exacerbated in the presence of an upper respiratory tract infection. Policies to reduce hospital acquisition of MRSA include documenting and isolating those patients who are known to be positive. Screening, on admission, patients transferred from other hospitals, or with recent in-patient stays, before placing them in an open bay will identify the majority of colonized individuals. All patients admitted to ITU should be swabbed from the throat and anterior nares and, ideally any wound sites, as part of an on-going prevalence study.

MRSA is generally treated with the intravenous glycopeptide antibiotics, vancomycin or teicoplanin. MRSA bacteraemia should be treated with 2–4 weeks of intravenous therapy as it is usually presumed that an endovascular source of infection has been established. Oral agents such as trimethoprim-sulfamethoxazole, rifampicin, doxycycline and fusidic acid may have a role depending on the susceptibility pattern of the strain. The role and efficacy of decolonization remains controversial, but treatment with topical mupirocin for up to 5 days is currently the protocol of choice.

VISA and VRSA

Staphylococcus aureus sensitivity to vancomycin varies: vancomycin-intermediate *S. aureus* (VISA) and vancomycin-resistant *S. aureus* (VRSA) occur.

[18] Wyllie *et al.* BMJ (2005) 331: 992.

[19] Boyce *et al.* Infect Control Hosp Epidemiol (1997) 18: 622–627.

Spread of the *vanA* gene from the vancomycin-resistant enterococci (VRE) to *S. aureus* was reported in 2002. An isolate of *S. aureus* was identified in a 40-year-old American diabetic with peripheral vascular disease and chronic renal failure, who had been treated for chronic foot ulcers with multiple antibiotic courses, including vancomycin. Although isolates with intermediate resistance have been previously reported from countries such as the US, UK and Japan, this was the first reported case of high-level resistance of *S. aureus* to vancomycin.[20]

A further three cases have been described in the US, all of which are associated with the *vanA* gene. Treatment options are limited, but agents with some activity include linezolid, quinupristin-dalfopristin and trimethoprim-sulfamethoxazole. VRSAs and VISAs are still uncommon but this should not lead to complacency in view of the dramatic and almost exponential rise in MRSA prevalence over the last 15 years. Unfortunately, VISAs are difficult to identify using standard disc diffusion techniques. More complex methods such as broth dilutions and agar-gradient diffusions are required and this may lead to under-reporting in the absence of a coordinated surveillance program.

Vancomycin-resistant enterococci (VRE)

Enterococci, also known as group D Streptococci, are Gram-positive cocci and are part of the normal bowel flora. The two most common species are *Enterococcus faecalis* and *Enterococcus faecium*, and they are a common cause of nosocomial infection, particularly of prosthetic devices. *E. faecalis* is normally susceptible to ampicillin, and *E. faecium* to vancomycin, but there has been spread, especially in American hospitals, of a strain of *E. faecium* with high-level resistance to vancomycin. Although intrinsically resistant to multiple antibiotics, the enterococci have traditionally been sensitive to vancomycin. However, acquired resistance is now well documented in the form of acquisition of the *van* resistance genes. There are at least six forms of the *van* gene, although it is *vanA*, *vanB* and *vanC* that are primarily responsible for the rise in vancomycin resistance. The genes facilitate variation of the peptidoglycan structure of the enterococcal cell wall, removing the vancomycin binding site and rendering the drug inactive.

Enterococci are increasingly responsible for colonization and infection in hospitals, as they are resistant to many groups of antibiotics. The reservoir for enterococci is generally the gut and transmission is a result of either direct or indirect (e.g. staff or fomites) contact. There has even been a report of an

---

[20] CDC MMWR (2002) 51: 565–567.

ITU-based outbreak resulting from colonization of the handles of rectal thermometer probes. The most significant risk factor for acquiring VRE is previous therapy with antibiotics, particularly vancomycin and cephalosporins. Limiting the use of antibiotics – particularly in the ITU – is an important measure in VRE control. The rise in VRE reports is of concern given the possibility – as described above – of transfer of the *vanA* gene to *S. aureus*, resulting in VRSA.

Enterococci, including VRE, have low virulence and, reassuringly, infection with VRE only varies from other enterococci in regards to the necessary antibiotics. VRE infection is often associated with high mortality, however this is more likely to be a representation of a more vulnerable patient group prone to this infection. Although classically associated with prosthetic device infection and endocarditis, the most common VRE infections are bacteraemia and UTI. Although most cases are of colonization only, 10% will suffer a serious invasive infection. In this scenario, few therapeutic options are available, especially if the organism is also teicoplanin resistant. Recently, two agents with activity against resistant Gram-positive bacteria including VRE have been developed: dalfopristin-quinupristin and linezolid. Both agents should be reserved for special cases following the advice of an infectious disease physician or clinical microbiologist.

Extended-spectrum beta-lactamases (ESBL)

The extended-spectrum beta lactamases (ESBL) are enzymes which were first identified over 20 years ago in relation to nosocomial infections, particularly in conjunction with vulnerable patients such as those on intensive care units. First identified within strains of Klebsiella, these enzymes confer resistance to cephalosporin antibiotics such as cefuroxime, ceftazidime and cefotaxime. Since 2003, a new strain of ESBL activity has been detected in strains of *E. coli* (CTM-X) conferring resistance to penicillins and cephalosporins in infections from both hospitals and the community. Often associated with urinary tract infections, these CTM-X β-lactamases are resistant to all available oral and many intravenous antimicrobial agents and require therapy with more powerful agents such as the carbapenems. Microbiology laboratories need to be alert to the problem of CTM-X ESBL, as it is possible for isolates to be missed if not specifically tested for. The *E. coli* CTM-X isolate is a growing and worrying problem as not only are the bacteria resistant to many of our first-line antibiotics, but they are associated with higher degree of morbidity and mortality.[21]

....

[21] Livermore *et al.* J Antimicrob Chemother (2005) 56: 451–454.

SEPSIS AND SEPTIC SHOCK

The term 'sepsis' refers to infection in conjunction with a systemic inflammatory response. SIRS – or the 'systemic inflammatory response syndrome' – is a specific physiological state, the recognition of which permits more accurate diagnosis and guides management of severe infection. It should also be remembered that SIRS itself may not be due to infection, the most frequently quoted alternative being pancreatitis. Typical infective syndromes associated with SIRS are pneumonia, intra-abdominal sepsis, skin and soft tissue infection and urinary sepsis – the latter having the most favourable outcome. In England and Wales, there are approximately 21,000 cases of severe sepsis per year. Despite advances in critical care medicine, the mortality rate from severe sepsis is estimated to vary between 30 and 50%.

SIRS is defined as two or more of temperature dysregulation (> 38 or < 36°C), tachycardia (> 90 beats/min), tachypnoea (rate > 20/min) or deranged WBC count (> 12 cells/μl or < 4 cells/μl). If there is evidence of infection one can diagnose sepsis. If there is additional evidence of organ dysfunction (e.g. confusion, acute renal failure or hypoxia), sepsis can be described as 'severe'. In the presence of a systolic blood pressure less than 90 mmHg (or a mean arterial pressure < 70 mmHg), which does not respond to fluid resuscitation, the condition can be described as 'septic shock'.

A review of over 10 million cases of sepsis admitted to American hospitals in the two decades prior to 2000 revealed a change in the microbiological causation of sepsis. Gram-negative organisms (e.g. *E. coli*) have been replaced by Gram-positive ones (particularly *S. aureus* and *Streptococcus pneumoniae*) as the most common causes of sepsis. In third place, but with a 200% increase in frequency in the 20 years since 1979, is fungal sepsis, for example with *Candida albicans*.

The physiology underlying sepsis and SIRS has received much attention, particularly amongst intensivists. In essence, bacterial components such as endotoxins and lipoteichoic acid act on neutrophils and macrophages. This induces pro-inflammatory factors (e.g. TNF-α, IL-1 and IL-6) as well as counter-regulatory host responses (e.g. IL-4 and IL-10) that turn off production of pro-inflammatory cytokines. In sepsis, the pro-inflammatory reaction cascades out of control, with activation of complement, coagulation and widespread arterial vasodilatation. Circulatory abnormalities produce an imbalance between systemic oxygen delivery and oxygen demand, resulting in global tissue hypoxia, multi-organ dysfunction and, eventually, death.

The management of sepsis, particularly if severe or associated with shock, is complex and best left to those specialized in intensive care. In the first instance, management needs to be supportive to overcome tissue hypoxia and hypotension.

With access to invasive monitoring, the goals for the initial management of a septic patient are to achieve a central venous pressure between 8 and 12 cm H_2O, mean arterial pressure $\geq$ 65 mmHg, urine output $\geq$ 0.5 ml/kg/h and central venous (or mixed venous oxygen) saturation $\geq$ 70%.

Once the patient is stable, the septic focus, if there is one, must be identified. Thorough, but routine, microbiological cultures are often adequate. Three sets of blood cultures from different sites are ample. In undiagnosed cases of infection, imaging of the abdomen often reveals the focus, particularly post-operatively. Some foci will not be responsive to antibiotics. Prosthetic devices (particularly intravenous cannulae) need to be removed and collections drained. The sinuses should not be forgotten as a potential focus of infection in a sick patient.

Until a pathogen is identified, empiric antimicrobial therapy needs to be broad. Gram-positive cover is required and many units use vancomycin, in view of the increasing rate of MRSA. Cover for Gram-negative organisms includes the third generation cephalosporins (e.g. ceftazidime or cefotaxime), the carbapenems (e.g. meropenem) and anti-pseudomonal penicillins in conjunction with a beta-lactamase inhibitor. Where *Pseudomonas aeruginosa* is the suspected pathogen, dual therapy (e.g. with the addition of gentamicin) is often advocated to minimize the development of drug resistance.

Drotrecogin alfa (recombinant human activated protein C – APC) has been recommended by the Surviving Sepsis Campaign for the management of patients with severe sepsis on ITU with failure of more than one organ.[22] As of September 2004, NICE has endorsed this recommendation. Activated protein C is anti-inflammatory, promotes fibrinolysis and inhibits thrombosis. In sepsis, endogenous levels are reduced and therefore treatment with APC may act to reverse the sepsis-associated inflammatory response. The guidelines followed the multi-centre PROWESS trial, in which APC was administered to patients within 24 h of presentation with sepsis.[23] The trial showed a reduction in mortality at 4 weeks in patients receiving APC (24.8 versus 31.3%). Although APC is associated with increased risk of haemorrhage, in patients who are more severely unwell with an APACHE II (Acute Physiology, Age and Chronic Health Evaluation) score > 25 treatment is associated with a better outcome. In less severely unwell patients, the role of APC is not proven. Not surprisingly these outcomes come at a financial price – the estimated cost for each attributable year of life saved due to APC is approximately $24,000 US.

[22] Surviving Sepsis Campaign Guidelines, Crit Care Med (2004) 32:858–872.

[23] PROWESS Group, NEJM (2001) 344: 699–709.

Chapter 10

William Gelson and Graeme Alexander

HEPATOLOGY

Patients present acutely to hepatologists as a consequence of jaundice, acute liver failure or chronic liver failure with overt decompensation. In contrast, most clinic referrals to hepatologists are a consequence of abnormal liver function tests. Increasingly, patient referral is prompted by the presence of a mass (or masses) in the liver identified incidentally following liver or abdominal ultrasound, where prompt diagnosis is essential.

Jaundice

It is a surprising but consistent observation that patients are often unaware of the onset of jaundice, although family and friends observe these changes more often. Patients note other features of cholestasis, especially pruritus, much more commonly.

New-onset jaundice always requires investigation. Fast-track jaundice services are currently being established in many centres, often with direct referral to a clinical nurse specialist by general practitioners. Reliance on patterns of liver function tests to narrow the diagnosis has been superseded by radiology in conjunction with a much broader diagnostic armamentarium based on serology. Admission for investigation is rarely necessary except for specific procedures and where disease is very advanced.

There are very many causes of jaundice; in a recent audit of a fast-track jaundice service, the leading causes in order of frequency were gallstones, pancreatic carcinoma, metastatic disease, Gilbert's syndrome and drug-induced jaundice (see the table on page 219). It must be remembered that jaundice may be in evolution at presentation and the full clinical syndrome may not be manifest for several days.

When investigating jaundice, it is important to follow a structured approach. In most cases, the combination of liver ultrasound and a careful history will lead to a narrow differential diagnosis. Simple, specific questions can help focus the differential diagnosis even further. Is jaundice cholestatic with dark urine, pale stools and pruritus? Is it intermittent? Is it associated with pain? Is it progressive and associated with constitutional symptoms, particularly weight loss, suggestive of cancer? Was the onset related temporally to the introduction of new medication? Has it been a recurrent problem, perhaps dating back years and exacerbated by intercurrent illness? Was the patient jaundiced at birth? General questions should include risk factors for liver disease, especially excess alcohol consumption and intravenous drug use, previous medical history, drug history, travel history, contact history and family history. The main benefit of examination is in the diagnosis of malignancy.

Jaundice should be evident to experienced clinicians and does not necessarily need to be confirmed biochemically before embarking upon an ultrasound, which (with Doppler studies) is the most useful initial investigation. The presence or absence of dilated extrahepatic or intrahepatic bile ducts guides the next investigative step. With dilated biliary ducts, an obstructive lesion may also be apparent, such as stones or malignancy. Hepatic vein thrombosis, cirrhosis with or without portal hypertension, fatty infiltration, malignant infiltration, gallstone disease and pancreatic tumours may all be visualized at ultrasound. Ultrasound appearances will also guide further investigation.

Where there is biliary duct dilatation, with gallstones identified within the bile ducts, normal practice would be to confirm the diagnosis at endoscopic retrograde cholangiopancreatography (ERCP) when stones could be removed by balloon or basket with a covering sphincterotomy prior to cholecystectomy. However, not all patients are fit for an ERCP, especially the elderly. Biliary duct dilatation may be associated with a pancreatic mass, which should be further investigated with CT scanning, which may support the diagnosis and help with staging prior to the formulation of a definitive management plan. Endoscopic ultrasound may have a role, especially if biopsy of the mass is deemed important. Ultrasound appearances may suggest malignant infiltration of the liver, which should usually be confirmed by biopsy prior to oncology referral, as appropriate.

Ultrasound may reveal features of chronic liver disease with portal hypertension, in which case the jaundice represents hepatic decompensation, and knowledge of the aetiology (see page 230) is critical for subsequent management.

In the case of a normal ultrasound, the history becomes more critical in determining the next step. With symptoms suggestive of biliary tract disease or with cholestatic liver function tests, magnetic resonance cholangiopancreatography (MRCP) may be indicated. In the absence of symptoms suggestive of biliary tract disease or a history of exposure to new medication, especially if liver function tests suggest a hepatitic process, then a screen for acute hepatitis and chronic liver disease should be initiated. In addition, a split bilirubin (conjugated and unconjugated) should be requested specifically from the laboratory at this point. If the jaundice is largely unconjugated, screening tests for haemolysis should be undertaken. Unconjugated bilirubinaemia is most probably a consequence of Gilbert's syndrome. Unconjugated bilirubinaemia is common in healthy people (5%), and is often not noted by patients or family but picked up incidentally. A bilirubin > 80 μmol/l is exceptional and levels fluctuating between 20 and 40 μmol/l are more typical. The diagnosis can be confirmed by molecular techniques but this is required very rarely and is technically difficult. In practical terms, Gilbert's syndrome is defined as an unconjugated bilirubinaemia with a normal haemoglobin, normal haptoglobin and normal reticulocyte count. The association of an unconjugated bilirubinaemia with an abnormal haptoglobin and increased reticulocyte count points clearly to haemolysis, where the haemoglobin need not be reduced, but often is.

If this approach does not bear fruit then liver biopsy beckons, according to the need for a firm diagnosis, since jaundice in this context is likely to be important.

Aetiology of jaundice in a 'fast track' jaundice service

Aetiology	Prevalence (%)	Most useful first tests
Gallstones	27	Ultrasound
Pancreatic Cancer	15	Ultrasound/CT
Metastatic Cancer	10	Ultrasound and biopsy
Drug induced*	7	History
Gilbert's syndrome	7	Split bilirubin
Autoimmune hepatitis	5	Serology
Cholangiocarcinoma	5	Ultrasound/CT
Alcoholic hepatitis	5	History
Pancreatitis	3	Ultrasound and serum amylase
Cholecystitis	2	Ultrasound
Hepatoma	2	Ultrasound
Acute or chronic viral hepatitis	2	Serology
Nonalcoholic steatohepatitis (NASH)	2	
Primary biliary cirrhosis (PBC)	2	Serology
Unexplained	6	

* Flucloxacillin and co-amoxiclav accounted for > 90% drug-induced jaundice. This diagnosis is especially common in the elderly, in whom the jaundice may be severe, prolonged and occasionally fatal.

ACUTE LIVER FAILURE

Acute liver failure is rare in everyday clinical practice, but provides the greatest opportunity in liver disease for significant clinical error. Always discuss management with the local liver or liver transplant centre, and if only one test were to be performed, make it the prothrombin time and not liver function tests. An elevated prothrombin time is always an indication for thought.

Once termed fulminant hepatic failure, acute liver failure is a syndrome in which liver damage leads to encephalopathy, jaundice and coagulopathy (manifest as prolongation of the prothrombin time). By definition, this occurs within a short time frame and conventionally excludes patients with established liver disease, although some such patients prove (rarely) to have had subclinical Wilson's disease.

Acute liver failure is subdivided into three distinct entities by the time from the onset of jaundice to the onset of hepatic encephalopathy. This subdivision is useful because each subset has distinct clinical characteristics. Hyperacute liver failure is the development of encephalopathy within 7 days of the onset of jaundice, acute liver failure when the onset is from 1 to 5 weeks and subacute liver failure when the onset is from 5 to 12 weeks. Acute and hyperacute liver failure lead to similar grades of encephalopathy and derangement of prothrombin time. It is not possible to ascertain the natural mortality of each condition in current practice as most cases are considered for liver transplantation, but hyperacute liver failure has a far better prognosis compared to acute liver failure, while mortality is greatest for subacute liver failure (even though the latter carries a low risk of cerebral oedema and less marked derangement of prothrombin time).

The three commonest causes of acute liver failure requiring liver transplantation in the UK are seronegative hepatitis (confusingly termed 'non-A, non-B hepatitis'), often affecting middle-aged women; drug-induced liver disease, often affecting older patients; and paracetamol toxicity. Other important but rare causes of acute liver failure include viral hepatitis (A, B, D and E, but not C), herbal remedies, toxins, autoimmune liver disease, pregnancy-related liver disease, Wilson's diseases, Budd–Chiari syndrome, malignant infiltration (often not considered or missed) and ischaemic hepatitis.

There are three major strands to treating patients with acute liver failure: generic management of the liver failure, an early decision regarding transfer and transplantation and aetiology-specific management of the underlying liver condition.

Generic management involves meticulous measurement and correction of metabolic disturbances (glucose, potassium, phosphate and sodium), correction of thrombocytopenia when bleeding is present, prophylaxis against bacterial and fungal infection (antibiotics and antifungal agents as advised by microbiology locally), renal replacement as needed and haemodynamic support (vigorous fluid resuscitation, transfusion as required). The management of cerebral oedema involves measurement of intracranial pressure (either directly or by secondary measurements such as pupillary responses and blood pressure), nursing in a nonstimulatory, quiet environment at 10° in the head-up position, and giving mannitol as required. Coagulopathy *per se* should not be corrected unless the patient is bleeding actively, as the prothrombin time gives vital prognostic information.

Leaving the ethical dilemma of performing a liver transplant on an unconscious and perhaps unsuitable patient aside, the requirement for liver transplantation is based on the King's College Hospital criteria, on which the following table is based.[1] A common error is to look at transaminase levels, but these have no prognostic relevance.

Factors favouring liver transplantation over medical management

Paracetamol overdose	Other aetiology
pH < 7.3 despite fluid resuscitation	PT > 100 s
or all three of	or any three of:
• PT > 100 s • Creatinine > 300 µmol • Gd 3 or 4 encephalopathy	• Age < 10 or > 40 years • 'Non-A non-B', or drug-induced aetiology • Jaundice to encephalopathy time of > 7 days • Creatinine > 300 µmol • PT > 50 s

These criteria are indications for transplantation and not indications for transfer to a liver transplant unit. Patients should be transferred to liver transplant units well before evolution to liver failure. A useful prognostic marker for patients who have taken a paracetamol overdose is that if the prothrombin time in seconds exceeds the time from overdose in hours (assuming that more than 16 h have elapsed), then the patient falls within a poor prognostic group and should be considered for transfer.

---

[1] O'Grady *et al.* Gastroenterology (1989) 97: 439–445.

Clues in identifying the aetiology of acute liver failure

Viral	Exposure history, IgM to HAV, IgM anti-HBc, IgM anti-HDV, IgM or IgG HEV, EBV serology
Drugs and toxins	Exposure history, drug levels, eosinophil count
Autoimmune	ANA, SMA, LKM and high levels of IgG
Wilson's	Serum copper and caeruloplasmin
Malignancy	Imaging, histology
Pregnancy-related fatty liver	Ultrasound, uric acid, histology
Preeclampsia in pregnancy	Hypertension, proteinuria and oedema in pregnancy with HELLP (haemolysis, elevated liver enzymes and low platelets)

Paracetamol

Paracetamol overdose remains the commonest cause of acute liver failure in general medical practice in the UK. If an enthusiastic health economist were to assess the cost per QALY of combining methionine with paracetamol, the results would provide interesting reading. A significant number of deaths still occur in the UK each year and in about a third of such cases, an opportunity to intervene meaningfully has been missed.

When identified early, toxicity is avoided by treatment with N-acetylcysteine. At later stages, even after paracetamol can no longer be detected in plasma, N-acetylcysteine still modifies the course of acute liver failure beneficially. There are numerous examples, often tragic, when N-acetylcysteine is wrongfully withheld from patients, or not used for the correct duration. The treatment curves for the management of paracetamol poisoning rely completely on the history of the timing of the overdose, almost always ascertained from the patient themselves, who may be an unreliable witness for a number of reasons. To avoid inappropriate nontreatment, either two separate paracetamol levels need to be taken 4 h apart or the patient treated empirically, especially if they are known to have ingested a significant amount (although even 6 g has been associated with acute liver failure). N-acetylcysteine has such a good safety profile that a very strong case for liberal use can be made. N-acetylcysteine should be given until paracetamol levels are undetectable and the PT is less than 25 s. The minimum duration of treatment is 20 h. Symptoms, especially right upper quadrant pain, suggest ongoing hepatic necrosis. Likewise, patients should not be discharged 'medically' until they are asymptomatic, the PT and creatinine are normal and they have an undetectable paracetamol level.

Pregnancy-related liver disease

Abnormalities of liver function are common in pregnancy and help from the medical team is often sought out of hours. Some liver diseases are more common or may present in pregnancy, including gallstones, primary biliary cirrhosis and Budd–Chiari Syndrome. Diseases unique to pregnancy include intrahepatic cholestasis of pregnancy, preeclampsia and acute fatty liver of pregnancy. Hyperemesis gravidarum may also cause mild elevations of bilirubin and aminotransferases. Intrahepatic cholestasis of pregnancy is thought to be secondary to heightened sensitivity to the effects of oestrogen on the uptake and secretion of bilirubin and bile salts in a genetically predisposed individual. The condition is relatively benign, although preterm labour and the incidence of foetal mortality are marginally increased. Agents such as ursodeoxycholic acid and cholestyramine (both safe in pregnancy) are used therapeutically.

Preeclampsia with liver involvement is a serious disorder, requiring prompt diagnosis and management and is characterized by the triad of hypertension, proteinuria and oedema. It begins late in the late second trimester and affects about 3% of all pregnancies. There is a spectrum of liver injury including the HELLP syndrome, the commonest manifestation, as well as the more rare complications such as hepatic infarction, haematoma and rupture. The pathogenesis is unknown. Endothelial dysfunction is important and leads to vasoconstriction and activation of the coagulation cascade. This causes ischaemic damage to multiple organs including the liver. There is increased mortality in mother and baby, and appropriate management (immediate delivery of the baby and the attached placenta) is lifesaving.

Acute fatty liver of pregnancy is a serious condition for both mother and foetus, in which hepatocytes are infiltrated by microvesicular fat, leading to profound liver dysfunction. Analogous conditions are Reye's syndrome and some forms of drug toxicity (such as sodium valproate and tetracycline). The condition occurs in approximately 1 in 1000 pregnancies in the third trimester. Again, the management is delivery.

Budd–Chiari syndrome

This is a condition in which thrombosis of the hepatic vein leads to liver congestion, damage and portal hypertension. The presentation may be acute, subacute or chronic. Cardinal features are abdominal pain, hepatomegaly, ascites, deranged liver tests and impaired synthetic function. Risk factors are coagulopathy (either primary or secondary) and local physical factors such as tumours causing venous stasis. Management is not evidence based, but includes the conventional management of portal hypertension, anticoagulation, TIPS shunts, angioplasty and if appropriate, transplantation. Hepatic encephalopathy is a poor prognostic sign and usually indicates the need for transplantation. There is usually an underlying coagulation defect which should be addressed: causes include deficiency of protein C or protein S, malignancy and, most commonly, polycythaemia rubra vera (the latter may not be fully manifest for up to a decade and may not be apparent because of iron deficiency).

Malignant infiltration

Carcinomatous, lymphomatous and amyloid infiltration of the liver can lead to liver failure. Liver biopsy should be considered to guide chemotherapy and avoid inappropriate liver transplantation.

Wilson's disease

Wilson's disease, a chronic liver disorder, can present as acute liver failure. In the absence of hepatic encephalopathy, patients respond occasionally to high-dose D-penicillamine or trientine. However, liver transplantation is almost invariably indicated.

CHRONIC LIVER FAILURE

Chronic liver disease is the more common variety of liver disease experienced in clinical practice. Its incidence, and that of cirrhosis, is increasing. In 2000, over 4000 deaths in England were caused by cirrhosis, 500 of them in men under 45 years of age.[2] Management focuses on treating the underlying disorder where possible, anticipating the complications, treating those complications when they arise and considering when to transplant in the event of progression despite best management.

Hepatic decompensation is often a late manifestation of liver disease as the liver displays an extraordinary degree of redundancy, requiring only 20% of its hepatocytes to function effectively. Hepatic decompensation can be acute-on-chronic, or chronic. Acute-on-chronic decompensation occurs due to a superimposed insult, such as sepsis, whereas chronic decompensation is directly related to the underlying hepatic pathology. Decompensation equates to failure of the liver to perform its normal physiological functions, which can be divided into synthetic, metabolic, immunological and haemodynamic.

---

[2] Chief Medical Officer, Annual Report 2001 (www.dh.gov.uk)

Synthetic function is assessed by the production of albumin and clotting factors; metabolic function by nutritional status, the presence of encephalopathy and serum bilirubin. Specific therapies for decompensation include correction of coagulopathy if the patient is bleeding, good nutritional support (including treatment of osteoporosis) and ensuring a regular bowel habit. Management of acute decompensation involves vigorous supportive measures with identification and management of the underlying cause for the decompensation. The only definitive management for chronic decompensation is liver transplantation.

Infectious complications are very common in liver disease. This is probably multifactorial. Firstly, the liver fails to clear antigen from the portal circulation. Secondly, nutritional and metabolic disturbances lead to immune cellular dysfunction, affecting all aspects of the immune system. Thirdly, the liver fails to produce elements of the humoral immune system such as complement and albumin. When a systemic infection is established, acute hepatic decompensation develops leading to a further decline in immunological function and worsening infection. This vicious cycle must be stopped early with broad spectrum antimicrobial agents initially, until a causative organism is cultured and sensitivities are known.

Haemodynamic decompensation is progressive and probably stepwise. According to the peripheral vasodilatation hypothesis, the important steps are cirrhosis, portal hypertension, splanchnic arterial vasodilatation, reduced effective arterial blood volume, activated vasoconstrictor systems and renal vasoconstriction.[3] This leads to a low systemic vascular resistance, a decrease in central blood volume (with increased splanchnic blood volume, activation of both the renin–angiotensin axis and the sympathetic nervous system, and vasopressin production). The important clinical consequences are salt and water retention leading to ascites and hyponatraemia, varices, systemic hypotension and the hepatorenal syndrome.

Ascites

The presence of ascites complicating cirrhosis is a poor prognostic sign, carrying a 2-year survival of just 50%.[4] Patients in this group should therefore be considered for transplantation. Ascites should be tapped at initial presentation,

[3] Schrier et al. Hepatology (1988) 8: 1151–1157.

[4] Fernandez-Esparrach et al. J Hepatol (2001) 34: 46–52.

or at the time of a clinical deterioration, to determine whether there is a superimposed bacterial infection. Samples should be sent for white cell/ neutrophil count, culture, cytology for malignancy (providing large volumes to be centrifuged to increase the diagnostic yield) and albumin concentration. The fluid may be blood stained.

Ultrasound for portal vein thrombosis, low hepatopetal portal blood flow or reversed portal blood flow (hepatofugal) is required and may explain the onset of ascites, while a high suspicion should be maintained for hepatocellular carcinoma in each patient with new onset liver failure. Urea, creatinine and electrolytes should be checked, as well as weight on admission and daily there- after. Experienced hepatologists monitor the urinary sodium at each change in management. Management strategies for ascites include salt restriction, diure- sis, fluid restriction, paracentesis and a transjugular intrahepatic portosys- temic shunt (TIPS).

Salt restriction is the first step, but can be counter productive since adherence to this advice often causes worsening of malnutrition. Most hepatologists advise patients not to add salt to meals and to avoid using salt in cooking. Beware preprepared meals, which have a high salt content. If a patient has high urinary sodium but is not responding to therapy it usually means that the patient is consuming salt, often inadvertently. Inspect the bedside table for the cause.

If sodium restriction is ineffective or if the ascites is voluminous, then diuret- ics should be commenced. Spironolactone, which antagonizes aldosterone is logical and the drug of choice, and progress is monitored by weight reduction. Weight loss of any amount is acceptable, but loss in excess of 1 kg per day may precipitate encephalopathy. Renal impairment, hyponatraemia and hyper- kalaemia complicate spironolactone therapy, and the drug must be withdrawn if they occur. Higher doses are more likely to cause problems: doses of greater than 200 mg are the domain of the specialist ascites enthusiast. If spironolac- tone at reasonable dose is ineffective, first ascertain whether there is a natriure- sis. If there is, determine the source of the extra dietary salt and address it. Some patients are intolerant of spironolactone (especially men who develop breast tenderness); amiloride and triamterene are alternatives but much less effective.

If the urinary sodium is low on spironolactone, then consider adding furosemide cautiously. This is even more likely to cause hyponatraemia and renal impairment, when again the drug should be withdrawn. Higher doses bring increased toxicity. A good rule of thumb is that furosemide in this group is for in-patients and experts. It is worth checking if the addition of furosemide induces a natriuresis. If it does not, it will not work.

Fluid restriction is not beneficial in the management of ascites except in the context of hyponatraemia. By inducing 'aquaresis', vasopressin 2 receptor antagonists may revolutionize the management of ascites in the future, perhaps obviating the need for TIPS shunting.

With progressive liver disease, ascites may become refractory to diuretics or more often diuretics cannot be prescribed without inducing electrolyte abnormalities. This is the time to stop prescribing them and consider alternative strategies.

When ascites is tense and causing discomfort or can no longer be controlled by diuretic therapy, it is managed by paracentesis and albumin replacement. Most such patients will require treatment at 2–3 week intervals. Albumin should commence before ascites is tapped and the total dose is determined by the volume of paracentesis. It is expensive. All patients in a programme of paracentesis should be considered for longer term and more definitive strategies including transplantation or TIPS shunt.

When ascites that is noncirrhotic in origin is drained, opinion is somewhat divided as to the role of albumin replacement: it seems rational to use albumin when there is hepatic infiltration but not when the ascites is essentially unrelated to the liver (as, for example, in advanced ovarian carcinoma).

Spontaneous bacterial peritonitis

A common complication of ascites is spontaneous bacterial peritonitis (SBP), when ascites becomes infected by enteric organisms, presumably due to bacterial transit from the bowel into a rich ascitic fluid culture medium at an optimal temperature in an immunocompromised host. It is an emergency that carries a very poor prognosis and it constitutes an indication for transplantation in appropriate patients. The diagnosis should always be entertained when a patient with ascites becomes acutely unwell. An ascitic fluid sample should be sent for microscopy and culture in blood culture bottles. A white cell count > 500 per ml (or a neutrophil count of > 250 per ml) is diagnostic and always necessitates the use of broad-spectrum antibiotics (such as cefotaxime or ciprofloxacin) until the identity and sensitivities of the causative organism are known. Culture is usually negative. Maintenance of adequate central volumes is critical and there is evidence for giving 1.5 g/kg human albumin at the time of diagnosis, followed by 1 g/kg on day 3, the efficacy of which may in part be due to the antibiotic effects of albumin.[5] Norfloxacin is indicated as long-term prophylaxis for all patients with ascites.

---

[5] Sort *et al.* NEJM (1999) 341: 403–409.

Variceal haemorrhage

The initial management of acute variceal bleeding is resuscitation (as discussed in Chapter Eleven). Splanchnic vasoconstriction with an agent such as terlipressin, with or without octreotide, is first line therapy in order to stabilize the patient prior to endoscopy for diagnosis and treatment. Endoscopy should be undertaken as soon as it is safe to proceed. Wherever possible, oesophageal varices are then managed by a course of endoscopic band ligation over a period of weeks: injection sclerotherapy is now regarded as second-best therapy. One could argue that all such cases should be managed in specialist centres, if only to ensure adequate nighttime cover.

For massive life-threatening haemorrhage, balloon tamponade via a Sengstaken Blakemore tube can be considered. Failure to control bleeding should lead to consideration of a TIPS or surgical decompression of portal hypertension. Gastric varices sometimes respond to tissue adhesive therapy, but usually require a TIPS shunt. Variceal haemorrhage *per se* is not an indication for liver transplantation but as with each manifestation of liver failure, transplantation should always be discussed.

One should not be shy of endotracheal intubation to protect the airways during haemorrhage and endoscopic management.

Bacterial infection is a common association of variceal haemorrhage and some argue that it may be a precipitating cause. Blind antimicrobial therapy is indicated. So too are measures to reduce acid secretion and reduce the risk of bleeding from banding-induced ulcers. Proton pump inhibitors and sucralfate are both effective and some physicians use both.

As with ascites, bleeding varices may be related to reduced portal blood flow or the evolution of a hepatocellular carcinoma, so liver ultrasound and serum alpha-fetoprotein should be requested. Liver ultrasound of the portal vein should be undertaken as soon as possible (bearing in mind the experience of the operator), since this will determine if a TIPS shunt would be possible if needed in an emergency.

Once stable, patients are entered into a secondary prevention programme. This is usually endoscopic with weekly banding until variceal obliteration is achieved, after which time surveillance endoscopies can be spaced out progressively.

There is a clear role for primary and secondary prophylaxis of both oesophageal and gastric varices with non selective beta blockade, a decision usually made after endoscopy, which determines the risk of haemorrhage.

Hepatorenal syndrome

This is a disorder best managed in specialist units unless a decision has been made to manage conservatively. Type 1 hepatorenal syndrome (HRS) is characterized by rapidly progressive renal impairment, most commonly precipitated by SBP. Without treatment it has a very poor prognosis with a median survival of less than 2 weeks, with almost 100% mortality at 10 weeks. Type 2 HRS is characterized by a slowly progressive reduction in glomerular filtration rate (GFR). These patients often have diuretic-resistant ascites and have a median survival of 3–6 months. HRS is a diagnostic label that is commonly used inappropriately. It is a diagnosis of exclusion, with the key being reduced GFR in the absence of other causes of renal failure. The International Ascites Club has produced guidelines to aid the diagnosis.[6] A major factor is the presence of renal impairment with low urinary sodium despite obtaining central venous pressure-proven euvolaemia. This usually involves stopping diuretics and providing fluid support. Established management of HRS involves maintaining euvolaemia with albumin and splanchnic vasoconstriction with terlipressin.[7] The latter may induce ischaemia in the extremities as well as in the territory of the cerebral or coronary vessels. Definitive management is liver transplantation.

The choice of fluid in patients with chronic liver failure is a matter of constant debate. In the acutely ill patient, albumin is probably the best choice. It has beneficial oncotic and antibiotic properties, and is a free radical scavenger and transporter. It also avoids additional salt and water loading. 5% dextrose is likely to be the best maintenance fluid in a less acute setting, given the salt overload of chronic liver failure.

Screening in chronic liver failure

Patients at risk of hepatocellular carcinoma (cirrhotic patients with hepatitis C, alcoholic liver disease, haemochromatosis or nonalcoholic fatty liver disease and all patients with chronic hepatitis B) undergo six monthly ultrasound and assay of serum alpha-fetoprotein. Although adopted widely, the evidence to support this practice has yet to be garnered.

In many centres, variceal screening with upper GI endoscopy is offered to all patients, although in others, it is reserved for the subset with low platelets and an enlarged spleen, or patients with splenic varices, recanalization of the umbilical vein or reversed flow in the portal vein. If small varices are found at endoscopy, they are not treated, but repeated endoscopic screening is offered. Large varices are treated as part of a primary prevention programme by means of either banding or effective beta blockade.

---

[6] Arroyo et al. Hepatology (1996) 23: 164–176.

[7] Ortega et al. Ibid (2002) 36: 941–948.

DEXA scanning at 2-yearly intervals assesses for osteopaenia/osteoporosis which should be treated. Annual testosterone and vitamin D levels allow appropriate replacement therapy to be considered.

Causes of chronic liver disease

A crude idea of the causes of chronic liver disease and their frequency can be gained from the study of those undergoing liver transplantation. In the UK in the past 5 years, about 25% of transplants have been for cirrhosis due to alcohol-related liver disease (ALD); this under represents the burden of ALD nationally since only those patients capable of prolonged abstinence are considered for liver grafts. 15% of liver grafts are for hepatitis C virus (HCV)-related cirrhosis or hepatocellular carcinoma, 12% for primary biliary cirrhosis (PBC), 10% for primary sclerosing cholangitis (PSC), 6% for cryptogenic cirrhosis and 2% for hepatitis B virus (HBV)-related cirrhosis or hepatocellular carcinoma. Rarer causes of chronic liver disease include autoimmune hepatitis (AIH), α-1 antitrypsin deficiency and haemochromatosis.

It is important for all patients with chronic liver disease to have a complete liver screen. Many patients have more than one cause of liver damage and many carry an incorrect label, which could compromise active treatment and eligibility for liver transplantation. The most common scenario is the under-investigated patient who consumes alcohol in excess.

A liver panel to screen for chronic liver disease

Alcohol-related	Record of units consumed per week, with a collateral history, mean corpuscular volume, IgA level
Chronic viral hepatitis	HBsAg (if positive, HBeAg and HBV DNA) and anti-HCV antibody (if positive HCV RNA)
PBC	Antimitochondrial antibody, anti-PDH and IgM level
Autoimmune hepatitis	Antinuclear, anti-smooth muscle antibody, anti-liver/kidney microsomal antibody and IgG level
Non-alcohol-related fatty liver disease	BMI and markers of insulin resistance
Haemochromatosis	Ferritin/transferrin saturation and if abnormal C282Y and H63D mutation analysis
Wilson's	Caeruloplasmin and if abnormal slit lamp, serum copper, urinary copper (pre- and post-D-penicillamine) and tissue copper
α-1 antitrypsin deficiency	α-1 antitrypsin level and if low, phenotype
PSC	pANCA and consider MRCP and liver biopsy
Other	Ultrasound scan to assess for portal hypertension, Budd–Chiari syndrome, liver lesions and infiltrative disorders

Alcohol-related liver disease

Alcoholic liver disease (ALD) is the most common liver disease encountered in clinical practice. Abstinence is the key, and requires experienced coordinated multidisciplinary teams to address these complex issues. Identifying patients likely to achieve long-term abstinence is never easy, but maintaining employment, home and partner help enormously. In contrast, social isolation is a poor prognostic sign.

Although it is well known that the amount of alcohol consumed is related to the development of ALD, there is considerable variability in susceptibility.[8] Research into this area is sparse perhaps because of the stigma attached to alcohol. Of the few risk factors that are known, being overweight, female and having coexistent HCV are important. The diagnosis of ALD relies on a compatible history, compatible blood results and the exclusion of other causes of liver disease. Any diagnostic doubt necessitates liver biopsy.

Alcohol can lead to four hepatic entities: fatty liver, alcoholic hepatitis and chronic liver disease with cirrhosis, with or without superimposed hepatocellular carcinoma. The fatty liver can be an acute phenomenon, after a drinking binge, or can persist chronically with ongoing alcoholic insult, leading to chronic liver disease. Chronic liver disease with cirrhosis has been discussed already. Abstinence is absolutely vital and is achievable. 30% of patients who enter a liver service with chronic ALD stop consuming alcohol and can experience marked improvement in liver function for up to 2 years. Support is the most important component, with pharmacological agents such as acamprosate having only a subsidiary role.

Alcoholic hepatitis presents with jaundice and occurs on a background of alcohol-related liver damage, often after a heavy binge. It is characterized histologically by a neutrophil-rich infiltrate. The clinical syndrome can be mistaken easily for sepsis and encompasses weakness, anorexia, confusion, abdominal pain, jaundice, elevated inflammatory markers, renal impairment and variable features of hepatic decompensation and chronic underlying liver disease. Prognosis is determined by the Maddrey Discriminant Function (DF), defined as shown:

$$\frac{\text{Total bilirubin (in } \mu\text{mol}) + 4.6 \times (\text{PT in seconds} - \text{control PT in seconds})}{17}$$

---

[8] Bellentani *et al.* Gut (1997) 41: 845–850.

Untreated, patients with a DF greater than 32 have a 30-day mortality rate of 33% and a 6-month mortality rate of 50%. Patients with a DF less than 32 have a greater than 90% chance of surviving 6 months.

The mainstay of treatment is supportive with prophylactic broad-spectrum antibiotics, fluid resuscitation, careful use of diuretics, avoidance of both alcohol and an alcohol-withdrawal syndrome, nutritional support and vitamin replacement. Complications such as renal failure and sepsis should be addressed appropriately.

The role of corticosteroids has been contentious for years. Recent meta-analyses arrived at different conclusions. What is clear is that corticosteroids are not indicated for patients with bleeding or active sepsis. Pentoxiphylline was shown to be effective in one randomized controlled clinical trial and has been adopted by some centres on the basis of that solitary study, perhaps because it has low toxicity and is inexpensive. The absence of confirmatory studies is odd.

Chronic viral hepatitis

HBV and HCV have a combined prevalence of about 2% in the UK. HBV is contracted sexually or by blood–blood contact. More than 95% of immune competent patients clear HBV (loss of HBsAg with development of anti-HBs and anti-HBc), unless the disease is contracted in childhood, when 10% or less clear it. The patients who do not clear the virus develop a protracted relapsing/remitting chronic hepatitis. Untreated, 30% of men become cirrhotic and at least 10% of those develop HCC, usually as a consequence of cirrhosis. Once cirrhosis has developed, 25% decompensate within 5 years.

HCV is contracted by blood–blood contact. Sexual transmission is reported but is rare. Between 5 and 10% of patients probably develop an acute hepatitis, usually unnoticed, about 6 weeks from HCV exposure. Around 15% remain HCV RNA negative after exposure and are considered to have recovered, but there is no clear serological profile to indicate acquired immunity. 85% evolve to a chronic hepatitis, which is progressive rather than relapsing and remitting. 20% of the patients with chronic HCV develop cirrhosis between one and three decades later. Risk factors for rapid progression are smoking, older age at the time of infection, high BMI, concomitant alcohol abuse, being male and immune deficiency (HIV co-infection in particular). Cirrhotic patients have a 25% risk of death in 5–10 years. The annual risk of hepatocellular cancer in HCV with cirrhosis is 3 to 5%. It is rare in the absence of cirrhosis.

The presence of serum HBsAg, HBeAg or HBV DNA, or HCV RNA, confirm chronic infection with HBV and HCV respectively. Activity of HBV can be ascertained by a combination of raised aminotransferases and interface hepatitis on liver biopsy in a viraemic patient. Activity of HCV can only be ascertained confidently by assessing the grade and pattern of inflammation on liver biopsy.

NICE currently advise treating HCV-infected patients with at least moderate disease as determined by liver biopsy. Treatment is with pegylated interferon-α and ribavirin. Patients with HCV genotypes 1 and 4 are treated for 48 weeks and types 2 and 3 for 24 weeks. Favourable treatment outcome is predicted by short duration of HCV infection, younger age, mild disease, low RNA viral load, having genotype 2 or 3 and demonstrating low hepatic iron on biopsy.

Treatment of HBV is more complex. There are recent NICE guidelines.[9] The options are a short course of interferon-α or oral antiviral therapy. Interferon-α has the huge potential advantage of permanent viral clearance, but is only effective in the minority with active disease (female patients with liver biopsy evidence of interface hepatitis, low level HBV DNA and a high ALT have the best chance of responding). Antiviral agents that suppress viral replication, such as lamivudine and adefovir, are better tolerated than interferon but they have to be taken long term, possibly for years. They are first choice for those receiving immune suppression and those with chronic liver failure. Both lamivudine and adefovir inevitably induce resistant mutations (more commonly with the former). With newer drugs on the horizon it is probable that a combination of oral antiviral agents will be recommended in due course.

Biliary disorders

Primary biliary cirrhosis (PBC) is a disease that usually presents in middle age and affects women nearly ten times more frequently than men. The diagnosis can be made serologically in most cases. Characteristically, the alkaline phosphatase or γ-glutamyl transpeptidase is more than twice the upper limit of normal, and the patient is antimitochondrial antibody and anti-PDH positive (pyruvate dehydrogenase - the major mitochondrial autoantigen). These antibodies have in excess of 95% specificity and 98% sensitivity, obviating the need for biopsy except in unusual circumstances.

The disease is usually characterized by a progressive increase in the alkaline phosphatase with worsening pruritus and later by progressive jaundice. In addition to the features of decompensated liver disease, the major symptoms are of malaise and lethargy. Hyperlipidaemia, which probably does not accelerate atherosclerosis, is a feature, as is osteoporosis, which must be screened for

---

[9] TA096, February 2006 (www.nice.org.uk)

and treated accordingly. Co-existent autoimmune disorders also occur. HCC is rare and it is a matter of debate whether the cost of screening for HCC is warranted in this group: the authors recommend this. Ursodeoxycholic acid is first-line therapy for pruritus with alternatives including cholestyramine, rifampicin, MARS (extracorporal albumin dialysis) and UV light. There are contradictory data concerning the effect of ursodeoxycholic acid on long-term outcome.

Timing transplantation in PBC involves balancing the patient being well enough to survive the procedure, but being sick enough to merit it. Currently, a bilirubin of between 100 and 150 µmol/l or decompensation prompts consideration of transplantation. Chronic pruritus and malaise are important considerations in some patients, but the gravity of liver transplantation must be emphasized to patients before proceeding. At present, 1-year survival post transplantation is in the region of 92%, and 5-year survival 71%.

Primary sclerosing cholangitis (PSC) is strongly associated with inflammatory bowel disease, and negatively associated with smoking. Whereas PBC is a disease of solely the intrahepatic bile ducts, PSC predominantly affects the large intrahepatic and extrahepatic ducts. The presence of pANCA has 70% sensitivity and 90% specificity. Biliary imaging is vital diagnostically: this must be by MRCP unless a biliary procedure is indicated, when ERCP can be utilized. ERCP is a potentially life-threatening investigation and should not be undertaken when there is a viable alternative. Liver biopsy stages the disease.

Management of PSC involves detection and management of complications until transplantation becomes necessary. If patients do not have clinical inflammatory bowel disease then colonoscopy is required at initial assessment to ensure that it is absent, and patients should also be entered into an appropriate colorectal cancer screening programme. They are at heightened risk of colorectal cancer even in the absence of inflammatory bowel disease. Screening and treatment for osteoporosis is also important. Ursodeoxycholic acid may help pruritus and decrease the risk of cholangiocarcinoma. Episodes of cholangitis are treated with antibiotics and in jaundiced patients, the stenting of dominant strictures can be considered. The risk of cholangiocarcinoma in PSC is high. Screening can be carried out by measurement of CA 19-9, which has low specificity. Whether screening is useful is uncertain since there are few effective therapies should a tumour develop.

Other aetiologies

Autoimmune hepatitis (AIH) is characterized by an ALT of more than 5 times normal, an IgG of more than double normal or a positive smooth muscle antibody and compatible liver histology.[10] Treatment is with prednisolone and azathioprine. Azathioprine is introduced when the bilirubin normalizes and prednisolone is then gradually reduced. The disease is monitored by ALT and IgG levels. At between 2 and 4 years, minimal activity on biopsy allows for prednisolone withdrawal. Azathioprine is used in the long term to avoid disease recurrence.

On the basis of epidemiological and longitudinal studies, it is now well recognized that cryptogenic cirrhosis is predominantly caused by nonalcoholic fatty liver disease (NAFLD). NAFLD is a spectrum of liver disease characterized by insulin resistance that begins with fat accumulation (hepatic steatosis) and progresses through steatohepatitis (NASH) and fibrosis to cirrhosis. The degree of inflammation and fibrosis on biopsy is important. Hepatic steatosis is relatively benign: indeed, 25% of Americans have it. However, of patients with steatohepatitis, 10% will go on to get fibrosis and 30% of patients with fibrosis develop cirrhosis in 10 years.

Many patients with NAFLD die with, rather than of, their liver disease. In one series of 420 patients diagnosed with NAFLD between 1980 and 2000, 13% had died at follow up in 2005.[11] The relative risk of death was 1.32, but liver disease was only third on the list of cause of death, behind malignancy and ischaemic heart disease.

Risk factors for NAFLD are central obesity, type 2 diabetes and hypercholesterolaemia. NAFLD can also be secondary to some drugs, hereditary metabolic defects and malnutrition. Management involves weight loss, exercise and optimal management of all features of the metabolic syndrome. Metformin, glitazones and statins may be beneficial.

Genetic haemochromatosis is common, with a recessive HFE gene mutation frequency of 10% and an incidence of approximately 1 in 400. The clinical syndrome of diabetes, hypogonadism, bronze skin, arthralgia and liver disease is caused by iron deposition in the pancreas, pituitary, skin, joints and liver respectively. Not all homozygous patients with HFE gene mutations develop haemochromatosis and this is explained by the contributions of other proteins involved in the metabolism of iron. In those that do develop disease, clinical features can vary. Women are protected from iron overload between menarche and menopause.

---

[10] Czaja *et al.* Hepatology (2000) 31: 1194–1200.

[11] Adams *et al.* Gastroenterology (2005) 129: 113–121.

A ferritin of greater than 200 µg/l and transferrin saturation of greater than 50% is seen in 90% of patients with genetic haemochromatosis. Transferrin saturation is particularly important as, being an acute phase protein, ferritin is elevated in many clinical contexts including most chronic liver diseases. Assessment of HFE genotype by testing for the common mutations (C282Y and H63D) is the next step. Liver biopsy is only indicated if there is diagnostic doubt or to identify cirrhotic patients so that they can have appropriate screening. Homozygotes with the C282Y mutation who have normal LFTs, no hepatomegaly and a ferritin of less than 1000 µg/l will not have cirrhosis (100% negative predictive value) and do not require biopsy.

Management of haemochromatosis is by venesection. A unit of blood is taken weekly until ferritin and transferrin saturation starts to fall. Once this occurs, venesection can be progressively spaced until the ferritin normalizes (< 50 µg/l) and transferrin saturation is below 50%. Patients then require maintenance venesection, which usually occurs between 2 and 4 monthly.

ABNORMAL LIVER FUNCTION TESTS

Elevated liver tests are a common indication for referral to the liver clinic. History and examination help to identify the presence of chronic liver disease, features of biliary pathology, potential drug and hereditary causes, risk factors for liver disease and whether the patient is actually unwell. Investigations help to assess disease severity (PT, albumin and bilirubin), identify patients with chronic liver disease (ultrasound, platelets and biopsy) and identify a cause (full liver screen, ultrasound with Doppler flows and biopsy).

The indication for biopsy is clear cut when a patient is unwell and the aetiology unclear following a liver screen, or when disease severity needs to be ascertained. When these criteria are not met and the patient is obese, the underlying diagnosis is often hepatic steatosis. Although diagnosis of hepatic steatosis can only be determined histologically, it is often appropriate to take the pragmatic approach of taking a liver biopsy only if liver tests remain abnormal despite weight reduction.

With deranged liver function tests in the inpatient setting, there are three groups of causes: acute liver disease, underlying chronic liver disease and, as is most common, deranged tests as a secondary phenomenon. Relevant liver screens, as discussed earlier, determine aetiology of acute and chronic liver disease. Within these groups it is vital to identify acute liver failure and hepatic decompensation, due to their significant associated morbidity and mortality. Common secondary phenomena are cardiac failure, sepsis and drug toxicity, and once these are addressed, calm (in relation to the liver tests) should be restored.

LIVER LESIONS

These can be divided into neoplastic, infective and tumour-like lesions. As usual, neoplastic lesions can be benign or malignant, with malignant lesions being either primary or metastatic. Infective lesions are bacterial, amoebic or parasitic. Tumour-like lesions fall on the disordered development/proliferation spectrum.

Lesions are almost always diagnosed radiologically (and occasionally coincidentally) with ultrasound often being the initial modality. Imaging with CT scanning, MRI scanning and angiography can be used to evaluate lesions further. Microbiology and cytology of cyst contents, along with histology, after radiologically guided biopsy are often necessary to clinch a diagnosis. Serological tests are important. Examples are hydatid serology, amoebic serology, CA19-9 for cholangiocarcinoma, CEA for gastrointestinal primaries and alpha-fetoprotein for hepatocellular carcinoma (HCC). Other blood tests may be helpful, for example neutrophilia and eosinophilia in association with bacterial and amoebic abscesses respectively. A patient's exact investigations are tailored to clinical context. For example, in a patient with HCV cirrhosis and a liver lesion, tests for HCC would be appropriate, whereas in a patient presenting with swinging fevers and a hypoechoic mass after a recent diverticular abscess, investigations would be for a pyogenic abscess.

The options for the management of neoplastic lesions are resection, transplantation or a conservative approach. Common examples are hepatic adenomas which are resected because of their malignant potential, HCC which is managed with transplantation (if certain good prognostic criteria are fulfilled) and metastatic adenocarcinoma which can occasionally be resected, but is usually managed with chemotherapy and/or a palliative approach. Pyogenic abscesses are drained and the patient is given appropriate parenteral antibiotics. Amoebic abscesses are treated with metronidazole and Hydatid cysts are excised. Tumour-like lesions such as focal nodular hyperplasia and haemangiomas do not usually require treatment, as they are benign.

Chapter 11

William Gelson and Anthony Ellis

GASTROENTEROLOGY

The bleeder

Where is the bleeding patient? In the bleeding unit. No longer a conversation between mildly irritated consultant and over-worked junior doctor but an example of how management has changed in the patient presenting with haematemesis or melaena. In hospitals with specific clinical areas identified for the management of such patients, mortality has fallen. This is most likely because of improved resuscitation, monitoring and overall care, rather than any single medical or surgical advance in treatment.

Acute upper GI bleeding continues to be the most common gastroentero-logical emergency faced by on-call physicians. The annual incidence varies between 50 and 150 per 100,000, according to the local socioeconomic milieu. One might have expected to see a fall in incidence with time due to the more widespread use of proton pump inhibitors and other antacids. However, an ageing population and the more widespread use of anti-platelet agents mitigate against this. A study from the Netherlands demonstrated a fall in inci-dence from 61.7 to 47.7 per 100,000 between 1993 and 2000 which, after correction for age, represented a 23% decrease in hospital admissions for upper GI bleeding.[1] A study looking specifically at bleeding related to prescription of anti-platelet agents demonstrated a rise in incidence from 19 per 100,000 in 1996 to 39 per 100,000 in 2002.[2] The overall mortality continues to be significant at around 11%, rising to 33% in those for whom a

[1] Van Leerdam *et al.* Am J Gastro (2003) 98: 1494–1499.

[2] Taha *et al.* Aliment Pharmacol Ther (2005) 22: 285–289.

bleed has complicated a hospital admission for another indication. Mortality rises rapidly with age.

Initial assessment of the patient with a GI bleed should be synchronous with early resuscitation to stratify both the amount and timing of the bleeding, elucidate a cause and facilitate early treatment. The history should include details of recent NSAID usage, illness, previous dyspepsia, alcohol consumption and any pre-existing liver disease. A patient who has a history of an aortic aneurysm repair merits special attention due to the possibility of an aorto-enteric fistula (where abdominal CT becomes the priority following resuscitation). Examination principally evaluates the degree of cardiovascular instability and the presence of any co-morbidity known to affect outcome. Urgent investigations following admission include a full blood count, prothrombin time, urea and electrolytes, and liver function tests. The blood bank will be grateful for an early specimen too.

A validated scoring system can be used to help categorize patients according to their risk of death: the Rockall score.[3] It is simple and practical to use, helping to identify those most and least likely to survive, and by extension, those needing more active intervention. It also identifies those patients suitable for safe, early discharge (with a score of zero pre-endoscopy, 2 or less post-endoscopy).

Rockall scoring system for rebleed and death following admission with gastrointestinal bleeding

Pre-endoscopy score	0	1	2	3
Age	< 60	60–79	≥ 80	
Shock	None	Pulse > 100 and Systolic BP > 100	Pulse > 100 and Systolic BP < 100	
Co-morbidities	Nil major		Cardiac failure, ischaemic heart disease or other major co-morbidity	Renal/liver failure, disseminated malignancy
TOTAL =				

[3] Rockall *et al.* Gut (1996) 38: 316–321.

Rockall scoring system for rebleed and death following admission with gastrointestinal bleeding—cont'd

Post-endoscopy score	0	1	2
Diagnosis	Mallory Weiss tear or no lesion/blood	All other diagnoses	Malignancy of upper GI tract
Major stigmata of recent haemorrhage	None or dark red spot		Blood in upper GI tract, adherent clot, visible or spurting vessel
TOTAL =			

Prior to endoscopy, the minimum score is zero and the maximum seven. The maximum score following endoscopy rises to eleven. Mortality can be predicted as shown in the table below.

Predicted mortality by Rockall score

Score	Pre-endoscopy (%)	Post-endoscopy (%)
0	0.2	0.0
1	2.4	0.0
2	5.6	0.2
3	11.0	2.9
4	24.6	5.3
5	39.6	10.8
6	48.9	17.3
7	50.0	27.0
≥ 8	n/a	41.1

For those patients in whom an in-patient stay is required (any score other than zero pre-endoscopy), the main principle of management is vigorous resuscitation in those with haemodynamic instability prior to endoscopic assessment. All too often, a patient attends for endoscopy with a pulse of 120 and a tiny blue cannula in the back of the hand. Endoscopy is often seen as the mainstay of treatment: it is not. The rule of two brown cannulae in big veins should always be adhered to. Remember – 'grey is good but brown is better!'

The initial resuscitation of a patient with GI bleeding is similar whether the source is thought to be from peptic ulceration or bleeding varices. The choice of fluid is less important than getting it in quickly. The most readily available fluid is 0.9% saline but Hartmann's solution is a suitable alternative especially if bleeding is thought to arise from varices. The aim is to reduce the pulse and improve blood pressure. After 2 l of crystalloid have been infused, plasma expanders may be used in addition if blood is not yet available. In those patients with cardiac disease, a central line may be useful to guide resuscitation. In all cases, coagulation defects should be sought and treated. Those patients with more than two poor prognostic factors (such as age greater than 60 years, shock and significant concomitant disease) should be catheterized and urine output monitored hourly, along with pulse and blood pressure, preferably on a High-Dependency Unit.[4]

Most bleeding stops with resuscitation and the body's natural haemostatic mechanisms, and endoscopy within 24 h is usually adequate. Continued bleeding, re-bleeding or bleeding varices (see Chapter Ten) should prompt emergency endoscopy. Frank haematemesis and labile vital signs, despite adequate resuscitation, suggest continued bleeding or re-bleeding. If competently assessed, the central venous pressure is also a helpful indicator.

Endoscopy is important for diagnosis, risk stratification and haemostasis, but it should only be undertaken by endoscopists *au fait* with the therapeutic procedures that may be required: mortality and re-bleeding are not reduced by simply having a look with a diagnostic endoscope. Haemostatic approaches for bleeding ulcers include adrenaline injection, thermal coagulation and glue. Adrenaline injection will achieve haemostasis in 95% but re-bleeding will follow in 15–20%.[5] The injection of alcohol or other sclerosants in addition to adrenaline does not produce any further benefit. Thermal haemostasis, using either a heater probe or bipolar probe, provides additional benefit and is used where available. Occasionally, mechanical clips can be deployed onto a large bleeding vessel.

Although bleeding ulcers (gastric, duodenal and occasionally oesophageal) or varices are most commonly found, the endoscopist will occasionally identify a more unusual cause of bleeding, such as a Dieulafoy lesion or gastric antral vascular ectasia (GAVE). A Dieulafoy lesion is an aberrant, abnormally large and tortuous submucosal artery, protruding through the mucosa. Such lesions can be hard to spot unless actively bleeding, accounting for up to 5% of major upper gastrointestinal bleeds. GAVE is characterized endoscopically

---

[4] Rockall *et al.* Gut (1996) 38: 316–321.

[5] Chung *et al.* BMJ (1988) 296: 1631–1633.

by thickened, red vascular folds radiating longitudinally from the pylorus to the antrum, said to resemble the stripes on the skin of a ripened watermelon. Such lesions are best treated by argon plasma coagulation.

If endoscopy fails to obtain haemostasis in non-variceal bleeding, then surgical intervention will be required. If a patient is stabilized with initial endoscopic therapy but re-bleeds, it is reasonable to attempt a 'second bite of the cherry' with a further endoscopy, especially if the first procedure was made difficult due to a stomach full of blood obscuring views. Re-bleeding after a second endoscopic procedure should result in consideration for surgery. In all cases of significant bleeding, the surgical team should be made aware of the patient in order that timely assessment can take place, preferably during daylight hours rather than just at the point that the surgical team are tucking into their late dinner!

The stability of a blood clot is reduced in an acid environment and if the gastric pH is below 6.0, platelet aggregation is inhibited and clot lysis occurs. Following endoscopy, high-dose PPI therapy should be given to those with stigmata of significant haemorrhage, who have received appropriate endo-scopic therapy.[6] Such treatment has been shown to reduce the rate of re-bleeding, transfusion requirements and the length of hospital stay. A suitable regimen is an IV bolus of omeprazole, followed by an infusion for 72 h. If a patient has required more than 4 units of blood, then they will also require calcium supplementation to counteract the hypocalcaemic effect of the citrate in the transfused blood.

Dysphagia

Causes of dysphagia are legion and include neurological disease, dysmotility, peptic stricture, achalasia, malignancy and structural abnormalities. The acute physician should be aware that almost 30% of elderly people acutely admitted to hospital have an element of dysphagia. Dysphagia complicates up to two-thirds of cases of stroke and is linked to the incidence of chest infection in this patient group. Over 50% of residents in long-term care facilities have feeding difficulties, dysphagia or both. Patients are best managed where there is networked access to a range of different disciplines: gastroenterology, speech and language therapy, nutrition, neurology and otolaryngology.

Underlying pathology can often be predicted from the history alone. The patient presenting with acute dysphagia, with or without symptoms of

---

[6] Lau *et al.* NEJM (2000) 343: 310–316.

limb weakness, should be assessed for evidence of a CVA. The patient with progressively worsening dysphagia of short duration in association with weight loss, on a background of Barrett's oesophagus, has oesophageal adenocarcinoma until proven otherwise. The young patient with longstanding non-progressive intermittent dysphagia with no worrying associated symptoms most likely has a motility disorder or achalasia.

Simple tests are useful initially. In those with a presumed CVA, a speech and language assessment is of paramount importance in order that the risks of aspiration can be assessed and nutrition tailored to the patient's needs. The presence or otherwise of the gag reflex is not a useful indicator of the patient's swallowing ability, and by extension the risk of aspiration.[7] For those that do need to undertake a more informal assessment, using a drinking straw as a 'pipette' delivers an appropriate volume of water. A full blood count will identify anaemia, deranged liver tests may raise suspicion of metastatic disease, and a chest radiograph may reveal a physical cause for dysphagia. Direct visualization of the oesophagus by endoscopy often follows, which is preferred to barium swallow by many because it can lead to tissue diagnosis and early definitive management. The only pitfall is the potential for perforation of a pharyngeal pouch, a diagnosis which should be considered in those patients who complain of dysphagia with associated halitosis, cough, gurgling in the neck or symptoms at the level of the thoracic inlet. A useful 'rule of thumb' is to investigate high dysphagia with barium initially and low dysphagia with an endoscopy.

A barium swallow is dynamic, allowing important information to be gathered not only with respect to anatomical abnormalities but also the motility of the oesophagus. The use of a bread swallow further improves the assessment in identifying dysmotility in the solid phase, which may not be as obvious when barium is used alone. Oesophageal manometry assesses peristalsis and is useful in confirming achalasia and studying dysmotility, especially in patients with persistent symptoms despite previous investigations having been negative.

Leaving neurological abnormalities to one side, the commonest causes of dysphagia are peptic stricturing (now less prevalent since the advent of PPIs), oesophageal malignancy, oesophageal dysmotility and achalasia. Peptic stricturing sometimes responds to treatment with a PPI alone, but dilatation is often required. The days of *bougienage*, a technique akin to forced sword swallowing, are largely over and most gastroenterologists use controlled radial expansion balloons which carry a much lower risk of perforation. Malignancy of the

---

[7] In Stroke: A Practical Guide to Management, Warlow et al. (Eds), Blackwell, Oxford, 1996.

oesophagus will be either squamous carcinoma or adenocarcinoma. Rarely, extrinsic compression from enlarged lymph nodes or gastrointestinal stromal tumours may present with dysphagia. All but the very early stages of mucosal malignancy do badly. Oesophagectomy, chemotherapy and palliation are the mainstays of treatment with the most appropriate package being decided at an MDT meeting.

Achalasia, a condition probably caused by the autoimmune destruction of Auerbach's plexus, was historically managed with a Heller's myotomy (which required a thoracotomy and/or a laparotomy with the associated morbidity and length of hospital stay). More recently, patients have been treated with balloon dilatation to good effect. The injection of botulinum toxin into the gastro-oesophageal junction is another alternative but the clinical response is short lived and repeat treatments are associated with a decline in efficacy. These shortcomings have restricted its use to the frail and elderly who are deemed unfit for pneumatic balloon dilatation or surgery.

Five-year follow-up studies suggest a significant failure rate of both balloon dilatation and botulinium toxin.[8,9] Surgery is now undertaken using laparo-scopic techniques. This has resulted in a much-reduced morbidity, mortality and hospital stay. We may be about to turn full circle and once again offer surgery as the initial treatment for achalasia in the young, fit patient.

Dysmotility can be difficult to treat. Full-dose PPI therapy should be tried initially (with or without a pro-kinetic such as metoclopramide or domperi-done). In some patients where spasm is significant, smooth muscle relaxants (such as nitrates and calcium channel blockers) can be useful. A further small but significant cohort will respond to treatment with psychotropic agents including amitriptyline.

Odynophagia is defined as pain on swallowing and this can be easily misconstrued by the patient or clinician as dysphagia. Any form of mucosal disruption from pharynx to gastro-oesophageal junction can cause it, as can oesophageal spasm. If elicited in the history, it has a good correlation with positive findings at endoscopy. Causes of mucosal disruption include infection (such as candidiasis), radiation and chemical insult (either exogenous or gastric acid). A gastroscopy will identify mucosal lesions, and barium swallow or oesophageal manometry will identify dysmotility syndromes. If mucosal disruption is to blame, specific treatments are instigated.

---

[8] Neubrand *et al.* Endoscopy (2002) 34: 519–523.

[9] West *et al.* Am J Gastroenterol (2002) 97: 1346–1351.

Dyspepsia

Definitions of dyspepsia vary. A reasonable one is 'abdominal pain or discomfort centred in the upper abdomen or epigastrium'. Dyspepsia is not in itself a disease entity, but is caused by a number of other conditions.

NICE has recently updated its guidance on the investigation and management of dyspepsia.[10] 'Alarm symptoms' are paramount: a patient with dyspepsia and one or more of GI blood loss, weight loss, dysphagia, vomiting, iron deficiency anaemia or an abdominal mass should be referred for an urgent upper GI endoscopy (under the '2-week wait rule' when the patient's journey starts in primary care in England).

The routine endoscopic investigation of patients aged under 55 years, presenting with dyspepsia and without alarm signs, is not necessary. However, in patients aged 55 years and older with new and persistent symptoms, in the absence of NSAID therapy, endoscopy is warranted.

Patients under the age of 55 years without alarm symptoms should at first be offered simple antacids and lifestyle advice (stop smoking, lose weight and eat sensibly). If these fail, a full-dose PPI should be tried for 1 month. A relapse prompts testing for Helicobacter pylori with the ^{13}C breath test with a treatment course for those patients found to be positive. Patients without evidence of H. pylori infection and those whose symptoms relapse after eradication, should be prescribed a PPI in sufficient dosage to control symptoms which can be continued as maintenance therapy. If symptoms continue despite these measures, an H_2 receptor antagonist may be added (especially in patients with nocturnal symptoms) although this particular strategy has only been studied in small numbers of patients.[11] A pro-kinetic can also be offered.

Causes of dyspepsia (which the NICE guidelines do not distinguish) include gastro-oesophageal reflux disease (GORD), peptic ulcer disease and functional dyspepsia. GORD is caused by a lax gastro-oesophageal sphincter mechanism that results in excessive exposure of the lower oesophagus to gastric acid. Characteristic symptoms are of a burning retrosternal chest pain, exacerbated by stooping, straining, weight gain, smoking and certain foods. Endoscopic abnormalities are seen in 38–68% of patients. 24-h lower oesophageal pH studies clinch the diagnosis. Management involves PPI therapy or anti-reflux surgery.

---

[10] CG017, August 2004 (www.nice.org.uk)

[11] Orr et al. Aliment Pharmacol Ther (2003) 17: 1553–1558.

Peptic ulcers are diagnosed endoscopically. They can be classified either by site (gastric and duodenal) or by association with NSAID usage. In those patients with no exposure to NSAIDs, 95% of duodenal ulcers (DUs) are caused by H. pylori infection as compared with 70% of gastric ulcers (GUs).

Patients with a DU and H. pylori infection (plus those who test negative in the presence of PPI treatment) should be given eradication therapy and treated for 4 weeks with a PPI. Eradication should be confirmed with the ^{13}C breath test after 12 weeks. Repeat endoscopy for these benign lesions is unnecessary.

Patients with a GU have a risk of underlying malignancy and should therefore have multiple biopsies during the first endoscopy. Patients should receive 8 weeks of PPI therapy and, if they are H. pylori positive, eradication therapy. Endoscopy should be repeated at 6 weeks and until complete healing is observed, to avoid missing a gastric cancer. Relapse after initial treatment should prompt repeat H. pylori testing before issuing maintenance PPI therapy as appropriate.

About 25% of GUs and 5% of DUs are NSAID-related. Up to 4% of patients on NSAIDs will develop ulcer-related complications, ranging from simple dyspepsia to death by exsanguination. The NSAID should of course be stopped and NSAID-related ulcers are otherwise treated as above. If it is felt that NSAID therapy is essential, it can be reinstated with PPI cover after ulcer healing. Although it is likely that cardiovascular mortality is equally high with some conventional NSAIDs, recent studies have very much marginalized the role of COX-2 inhibitors.

The major key to diagnosing functional dyspepsia is the presence of normal investigations with a symptomatic patient, in the absence of acid suppression. Functional dyspepsia is common, with a prevalence of at least 40% of patients undergoing investigations for dyspepsia. There are often underlying psychological factors. The most important aspects of management are support and reassurance. Anti-depressants are sometimes of benefit. Acid suppression has not been shown convincingly to be of more benefit in the management of functional dyspepsia than placebo.

A note of caution: with long-term PPI use, H. pylori can cause a pan-gastritis rather than an antral gastritis. This pan-gastritis – the same entity as is found in the Japanese H. pylori-infected population – may lead to an atrophic gastritis. Atrophic gastritis in turn predisposes to gastric adenocarcinoma. Worldwide, PPI sales are topped only by the sales of statins. By failing to eradicate H. pylori prior to long-term PPI use, we may risk a future epidemic of gastric adenocarcinoma.[12] Similar fears were raised in the 1980s with the H_2 receptor antagonists but to date appear unfounded.

....

[12] Raghunath et al. Aliment Pharmacol Ther (2005) 22 Supplement 1: 55–63.

Rectal bleeding

Rectal bleeding is a common symptom which, in most hospitals, is directed towards the department of surgery. Despite this, more and more cases seem to end up on medical wards as the on-call surgical junior outwits the junior physician into admitting the patient on the grounds that 'it may be medical'. The acute physician has to remain alert as thorough evaluation is needed due to the possibility of a background malignancy. Intermittent, longstanding bleeding is much less concerning than new onset bleeding. A change in bowel habit to looseness, increase in stool frequency, or lack of anal symptoms in association with bleeding are of concern, and should prompt urgent investigation. The history helps to pinpoint the origin of the bleeding. Fresh blood after defecation, or around the stool, suggests a rectal source; blood mixed with the stool, a distal colonic source and altered blood (or melaena), a proximal source.

Examination may reveal signs of malignancy, inflammatory bowel disease (IBD) or ano-rectal disorders such as haemorrhoids, fissures or fistulae. Digital examination of the rectum is mandatory and proctoscopy or rigid sigmoidoscopy is helpful in the rapid evaluation of the patient with overt rectal blood loss: however, this technique rarely forms part of the modern general physician's repertoire of practical skills. Whether further investigation is merited and which investigations are performed depends upon the initial assessment. On-going blood loss for which a cause has not been identified will require evaluation of the more proximal bowel. The colon may be investigated by means of colonoscopy or a combination of barium enema and flexible sigmoidoscopy. If blood loss is dark, it may be necessary to visualize the upper GI tract with a gastroscopy, or more rarely the small bowel by means of capsule enteroscopy or barium follow-through.

Occasionally rectal bleeding can be torrential. The initial management is appropriate resuscitation. Thankfully, most acute lower GI bleeding stops spontaneously. Identification of the source of bleeding can be difficult. Colonoscopy often reveals just blood and semi-fresh blood freely refluxes proximally, making it difficult to decide even which region of the bowel is the source of bleeding. Arteriography with the potential for embolization can be helpful, but bleeding must be at a rate of more than 0.5 ml/min. Rarely, a laparotomy with formation of a loop colostomy is used if the bleeding continues despite extensive investigation and a failure to identify the source.

Ano-rectal disorders are best managed by surgeons. Treatments for haemorrhoids include symptomatic approaches, banding and haemorrhoidectomy. For anal fissure, the Laud's stretch is now out of vogue, with nitrate creams, botulinium toxin and laxatives proving surprisingly effective.

For fistulae, various operative techniques, including seton sutures are curative: a seton suture involves passing a soft plastic tube through the fistula, tying the ends together and progressively tightening them over weeks, allowing migration of the suture through the skin in a cheese-wire fashion with healing behind by granulation. It sounds eye-watering but is effective.

Diverticulosis is very common, affecting one-third of the general population by the age of 45 years and two-thirds by 85 years.[13] Usually it is asymptomatic, but it can lead to pain and rectal bleeding. Complications include diverticulitis (managed with fluids and antibiotics), abscess formation and fistula formation (both managed surgically). Diverticulosis only occurs in Western populations. It is likely that low-fibre diets are to blame.

Arteriovenous malformations can be part of a syndrome (such as Osler–Weber–Rendu) or may occur sporadically. Once identified, these lesions can be treated with diathermy or laser at the time of colonoscopy (or in severe cases, with embolization).

Colorectal cancer (CRC) is the second commonest cause of cancer death in the UK. It is likely that most cancers evolve from a polyp that gradually becomes more and more dysplastic, with the progressive accumulation of somatic mutations. Although 75% of CRC cases are sporadic, several conditions predispose to CRC. These conditions are IBD (1% of cases), familial adenomatous polyposis (1%), hereditary non-polyposis CRC (5%) and family history (18%). If there is no family history of CRC, then the risk of developing it by the age of 79 years is 4%. If there is one first-degree relative over the age of 45 who is affected, the risk is 9%; with two it becomes 16% and with one relative less than 45 years of age, 15%. NSAIDs may protect against CRC, as might a high-fibre diet. Red meats, animal fats and smoking seem to enhance risk.

The majority of cancers occur in the distal colon with 60% in the rectum and sigmoid. Approximately 18% of tumours are found in the caecum and ascending colon. The remainder (22%) are distributed fairly evenly between. Several studies looking at tumour site have documented that the percentage of tumours occurring in the more proximal bowel appears to be increasing. This shift may be partly be explained by an ageing population who are more prone to developing right-sided tumours. In the future, screening may further alter the distribution of advanced tumours. Distal precancerous polyps and tumours will be identified by flexible sigmoidoscopy with synchronous

[13] Hughes, Gut (1969) 10: 336–344.

pathology in the more proximal bowel identified by subsequent colonoscopy. If flexible sigmoidoscopy is used alone then more proximal lesions will be missed until they become symptomatic or present with positive faecal occult blood. Both left- and right-sided lesions can cause pain, but left-sided lesions tend to cause bleeding, altered bowel habit and obstruction, whereas right-sided lesions are more likely to cause an isolated iron deficiency anaemia. Rectal lesions may cause tenesmus.

Any patient found to have a polyp or malignancy in the distal colon should undergo colonoscopic assessment of the whole bowel to identify synchronous lesions in the proximal colon. A CT scan of the abdomen and pelvis should also be arranged to assess disease spread. Local disease is managed surgically with adjuvant radiotherapy being dependent on local disease spread. Neoadjuvant radiotherapy prior to surgery is of benefit for some rectal lesions. If there are distant hepatic metastases, chemotherapy with 5-fluouracil, folinic acid and oxaliplatin is often the only option. Newer anti-angiogenesis agents (bevacizumab – a monoclonal antibody against vascular endothelial growth factor) are in the ascendancy and may improve prognosis to around the 20-month mark, although NICE is unpersuaded (see Chapter Thirteen). Some centres resect isolated hepatic metastases with an acceptable 5-year survival. Finding the correct balance between aggressive and sometimes unpleasant therapy and a conservative, palliative approach is vital, but often difficult.

As already alluded to, adenomatous polyps have malignant potential. When found, they must be removed. Most polyps are amenable to endoscopic therapy. Lesions are often small enough for a simple 'hot biopsy' – passing an electric current through the forceps producing heat. If larger, but pedunculated, a 'hot snare' is often effective. Large sessile polyps may have to be removed surgically if they cannot be removed endoscopically with endoscopic mucosal resection or by laser therapy. Endoscopic mucosal resection involves the injection of saline and epinephrine underneath a polyp prior to its snare-based removal.

Anaemia

The British Society of Gastroenterology (BSG) has issued guidelines on the management of iron deficiency anaemia.[14] Although generally useful, they are a touch didactic (as is often the way with guidelines), and a patient's history and anxiety levels may lead to a different approach. The guidance is summarized below.

---

[14] Guidelines for the management of iron deficiency anaemia, 2005 (www.bsg.org.uk)

If a patient who is less than 50 years of age has evidence of iron deficiency (low ferritin, microcytosis or hypochromia) but is not anaemic, then the advice is simply to give a course of oral iron therapy until 3 months after normalization of iron stores. Follow up bloods ensure anaemia does not ensue. If a patient is over 50 years of age, or if they are anaemic, the next step is coeliac serology. If this is positive, then a confirmatory small bowel biopsy should be undertaken. If negative, and the patient is a pre-menopausal woman, then upper and lower GI investigations are only performed in the presence of symptoms or of a positive family history: without symptoms, she should be given a course of iron and investigated only if she becomes transfusion dependent. If the patient is post-menopausal or male, then a 'top and tail' or 'double whammy' should be performed (our choice of words rather than those of the BSG). This involves an upper GI endoscopy and either colonoscopy or a barium enema. The major advantage of colonoscopy over barium enema is the potential for an early tissue diagnosis, avoiding the indignity of 2 tests, should a barium enema prove positive. However, waiting lists for colonoscopy are often longer. Some centres will complement a barium enema with a flexible sigmoidoscopy, as the sigmoid colon can be difficult to evaluate with barium alone. These investigations are often negative, in which case, dietary advice and a 3–6-month course of iron replacement are advised, with further investigations only becoming necessary if the patient's anaemia returns.

When an aetiology is identified, the commonest causes of GI blood loss are aspirin or NSAID use (10–15%), colonic carcinoma (5–10%), gastric carcinoma (5%), benign gastric ulceration (5%) and angiodysplasia (5%). The commonest causes of malabsorption are coeliac disease (4–6%), gastrectomy (< 5%) and H. pylori colonization (< 5%). The commonest causes of non-GI blood loss are menstruation (20–30%) and blood donation (5%).

The other variety of anaemia encountered by the gastroenterologist is megaloblastic anaemia caused by vitamin B12 or folic acid deficiency. B12 and folic acid are vital for normal erythrocyte development and deficiency leads to dyserythropoiesis and a macrocytic anaemia. B12 is absorbed in the terminal ileum, folic acid in the jejunum. B12 requires intrinsic factor for absorption. Intrinsic factor is produced by the gastric parietal cells and binds B12, allowing its absorption in the terminal ileum. Deficiency of intrinsic factor is often caused by autoimmune destruction of the parietal cells. Pernicious anaemia is related to other autoimmune conditions and is associated with blue eyes and premature greying. Antibody tests have now made the elegant Schilling test redundant.

After taking a dietary and medical history, a pragmatic approach for patients with B12 deficiency is to test for intrinsic factor and parietal cell antibodies, and to perform a coeliac screen (as villous atrophy can affect the terminal ileum). If the antibody profile suggests pernicious anaemia, the patient can simply have their B12 replaced. If the antibody profile suggests coeliac disease, or if the tests are negative, then an upper GI endoscopy should be undertaken. Gastric atrophy would be suggestive of pernicious anaemia. The next step would be a barium follow-through or colonoscopy with ileal intubation in those patients with symptoms of pain or bloating.

Important causes of B12 deficiency are poor intake (especially in vegans), pernicious anaemia, gastrectomy, diseases of the terminal ileum (Crohn's disease, TB, lymphoma, coeliac disease), *Diphyllobothrium latum* (the fish tapeworm) and removal of the terminal ileum at the hands of the surgeons. Females taking the oral contraceptive pill frequently have low levels of circulating B12 but normal tissue concentrations. Important causes of folic acid deficiency are poor intake (fruit and vegetables contain folic acid, which is removed by over-boiling), diseases of the jejunum (coeliac disease, Crohn's disease), bacterial overgrowth, surgical resection, increased requirement (pregnancy) and anti-metabolites (chemotherapy).

Replacement of folic acid is by mouth and that of B12 either by injection or orally at high dose. Folic acid must not be prescribed until a B12 level is known, as administration of folic acid in the presence of B12 deficiency can precipitate subacute combined degeneration of the cord.

Acute diarrhoea

Diarrhoea is the passage of loose or liquid stools more than 3 times daily, and/or a stool volume greater than 200 g in 24 h. Diarrhoea can be lethal. Indeed, infective diarrhoea accounts for approximately 11 million childhood deaths worldwide each year.[15]

When managing a patient with acute diarrhoea, the knee jerk reaction is simply to put up a drip. Although this is often adequate, a slightly more rigorous approach involves obtaining an underlying diagnosis, assessing diarrhoea severity, and treating the cause of the diarrhoea, whilst synchronously resuscitating the patient. Colitis must always be considered, because patients with colitis can go on to suffer toxic colonic dilatation, perforation and death.

The history should include a description of the stool, with particular emphasis on the presence of blood and mucus suggesting a colitis. Enquiry should be made into risk factors such as recent foreign travel, contacts with

---

[15] Parashar *et al.* Bulletin WHO (2003) 81: 236.

others affected by diarrhoea, consumption of potentially dubious food and recent changes in medication (such as proton pump inhibitors and NSAIDs – both of which can produce a microscopic colitis). A history of recently stopping smoking, a family history of inflammatory bowel disease (IBD), arthralgia, mouth ulcers or gritty eyes should raise the possibility of underlying IBD. Other important indicators of severity such as abdominal pain, constitutional symptoms and frequency of defaecation should be recorded.

Examination extends this assessment by gaining further information on constitutional state, abdominal tenderness and diagnostic clues such as arthropathy, circinate balanitis, erythema nodosum and iritis: admittedly a hunt only for the more patient physician.

Blood tests help to assess severity, abdominal X-ray identifies toxic dilatation and bowel oedema, and rigid sigmoidoscopy assesses the colonic mucosa both macro- and microscopically. The mandatory 3-stool cultures, and blood cultures (in the feverish patient), can identify an organism. Looking for *Clostridium difficile* toxin is imperative, particularly following recent antibiotics.

The commonest causes of acute diarrhoea are infective gastroenteritis (including *C. difficile*), IBD, drugs and constipation with overflow diarrhoea. More esoteric causes include bowel ischaemia, coeliac disease, malignancy, pancreatic insufficiency and endocrine or neuroendocrine disorders, all of which should be borne in mind if initial investigations are negative and severe symptoms persist. The management of drug-induced diarrhoea is simply to stop any offending agent and that of overflow diarrhoea, to prescribe laxatives and enemas.

Viral causes of gastroenteritis include Echo, Norwalk and adenoviruses. The latter tends to cause a general viral illness with upper respiratory tract involvement initially. Norwalk virus is the winter vomiting virus. It is caught by inhalation, making local epidemics in places such as hospitals common. Management of these conditions is supportive and preventative. Preventative management involves the isolation of cases and the rapid removal of egestia.

Bacterial causes of gastroenteritis include *Salmonella, Campylobacter, Staph aureus, Bacillus cereus, Yersinia, E. coli, Vibrio cholerae* and *Clostridium difficile*. *Shigella, Salmonella, E. coli, Campylobacter* and *C. difficile* can cause colitis. *Salmonella* is usually acquired by eating contaminated poultry, eggs or beef. *Campylobacter* is the commonest bacterial cause of diarrhoea worldwide and is transmitted by the faeco-oral route. It has interesting associations with Guillain-Barré and Reiter's syndromes. *Staph aureus* exerts its effects by toxin production. The toxin is quick to work and patients tend to vomit within hours of ingestion. An outbreak in one college of Cambridge University occurred after one of the kitchen hands contaminated food by mistakenly dropping his infected plaster in it. *E. coli* has many strains. The 0157/verotoxin producing strain is of particular interest as it can lead to haemolytic uraemic syndrome due to endothelial toxicity. *Bacillus cereus* is classically caught from contaminated rice with reheated takeaways often to blame. Cholera causes very watery diarrhoea, as the toxin leads to excessive small bowel secretions. It often occurs in situations when infected faeces contaminate water supplies.

Clostridium difficile colonizes the bowel as part of normal gut flora in 2–3% of adults and up to 70% of children. The normal gut flora attenuate *C. difficile* toxicity through competitive inhibition. Broad-spectrum antibiotics can destroy this equilibrium and allow the *C. difficile* to become pathogenic, causing pseudomembranous colitis. In this situation, *C. difficile* can spread rapidly via the faeco-oral route. In addition, because it is spore forming, *C. difficile* can persist effectively in the external environment. Interestingly, alcohol hand rub is insufficient to clean the skin after contact with *C. difficile* due to the presence of spores. There is no substitute for good old-fashioned hand washing in this situation.

Amoebi, such as *Entamoebi histiolytica*, can cause diarrhoea and should be considered in the returning traveller.

The mainstay of treatment for gastroenteritis is supportive. But for the treatment of *C. difficile*, antibiotic treatment is controversial. It often has no effect on complications or duration of symptoms and can prolong a patient's infectivity. Certainly, if there is suspicion of bacteriaemia and sepsis then antibiotics (ciprofloxacin being a reasonable choice in the first instance) are indicated. In addition, erythromycin shortens illness duration and shedding in *Campylobacter* enteritis, trimethoprim shortens the duration and shedding of *Shigella* (but does not prevent complications) and doxycycline helps to prevent the spread of cholera if both patient and contacts are treated. However, antibiotics appear to increase the likelihood of haemolytic uraemic syndrome in *E. coli* 0157 infection and prolong carrier state and risk of relapse in *Salmonella*.

It is often difficult to decide on how aggressive fluid support should be. If a patient has mild diarrhoea (1 to 5 stools per day), then oral fluids are usually adequate. If more than this, then intravenous supplementation is likely warranted.

Colitis is always a worry in the context of acute diarrhoea as it can progress to toxic dilatation and perforation. Patients with colitis should be carefully observed. Markers of severity are shown overleaf. Loperamide and other antidiarrhoeals should be avoided as they promote toxic dilatation and increase the chance of perforation.

Markers of severity of colitis
Stool frequency > 6 per day
Pyrexia or tachycardia
Haemoglobin < 10 g/dl
Toxic dilatation on abdominal film
Diffuse abdominal tenderness

As the challenge presented by *C. difficile* has grown, so has the range of specific treatments. Asymptomatic carriers do not require eradication. If diarrhoea is mild then cessation of the causative antibiotic may be the only necessary treatment. Otherwise, cessation of the antibiotic and metronidazole (oral or intravenous) or oral vancomycin therapy is indicated. Nearly all patients respond to this intervention, although up to 50% of patients relapse. Rarely, a toxic megacolon necessitates surgical intervention. Novel treatments for *C. difficile* include faecal transplantation (usually the stool of a related donor will be transferred by means of small bowel enema), intravenous immunoglobulin, cholestyramine (which binds toxins A and B), Brewer's yeast, bioactive yoghurt drinks and, in severe unresponsive disease, even steroids. Definitive evidence for these approaches does not exist. PPIs and chemotherapeutic agents may predispose to *C. difficile*. If diarrhoea persists despite appropriate therapy, a sigmoidoscopy should be performed in the first instance to investigate for an alternative aetiology.

Chronic diarrhoea[16]

Chronic diarrhoea is one of the commonest reasons for referral to a gastroenterology clinic. It is estimated to have a prevalence of between 4 and 5%. Although rather laborious, knowledge of its assessment is therefore important. The initial history attempts to get a handle – and only a handle – on whether the diarrhoea is functional or organic, and if organic, whether it is malabsorptive or colonic. An organic cause is suggested by diarrhoea that is continuous, nocturnal and of less than 3 months' duration. The absence of these, and symptoms compatible with the Rome 2 criteria (shown in the table overleaf) suggest functional diarrhoea.[17] The Rome 2 criteria are abdominal

---

[16] Guidelines for the Investigation of Chronic Diarrhoea 2nd Ed, 2003 (www.bsg.org.uk)

[17] Thompson *et al.* Gut (1999) 45 Supplement 2: 43–47.

pain or discomfort for 12 or more weeks in the past 12 months with two of: relief by defaecation; change in stool frequency and change in stool consistency. Malabsorptive diarrhoea classically causes malodorous and pale (steatorrhoeic) stools. Colonic diarrhoea causes liquid stool with mucous and/or blood.

Rome 2 criteria for functional diarrhoea

Abdominal pain or discomfort for ≥ 12 weeks in the last 12 months with two of:

- relief by defaecation
- change in stool frequency
- change in stool consistency

A comprehensive history and examination is key. A family history may point to coeliac disease or colonic cancer, and previous surgery to bacterial overgrowth or malabsorption. A drug history should be taken as NSAIDs, antihypertensives, PPIs, alcohol and antibiotics are all associated with loose stool. A past medical history of pancreatic disease, diabetes, thyroid disease or systemic sclerosis may be pertinent. A recent travel history may point to an infective causation. Anaemia, clubbing, lymphadenopathy, the presence of a goitre, pyoderma gangrenosum, dermatitis herpetiformis, abdominal masses and hepatosplenomegaly should all be sought on examination. General nutritional status is also important.

A standard panel of investigations should be undertaken to include a full blood count, liver function tests, C-reactive protein, ESR, calcium, vitamin B12, folic acid, iron studies, thyroid function tests, glucose and coeliac serology. The stool should be sent for microscopy, culture and evaluation for presence of fat (if malabsorption is considered likely).

If the history points towards a functional bowel disorder, the basic investigations are normal and the patient is less than 45 years old, then the diagnosis of an irritable bowel syndrome (IBS) is likely. Appropriate follow up prevents more sinister pathology from being missed. It is often the case, however, that this group of patients is exceedingly anxious and worried about underlying pathology, notably cancer. Basic investigations may not allay concerns, and in this circumstance, further negative investigations are often helpful. It is difficult to strike a balance between over-investigation and reassuringly providing a clean bill of health, but a frank discussion with the patient and the setting of an investigative ceiling is usually beneficial.

If the history, examination and basic investigations point towards an organic aetiology, then further investigation depends on the likely cause of the diarrhoea.

If it is felt to be malabsorptive, then the small bowel and pancreas should be investigated. If it is felt to be colonic, then unsurprisingly the colon is investigated. Of course, it is often difficult to distinguish the two, in which case the two can be investigated simultaneously.

The small bowel can be visualized both macro- and microscopically by means of an upper GI endoscopy and ileoscopy after colonoscopy, and radiologically with a barium follow through. Investigation of possible bacterial overgrowth with a hydrogen breath test can be helpful, as can a jejunal aspirate and culture. A therapeutic trial of metronidazole has its place. Enteroscopy, whereby the small bowel is investigated endoscopically (often with a paediatric colonoscope), is a difficult and sometimes uncomfortable investigation. The recent emergence of capsule enteroscopy is an advance, but comes without the benefit of biopsy and can lead to small bowel obstruction in stricturing Crohn's disease. Faecal elastase assesses pancreatic exocrine function and a CT pancreas is the initial test for macroscopic anomalies prior to a more detailed assessment with magnetic resonance cholangiopancreatography (MRCP). Colonic investigation is undertaken by means of sigmoidoscopy, colonoscopy, barium enema and CT colon according to local preferences and expertise.

If these investigations do not yield a diagnosis, the diarrhoea is suspected to be of a very high volume, the diarrhoea is suspected to be fictitious or there is a suspicion of laxative abuse, then inpatient assessment can be helpful. A stool frequency chart should be commenced and the stool weight recorded over a 24-h period. The patient should then be fasted for 24–48 h and observations continued. If putting a patient nil by mouth and onto a drip relieves the diarrhoea, functional disease is most likely. If there is genuine diarrhoea (which there often is not) which continues despite fasting, then stool and urine can be sent for laxative analysis. A gut hormone profile should also be sent (serum gastrin and VIP, and urinary 5-HIAA).

A small but significant group of patients with diarrhoea will have had a cholecystectomy prior to the onset of symptoms. Bile salt malabsorption can occur and the prescription of cholestyramine can evoke a miraculous response where all other strategies have failed. A further group of patients, particularly those with a structurally abnormal small bowel or dysmotility, will have small bowel bacterial overgrowth. Short courses of antibiotics such as metronidazole or tetracycline are effective but may need repeating from time to time.

Chronic constipation

Colonic neoplasms, particularly those in the distal colon can lead to constipation. An associated history of weight loss, rectal bleeding and relatively new but gradually progressive symptoms would be concerning, as would a palpable mass, cachexia, anaemia and raised inflammatory markers. Patients in these categories merit urgent investigation by means of colonoscopy or barium enema.

Other colonic disorders such as stricturing secondary to diverticulitis, colonic adhesions and IBD are important causes of constipation. IBD can lead to constipation proximal to an inflamed segment, which may necessitate the use of laxatives during a relapse.

Inadequate dietary fibre and dehydration are very common causes of constipation: simple dietary advice is the solution. Drugs are also common causes. Opiates are often to blame, and can lead to a vicious cycle whereby opiates lead to constipation, which leads to pain, an upping of the opiate dose and worsening constipation. The cycle needs to be broken, although this can be easier said than done. Other common drug causes are aluminium containing antacids, iron supplements, anti-cholinergics and anti-depressants.

On account of painful defaecation, ano-rectal disorders (such as fissuring, stenosis, haemorrhoids, anterior muscle prolapse and tumours) can result in constipation. Equally, pelvic floor dysfunction, usually a complication of difficult childbirth, can be to blame.

Endocrine and metabolic disorders that may cause constipation include hypothyroidism, hypercalcaemia, hypokalaemia, uraemia and diabetes: the latter through autonomic neuropathy. Other neurological disorders such as paraplegia, cord compression and multiple sclerosis are important causes, as is depression. IBS can be 'constipation predominant'.

One man's sluggish bowel may be very different to another's. A description of what the patient really means by 'constipation' is vital. Sometimes a patient is worried that they 'go too infrequently' and may be delighted to hear that having movements just 3 times a week is considered normal. Patients can define constipation as 'difficulty passing stool', which when it comes is normal. This suggests an ano-rectal problem. Any psycho-social stressors are very important. There is a high prevalence of past or recent physical abuse in the constipation-predominant IBS group.

After examination, basic investigations include blood tests for metabolic and endocrine causes and an assessment of the bowel (endoscopic or barium). If these are normal, it is then useful to assess bowel transit with radio-opaque markers and serial abdominal films. Some centres perform ano-rectal manometry to diagnose pelvic floor dysfunction.

If a cause for constipation is found, this should be treated, alongside the generic management of constipation. Biofeedback can be helpful in the management of pelvic floor dysfunction. This involves returning the physiological defeacation reflex to normality. To do this, visual and verbal feedback techniques are used to achieve anal relaxation, ano-rectal co-ordination and sensory conditioning: the mind boggles.

Constipation secondary to IBS should initially be managed with general measures such as eating plenty of fibre, maintaining hydration and taking regular exercise. The next step is a bulking agent such as Fybogel, then an osmotic laxative (perhaps lactulose) and finally, a stimulant, such as senna. Laxatives should only be used intermittently. This is especially pertinent for stimulant laxatives that can damage the enteric nervous system, leading to a 'cathartic megacolon' and worsening constipation. Occasionally, inpatient treatment to 'purge the colon' is helpful. This involves the use of strong laxatives (such as Picolax) along with enemas, much as when preparing a patient for colonoscopy. Such measures should only be undertaken by a specialist team as there are potential risks including perforation if an underlying pathology is present.

Inflammatory bowel disease

IBD is estimated to affect up to 0.3% of the UK population. It has a bimodal distribution, with the larger peak between 20 and 30 years of age and a more modest one between 60 and 80 years. The incidence is about one new case per 10,000 population per year, and the prevalence 4–10 per 10,000 population. 15% of patients have a relative with Crohns' disease (CD) or ulcerative colitis (UC), but the genetic influence appears less in patients with the latter.

The pathogenesis of IBD remains uncertain. Clinical and laboratory studies suggest the combination of a number of possible genetic and environmental factors including an autoimmune response to a luminal or mucosal antigen, a dysfunctional immune response to a commensal bacterium, or an infection with a pathogenic organism which remains in the intestinal tissues promoting a chronic inflammatory response. At present, it would appear that CD and UC are separate entities but Crohns' disease may well turn out to be several diseases with some common features but different outcomes, in terms of site affected, the response to treatment and the need for surgery.

Crohns' disease can affect any part of the GI tract. The commonest sites are terminal ileum (45%), colon (30%) and both (13%). Inflammation is patchy but affects the full thickness of the bowel with a lymphocytic and often granulomatous infiltrate. A positive pANCA is found in 15%. UC affects a variable amount of colon extending proximally from the rectum with occasional 'backwash' ileitis in the context of a pancolitis. The inflammation tends to be continuous but is more superficial than that found in CD, with a neutrophilic infiltrate confined to the mucosa and submucosa. pANCA positivity is found in about 70%.

IBD has several associations. Sacroileitis, ankylosing spondylitis and primary sclerosing cholangitis do not reflect disease activity. Uveitis and pyoderma gangrenosum have a modest correlation. Meanwhile, peripheral arthropathy and erythema nodosum strongly correspond with the activity of the underlying disease process.

Smoking increases the risk of CD (relative risk of 4), but protects against UC (odds ratio of 0.4), and it is not uncommon for patients to present with UC following smoking cessation. Patients with CD are more likely than the general population to have had an appendicectomy (although this may in part represent the effect of a diagnostic lead time), whereas patients with UC are less likely. NSAIDs exacerbate and activate IBD.

Investigations depend upon the presenting symptoms. Bloody diarrhoea is investigated by sigmoidoscopy or colonoscopy, right iliac fossa pain is investigated with barium follow-through or ileoscopy, and peri-anal fistulae prompt MRI scanning. Radiological investigations can detect mucosal abnormalities and structural abnormalities, but obviously cannot view the mucosa or obtain histological specimens.

Assessment of disease activity requires a combination of clinical observations and blood tests supplemented by bowel imaging. Anorexia, fever, tachycardia, and weight loss in conjunction with a low serum albumin, anaemia and raised inflammatory markers all indicate active disease. All patients should have a stool sample sent off for culture and a *Clostridium difficile* toxin assay.

Strictures cause colicky pain, mucosal inflammation causes diarrhoea (usually non-bloody) while fistulae and abscesses cause symptoms dependent upon their site. Colitis in UC tends to produce diarrhoea, cramping low abdominal pains and tenesmus.

Once a diagnosis has been made, the objective of medical management is to induce and maintain remission. The agents available are 5-ASA agents, steroids, immunomodulators, biological therapy, antibiotics and nutritional regimens.

5-ASA preparations can be given orally or rectally and the choice of formulation depends on the distribution of the disease. Rectal disease is best treated by suppositories, sigmoid disease by enemas and suppositories, and more proximal disease with oral preparations. Oral 5-ASA preparations may be activated by a change in luminal pH, breakdown by bacteria, or may simply be released over time as the tablet transits the bowel. The choice of oral ASA preparation may be tailored to the distribution of disease. Pentasa is released in a time-dependent fashion in both the small and large bowel. Asacol and

Salofalk release mesalazine at a pH of 7 and 6 respectively, resulting in drug release in the terminal ileum and beyond. Olsalazine (two ASA molecules joined by a di-azo bond) and balsalazide (a single ASA molecule bonded to an inert carrier) are both broken down by colonic bacteria, releasing ASA more distally in the colon.

Oral 5-ASA preparations are more effective in UC where they induce remission in mild to moderate disease in at least 50% of cases and decrease relapse rates from 70–80% to 20–30%.[18] For patients with CD, there is some evidence that 5-ASA preparations induce remission (number needed to treat 6–21) and can be useful in maintaining remission achieved with steroids in patients with small bowel disease.

Metronidazole and ciprofloxacin can be useful in the treatment of mild to moderate CD, particularly in patients with peri-anal disease and infective complications. Patients with stricturing disease with bacterial overgrowth will also benefit. In the long-term, patients should be monitored for the development of a sensory neuropathy.

Steroids are effective at inducing remission and can be given orally, rectally and intravenously. They should be used in the context of moderate to severe IBD. Although effective at maintaining remission, their side effect profile negates their long-term use. Newer steroid formulations such as budesonide (with an extensive first pass metabolism in the liver) can be useful in ileal CD with decreased systemic steroid side-effects.

Azathioprine or 6-mercaptopurine are used as steroid-sparing agents to maintain remission in both CD and UC but take up to 3 months to have their full effect thus requiring co-prescription with steroids for this period.

NICE provided advice on the use of infliximab in 2002.[19] Infliximab is a chimeric mouse–human antibody directed against TNF-α. It is useful in the management of carefully selected patients with CD and is being evaluated in the treatment of moderately active UC. NICE recommends the use of infliximab in patients with CD who fulfil three criteria, namely: bad Crohn's (often with systemic symptoms), resistance to other treatments (steroids and immunomodulators) and absolute or relative contraindications to surgery.

This advice is based on two trials. The ACCENT trial studied 545 patients with moderate or severe refractory CD.[20] Patients were initially treated with

---

[18] In Clinic Handbook: Gastroenterology, Wong et al. (Eds), Bios, 2002.

[19] TA040, March 2002 (www.nice.org.uk)

[20] Hanauer et al. Lancet (2002) 359: 1541–1549.

infliximab 5 mg/kg and then randomized to receive a further infusion at a dose of 5 mg/kg, or placebo at 2, 6, and 8 weeks. Thereafter, those patients receiving infliximab received 5 or 10 mg/kg every 8 weeks. Remission at 52 weeks, defined by successful weaning of steroid therapy, was achieved in 34% of patients in the 10 mg/kg group compared to 11% in the placebo arm. The second trial looked at patients with fistulating CD.[21] All patients received an induction regimen of infliximab 5 mg/kg at weeks 0, 2, and 6. At Week 14, patients were randomized based on clinical response, defined as a ≥50% reduction from baseline in the number of draining fistulae at both weeks 10 and 14, to receive maintenance dosing with either infliximab 5 mg/kg or placebo every 8 weeks. Patients who did not respond to the initial 3-dose induction regimen were randomised separately from these patients. At week 14, 65% (177/273) of patients were in fistula response. Patients randomized to infliximab maintenance had a longer time to loss of fistula response compared to the placebo maintenance group (>40 weeks versus 14 weeks, respectively). At Week 54, 38% (33/87) of infliximab-treated patients had no draining fistulae compared with 22% (20/90) of placebo-treated patients ($p = 0.02$). The fistulae often slowly recurred, and the role of maintenance therapy needs to be fully established.

Ciclosporin has a role in acute colitis, when intravenous steroids fail to induce a rapid remission. It should only be prescribed by specialists with an interest in IBD, due to the potential risks associated with infection and delays in surgery.

Elemental and polymeric diets can induce a remission in CD affecting the small bowel, but are not as effective as steroids. They do however improve patient nutrition and ease symptoms in those with severe stricturing disease.

Surgery is required in the management of some patients with IBD. Resection or stricturoplasty is required in patients with CD and small bowel involvement where medical treatment fails. In all cases, preservation of bowel is important to reduce the risk of a short gut syndrome at a later date. Patients with CD and fistulae may require laying open of fistulae, placement of seton sutures, drainage of abscesses and occasionally, formation of a stoma in order that medical treatment can be optimized. A close relationship between the physician and surgeon is essential. Patients with acute fulminant UC, or disease refractory to medical therapy, will require colectomy which although a major operation, is curative. Although an ileostomy is formed at the time of surgery, many patients go on to have an ileo-anal pouch formed, thus removing the

---

[21] Present *et al.* NEJM (1999) 340: 1398–1405.

need for a stoma in the long-term with the attendant psychological complications. Colectomy may improve small joint arthropathy associated with UC but has no effect on axial arthritides (sacro-ileitis and ankylosing spondylitis).

The setting in which patients are managed depends upon the presentation. If a patient presents with severe disease, then they must be investigated and managed in hospital. Truelove and Witts' criteria determine severe colitis: these are, bloody stool frequency of more than 6 stools per day with one or more of: pulse over 90, temperature greater than 37.8, haemoglobin of less than 10.5, and ESR more than 30. For non-colonic CD, high fever, persistent vomiting, evidence of obstruction, rebound tenderness, cachexia or evidence of an abscess necessitate admission. These criteria can be used for both first presentation and also for the patient with known IBD. When a patient is admitted, the activity and distribution of disease need to be determined and then, the disease needs to be controlled.

With ulcerative colitis, regular examination of the abdomen and of the vital signs, stool frequency and daily blood tests allows an objective measure of severity.

Assessing disease severity in acute ulcerative colitis

Feature	Mild	Moderate	Severe
Motions/day	<4	4-6	>6
Rectal bleeding	Small	Moderate	Large
Temperature	Apyrexial	Intermediate	>37.8°C on 2 of 4 days
Pulse rate	Normal	Intermediate	>90bpm
Haemoglobin	>11 g/dl	Intermediate	<10.5g/dl
ESR	<20mm/hr	Intermediate	>30mm/hr

A careful endoscopy (perforation is easy) allows a visual assessment of the colonic mucosa along with a biopsy, for histological confirmation. Abdominal films assess the extent of disease and pick up toxic dilatation (they should be performed daily until the disease is clearly settling).

The mainstay of the initial treatment of colitis is intravenous, and in some units rectal, hydrocortisone, along with heparin to reduce the risks of DVT (thromboembolism is a major risk in acute colitis). ASA compounds are avoided as they can occasionally be associated with nausea, vomiting and diarrhoea, which may cause difficulty in assessing response to treatment. A stool frequency of greater than 8 per day or a CRP over 45 mg/l on day 3 of parenteral steroid treatment suggests a likely need for colectomy that admission (occurring in around 85% of patients). At this stage, ciclosporin rescue therapy can be considered: if ineffective, colectomy is currently the only option. In 70% of cases of acute colitis, remission is obtained and patients can be discharged on a reducing course of oral prednisolone and 5-ASA with early outpatient review.

Inpatient management of CD depends on the site and type of the disease. In general, patients are managed with intravenous fluids to correct dehydration, intravenous hydrocortisone, oral metronidazole and oral ciprofloxacin. Investigations should include an abdominal ultrasound and a CT scan if ileal or colonic disease is suspected, a flexible sigmoidoscopy if diarrhoea is a prominent symptom, and a pelvic MRI in the presence of perineal disease.

Irritable bowel syndrome

IBS is a functional disorder in which there is abdominal pain that is related to defaecation in association with a change in bowel habit. IBS tends to fall into constipation predominant, diarrhoea predominant or an alternating pattern. It is thought to affect 5% of men and 13% of women in the United Kingdom and it accounts for around 50% of all gastroenterology referrals, although less than half of those with symptoms consistent with IBS seek the advice of their GP, who then refers only 20% of these patients. The diagnosis is likely when the Rome 2 criteria (which were discussed earlier) are satisfied.

The pathophysiology of IBS is poorly understood, as is clear from the vast range of putative explanations offered up: it is likely to be multi-factorial. There may be increased visceral sensitivity and either heightened or abrogated autonomic motor activity. This may in turn be due to disordered transmission at the level of either the enteric nervous system itself, or the spinal cord. In addition, the brain may process afferent enteric information incorrectly. Abnormal digestion and absorption may be important, and carbohydrate intolerance and functional bile salt malabsorption might contribute to symptoms. IBS can complicate an episode of gastroenteritis. Underlying psychological symptoms are common in IBS and somatization as a result of these is likely to be important. The incidence of major adverse life events is high in this group of patients.

Diagnosis depends upon whether diarrhoea or constipation predominates, or both co-exist. The investigation of each has already been discussed. To re-iterate, in the face of a classic history and normal basic investigations, there is no need to subject a young patient to invasive tests. If, however, there are any worrying features then full investigation is warranted. In addition, investigations are often (justifiably) performed to provide reassurance so that patients can rationalize symptoms.

Successful management always involves engaging with the patient. Exploration of the patient's agenda is important, followed by explanation and reassurance. Symptomatic treatments are often efficacious. Examples are anti-spasmodics (such as mebeverine or hyosine) for pain, loperamide for diarrhoea, and laxatives and fibre for constipation. Diet diaries are helpful in an attempt to identify aggravating factors such that they can be avoided. A therapeutic trial of cholestyramine to bind bile salts may be helpful for diarrhoea-predominant IBS. Anti-depressants including amitryptiline, venlafaxine and citalopram have proven efficacy, although whether the mode of action is central or enteric is unclear. Serotonin is an important gut neurotransmitter, and there is some benefit in its modulation. The $5HT_4$ partial agonist, tegaserod, has some benefit in constipation-predominant IBS, presumably due to an improvement in peristalsis. The $5HT_3$ antagonist, alosetron, slows colonic transit and elevates the sensory threshold. Unfortunately, alosetron has been associated with gut ischaemia and has therefore been withdrawn! Its efficacy is prompting development of more drugs of this class.

Patients with bloating as their main symptom may benefit from a diet reducing the intake of wheat products, brassicas (broccoli and such) and legumes. These foodstuffs contain carbohydrates which may be broken down by colonic bacteria producing gas, distension, and pain.

Coeliac disease

Coeliac disease, caused by gluten sensitivity, is the commonest cause of malabsorption in people of northwest European descent. The prevalence in Great Britain has been put at between 0.5 and 1 %. There is a genetic predisposition and linkage to several HLA polymorphisms has been found, the commonest being HLA B8 DQW2.

Patients may present at any age. There is one peak between 9 months and 3 years, another in the third decade and a smaller one between the fifth and sixth decades. Presentations are varied. The commonest are with gastrointestinal symptoms (predominantly diarrhoea and abdominal pain) and the complications of malabsorption. These include deficiencies of iron, B12 and folate, weight loss and osteoporosis. Several conditions are associated with coeliac disease including dermatitis herpetiformis, autoimmune thyroid disease, primary biliary cirrhosis, primary sclerosing cholangitis, autoimmune liver disease, type 1 diabetes, arthritis, microscopic colitis and Down's syndrome.

Diagnosis is based upon serology and duodenal biopsy. Recently, an ELISA for IgA/IgG to anti-tissue transglutaminase (TTG) has become available that has a reported sensitivity of almost 100% and a specificity of 95-97%, although anti-endomysial antibodies are more commonly measured. As up to 4% of patients with coeliac disease have selective IgA deficiency and TTG and anti-endomysial antibody tests rely on IgA being present, IgA levels should be measured at the time of testing. Anti-gliadin antibodies, although less sensitive, are not therefore entirely redundant as, being IgG themselves, they remain reliable in the presence of IgA deficiency. Histological changes in coeliac disease include an increase in intraepithelial lymphocytes, crypt hypertrophy and villous atrophy.

Management is with a gluten-free diet and specific treatment of the complications. Gluten is found predominantly in wheat, barley and rye. Adhering to a gluten-free diet is difficult and dietetic, gastroenterological and Coeliac Society support are helpful. DEXA scanning picks up osteoporosis: this should be treated appropriately. Any dietary deficiencies should also be corrected.

When the condition is stable, annual follow-up is recommended. This is (perhaps unfashionably) for patient support but also to check that the disease is adequately controlled with screening tests for malabsorption (full blood count, B12, folate, iron, calcium, liver tests). The BSG advises an initial follow-up biopsy to ensure that the villous atrophy has resolved off gluten. Many physicians will only biopsy if symptoms remain, but it should be kept in mind that there are other causes of villous atrophy including tropical sprue, HIV and giardiasis.

Some patients develop coeliac disease that is apparently refractory to dietary modification. Although compliance is often the problem, the possibility of another diagnosis or a complication (such as ulcerative jejunitis or small bowel lymphoma) should be kept in mind. Truly refractory coeliac disease can be managed with prednisolone and azathioprine.

The complications of untreated coeliac disease are pretty staggering (as shown below) but after 5 years of successful treatment, the risks rescind to baseline.[22]

Sequelae of untreated coeliac disease

Condition	Relative risk
Small bowel lymphoma	60 to 876
Small bowel adenocarcinoma	7 to 240
Mouth and pharyngeal cancer	9.7
Oesophageal carcinoma	12.3
Non-Hodgkin's lymphoma	42.7

[22] In Clinic Handbook: Gastroenterology, Wong et al. (Eds), Bios, 2002.

Nutrition

Up to 40% of patients admitted acutely to hospital are undernourished and their nutritional status tends to deteriorate further during their inpatient stay. Loss of body weight leads to apathy, depression, fatigue and sadly, a loss of the will to recover. Poor nutrition leads to increased risk of chest infection (perhaps because of respiratory muscle fatigue), impaired cardiac function, impaired immune function and longer hospital stays. This results in substantial health care costs. In the United Kingdom, the daily budget for a patient's food is between £2.20 and £3.70, to include three meals, snacks and drinks. Optimizing nutrition on such a shoestring is a challenge.

Assessment of nutritional state is important. It is often performed rather poorly. There are no absolute tests of nutritional status, but taken together, the following provide a good guide, being useful in both assessing nutritional status and monitoring response to treatment. The first measure is that of general appearance. Assessment is often subliminal, but specifics are a thin appearance, unusual prominence of the underlying bones and muscle wasting. Most physicians can remember how to calculate the Body Mass Index and like all skills, this should be practised. Hypoalbuminaemia (which should be confirmed by blood testing) is most commonly a reflection of underlying infection, appearing only in the very advanced stages of malnutrition and should not be the first trigger for a look at the patient's nutritional state. Mid-arm circumference provides an estimate of muscle and fat stores. Triceps skin-fold thickness provides an indirect assessment of fat stores. Centile charts can be used for stratification.

Malabsorption and nutritional deficiencies

Deficiency	Symptoms, signs and test abnormalities
Iron	Microcytic anaemia, angular stomatitis and glossitis
Vitamin A	Dry eyes and skin, night blindness and keratomalacia
Vitamin D	Proximal muscle weakness, bone pain and osteomalacia
Vitamin K	Elevated prothrombin time and bleeding tendency
Vitamin B1 (thiamine)	Beriberi: Wernicke's encephalopathy (nystagmus, lateral rectus palsy and altered mental state) and Korsakov's psychosis (retrograde amnesia, impaired learning and confabulation)
Vitamin B2 (riboflavin)	Inflamed oral mucous membranes, angular stomatitis, glossitis and normocytic anaemia
Vitamin B3 (niacin)	Pellagra (photosensitive dermatitis, diarrhoea and dementia)

Continued

Malabsorption and nutritional deficiencies—cont'd

Deficiency	Symptoms, signs and test abnormalities
Vitamin B6 (pyridoxine)	Peripheral neuropathy and sideroblastic anaemia
Vitamin B12	Megaloblastic, macrocytic anaemia, glossitis and subacute combined degeneration of the cord (degeneration of both the corticospinal tracts and the dorsal columns)
Folic acid	Megaloblastic, macrocytic anaemia and glossitis
Vitamin C	Scurvy, anaemia and osteoporosis

If a specific vitamin deficiency is uncovered, then this should be treated, and of course empirically treated in the case of vitamin B1 in those with alcohol dependency.

The BSG has provided guidelines on inpatient nutrition.[23] Assuming that feeding is felt to be in a patient's best interests (ethically speaking), then the groups of patients who require nutritional support are: patients who are severely malnourished *per se* (a BMI of less than 18.5 is a useful marker), patients who have had more than 10% unplanned weight loss in the last 3 to 6 months and patients who are acutely unwell and unlikely to eat, or who have not eaten for more than 5 days.

A multidisciplinary team approach is sensible. Nutritional support is given enterally wherever possible. If this can be done by mouth then it should be, if not then by nasogastric tube in the short-term or by gastrostomy or jejunostomy in the longer-term. The long term use of nasogastric tubes is made difficult by displacement, blockage and occasionally worse. Feeding is by polymeric diet containing vitamins and minerals, energy in the form of carbohydrate and fat, nitrogen in the form of protein, and water and electrolytes. The amount of feed is tailored to a patient's nutritional and disease state.

Complications include regurgitation and aspiration, diarrhoea and metabolic disturbances. The latter can be caused by the refeeding syndrome, which is characterized by hypophosphataemia, hypokalaemia, hypomagnesaemia and altered glucose metabolism. Patients particularly at risk are those with complete starvation of more than 7 days duration and with a 20% loss of body weight in less than 3 months. Electrolyte disturbances can be dangerous, even fatal. Indeed, it was the phenomenon of refeeding that caused the deaths of

---

[23] Guidelines for enteral feeding in adult hospital patients, 2003 (www.bsg.org.uk)

many of those liberated from the Concentration Camps. All patients should have their electrolytes checked and corrected before feeding, and monitored during feeding. Those patients particularly at risk should have their feed started slowly, building up to the full rate over a week. Most dietetic departments and pharmacies produce a protocol between them.

One does well to remember that overall prognosis following gastrostomy insertion, particularly in the elderly, is often poor. Although this largely reflects underlying illness, it also reminds one that PEG insertion is not to be undertaken lightly. In a study of 674 elderly patients, mortality was 18% at 30 days, 44% at 6 months and 73% at 2 years.[24]

If a patient cannot take feed enterally, then total parenteral nutrition (TPN) via a central vein is required. Examples include major gastrointestinal surgery or intestinal failure secondary to multiple bowel resections for Crohn's Disease. Energy is supplied through glucose and a fat emulsion, and nitrogen through amino acids. Vitamins and minerals are also added, as well as heparin and corticosteroids to prevent coagulation and thrombophlebitis. Complications are common. Particular problems include line infections, line blockage and electrolyte disturbance. The latter necessitates daily blood tests. In the long-term, TPN can cause cirrhosis of the liver.

The areas of nutrition and feeding are ethical minefields. In essence, tube feeding and parenteral nutrition are medical treatments in law. Starting, stopping or withholding treatment is a medical decision, which should involve taking the wishes of the patient into account, or failing that, their 'best interests'. Discussions with relatives and carers are therefore invaluable (and advisable). Comprehensive advice on this area is provided in a leaflet produced by the General Medical Council.[25] Increasingly though, the Courts may be involved.

Screening

Many of the issues surrounding screening and surveillance in gastroenterology are unresolved. The World Health Organization has laid down several criteria that must be satisfied before a screening programme can be instituted: the condition in question has to be important; it has to have a natural history that is understood such that it can be identified at an early or pre-malignant stage; and there must be ethical, acceptable, safe and effective procedures for the detection and treatment of the condition at an early stage. In addition, there

[24] Rimon *et al.* Age Ageing (2005) 34: 353–357.

[25] www.gmc-uk.org

must be sufficient resources to institute a screening programme, which must be cost effective for the health service overall.

Screening for colorectal cancer (CRC)

In relation to CRC, there is no doubt that it is an important disease. 16,000 deaths are attributable to CRC annually in the UK. The natural history is well understood: most cancers evolve from an initial polyp that gradually becomes more and more dysplastic with the progressive accumulation of somatic mutations. This process probably takes 10–15 years. Polyps are usually treatable endoscopically, allowing for the acceptable and effective management of the pre-malignant condition. Also, 5-year survival dips markedly from the early to late stages of the disease, making early detection a real bonus: if caught at Dukes' stage A, the 5-year survival is 90%; compared with 3% for Dukes' stage D (metastatic) disease. Management of early CRC involves major surgery. However, this is acceptable given the mortality benefit that ensues. A screening test is doubtless desirable but the precise form it should take arouses much strong feeling in gastroenterological circles.

Options include colonoscopy, sigmoidoscopy, barium enema, faecal occult blood testing, faecal DNA testing and CT colonoscopy. Colonoscopy is considered by many to be the gold standard as it involves the visualization of the whole colon. However, it is expensive and moreover, it has the notable drawback of a perforation rate of 0.5%. This renders it utterly useless as a publicly funded primary screening tool.

Because CRC occurs more commonly in the distal colon, sigmoidoscopy is a possibility and its potential use in screening has been evaluated in the UK.[26] 354,262 adults between 55 and 64 years of age were approached and offered flexible sigmoidoscopy as a screening tool. Perhaps surprisingly, 55% responded and 71% of these were randomized to screening. At an initial interview, 5% of these individuals were classified as high risk and therefore referred direct for colonoscopy. Of the remainder, distal adenomas were detected in 12.1% and distal cancer in 0.3%. Most of these were Dukes' A. Patients with distal adenomas went on to have colonoscopy and a significant proportion of these had proximal (synchronous) adenomas. These figures are impressive and sigmoidoscopy has a much lower perforation rate of 1 per 1000. However, the question of whether to offer further screening to patients with a normal sigmoidoscopy at initial screening remains unresolved.

26 UFSST Investigators, Lancet (2002) 359: 1291–1300.

Faecal occult blood testing has been systematically reviewed as a screening tool and results in a 16% reduction in CRC mortality (when non-compliance is taken into account). It is relatively inexpensive, and fairly uncomplicated, with an effective 'complication rate' of 0.006% overall (as positive testing results in colonoscopy).

Currently, plans are afoot to commence population screening in the United Kingdom with faecal occult blood testing for patients aged 60–65 years. The programme is due to be rolled out nationwide by 2009. Patients with positive results will be directed to further investigation, most likely colonoscopy. New techniques such as virtual CT colonoscopy and faecal DNA testing may evolve as alternative screening tools in the future. Both techniques are non-invasive and would have greater patient acceptability than colonoscopy. Time will tell as to whether these or other investigations will become widely available and cost-effective in the future.

There are many well known risk factors for CRC, including patients with a family history of CRC, acromegaly, a genetic predisposition, primary scleros-ing cholangitis, IBD, previous CRC, ureterosigmoidostomy and known colonic adenomatosis. Such patients will require surveillance and are not to be confused with the population being offered screening.

Barrett's oesophagus

The other condition that lends itself to screening and surveillance is Barrett's oesophagus.[27] Barrett's (or 'columnar lined') oesophagus occurs where any portion of the normal squamous lining has been replaced by a metaplastic columnar epithelium, which is macroscopically apparent. A visual suspicion must be confirmed histologically. Barrett's oesophagus is a pre-malignant condition. Important clinical risk factors for progression to cancer are male gender, age > 45 years, segment length longer than 8cm, long history of reflux, early onset of symptoms, mucosal damage and uncommonly, a family history. Symptomatic control of reflux is thought to be of benefit but it is known that reflux can occur in the absence of symptoms. Sufficient acid suppression should be given to control any symptoms. Patients diagnosed with Barrett's should have the implications of the diagnosis made clear to them. The efficacy of screening for such patients is currently unproven but if the patient is agreeable, surveillance is usually offered at 2 yearly intervals. At endoscopy, quadrantic

---

[27] Guidelines for the diagnosis and management of Barrett's columnar-lined oesophagus, 2005 (www.bsg.org.uk)

biopsies should be taken at 2 cm intervals, together with biopsies of any visible lesion. A health economic model based on NHS costings estimates that a programme of 2 yearly surveillance costs £19,000 per life saved. This is comparable to other health care interventions, although some optimistic assumptions were made in the modelling. Low-grade dysplasia should be managed by extensive re-biopsy after intensive acid suppression. If low-grade dysplasia persists, then surveillance should continue at 6 monthly intervals. If high-grade dysplasia is demonstrated on two sets of biopsies, then carcinoma will be present in approximately 40% of cases and oesophagectomy in a specialist centre is recommended. In patients unfit for surgery, endoscopic ablation with argon plasma coagulation or photo dynamic therapy should be considered.

Chapter 12

Fiona McCann and Lorraine Hart

RESPIRATORY MEDICINE

Dying for a cigarette

Unlike cardiology, where the bread and butter conditions have a well-developed evidence base and are generally seen as rather trendy, respiratory medicine is much less flashy. Respiratory patients often get a raw deal from their doctors as many are assumed to have 'brought it upon themselves' by smoking. Such prejudice is unlikely to benefit either patient or physician. It is important for the general physician to understand why people smoke and to be sufficiently informed to advise patients on how best to stop.

Around 13 million people in the United Kingdom smoke and 120,000 are said to die each year in England as a result. This is despite the fact that the UK, aside from Norway, has the highest priced cigarettes in Europe. Smokers seem to find ways around this – in 2004, over 10 billion cigarettes were smuggled into the UK, depriving the Exchequer of approximately £3 billion in tax revenue (sufficient money for an additional 75,000 senior nurses).[1] Smoking increases the risk of pneumonia and pneumothorax as well as the more obvious lung conditions. The commonest time for people to start smoking is in their youth, particularly if their parents smoke. However by the time smokers reach the age of 20, 80% regret picking up the habit. The problem at this stage is that the nicotine in cigarettes is as addictive as cocaine or heroin and this addiction can take hold within 3 weeks. Smoking is a very effective drug delivery system and the nicotine peak arrives in the bloodstream within minutes. Withdrawal can be extremely unpleasant, giving rise to symptoms of anxiety, restlessness, hunger and craving.

The main problem with smoking cessation is that none of the nicotine replacement devices can deliver the drug as effectively as a cigarette can. It is

---

[1] Chief Medical Officer, Annual Reports. Crown Copyright, London, 2002 and 2004.

not, of course, nicotine itself which is harmful, rather the other noxious chemicals bound up within the cigarette, such as tar and carbon monoxide. The admission of a patient to hospital is a golden opportunity to deliver smoking cessation advice to a captive audience. Around 40–50% of all acute admissions involve smokers, of whom at least a quarter are likely to have been admitted with conditions related to their smoking. The recommended strategy for helping patients quit smoking is the 'AAAAA' plan. 'Ask' is a key part of a clinical history and it is vital to ask every patient about their smoking and to document this in the medical notes. It is useful to document not only smoking status but also a 'pack year history'. A roll-up equates to approximately two cigarettes and a cigar, three or four. Two ounces of tobacco per week is equivalent to approximately 20 cigarettes per day. 'Advise' each patient who smokes in a non-judgmental and personalized way to stop. 'Assess' the patient's willingness to stop smoking and if willing, 'assist'. Stopping smoking is done most effectively with the aid of nicotine replacement therapy (NRT). The table shows the rate of smoking cessation according to the intervention offered:[2]

Smoking cessation success rates

Intervention	Long-term abstinence (%)
No intervention – willpower only	3
Brief opportunistic advice from doctor	5
• plus NRT	10
Intensive support from specialist	10
• plus NRT	18

Given the prevalence of smoking, even brief opportunistic advice from doctors will have an impressive impact on the total number of smokers who successfully quit. The use of nicotine replacement doubles success rates and in combination with a support group, the rates are still better. NRT is available in the form of gums, inhalators, nasal sprays, sublingual tablets, lozenges and patches. There has been massive expansion in NHS stop smoking services in recent years, although their impact seems to vary dramatically between primary care trusts.[3] Side effects of NRT include sore throat, hiccups, headache, nausea and palpitations but these will all be more prominent if the

[2] West *et al.* Thorax (2000) 55: 987–999.

[3] Department of Health, Choosing Health – making healthier choices easier. Crown Copyright, London, 2004.

patient continues to smoke.[4] Patients should set themselves a 'quit date' and tell as many people about this as possible. They should then take nicotine replacement for up to 8 weeks. Caution should be taken in a patient who has unstable coronary disease or who is pregnant, particularly if the patient continues to smoke whilst on NRT. NICE guidelines do not specify how to prescribe the NRT but one common practice is use a nicotine patch for a basal nicotine level (dose dependent on number of cigarettes smoked per day) combined with a fast release 'bolus' nicotine delivery system, such as the inhalator, gum or sublingual tablets. An alternative to nicotine replacement is bupropion that may be more effective but tends to have more side effects. NICE do not recommend combining NRT with bupropion.[5]

The main hurdle to assisting patients with their smoking is that many hospitals will not allow the prescription of NRT on-formulary. This is a somewhat shortsighted view. The acute admission offers a good opportunity to highlight the dangers of smoking and often scares people into wanting to stop. Spending time with a patient only to have to tell him to visit his GP for a prescription is squandering a considerable opportunity. The alcohol withdrawal parallel–that an elective dry-out is likely to be accompanied by improved motivation and therefore success – may or may not hold true. In reality, the cost of prescribing nicotine replacement is money well spent with the cost per year of life saved considerably less than that spent on aspirin post myocardial infarction.[6] Finally, once the patient has been prescribed NRT and advised about a plan it is important to 'arrange' follow up, the fifth aspect of the AAAAA plan.

The 'AAAAA' plan

Ask
Advise
Assess
Assist
Arrange follow-up

Smoking-related diseases have had a very lowly position in the media and on the international list of research priorities until recently. Smokers often come from low socioeconomic groups with little political influence. However, times are changing and smoking cessation has been a big topic for debate in recent years.

---

[4] Molyneux, BMJ (2004) 328: 454–456.

[5] TA039 (March 2002) www.nice.org.uk

[6] Parrott *et al.* BMJ (2004) 328: 947–949.

Government strategies to reduce the burden of smoking-related diseases have been steadily incremental with the ban on television advertising in 2003, the full ban on sports sponsorship from July 2005 and now the ban on smoking in all public places in England, set to come into force in the summer of 2007. It has been shown in other countries, such as Norway and Canada, that consumption of cigarettes falls considerably when such bans are implemented.

Working out wheeze

The patient arriving in hospital short of breath or wheezy can provide a difficult diagnostic challenge. More often than not, a scattergun approach is taken involving liberal administration of bronchodilators, steroids and antibiotics. Wheezy patients will broadly separate into three groups: those with asthma, those with chronic obstructive pulmonary disease and those with another diagnosis.

Asthma is a common condition and its management is familiar to physicians. However, it continues to cause up to 1000 deaths a year in the United Kingdom.[7] Most asthmatics will have had symptoms as children that may have then remitted for a time. A small percentage will develop asthma *de novo* as adults (4–8% of those above 65 years of age).[8] Occupational exposures may be the cause of late-onset asthma on occasion and it is important to take a detailed occupational history. It can be difficult to link symptoms with work as there may be a long history, with insidious onset of symptoms. Any suggestion of occupational causation should prompt referral to a specialist. Some researchers have proposed that chlamydia infection has a role in the causation of adult-onset asthma and in some trials, the use of macrolides has proved beneficial (although this may be an anti-inflammatory property rather than an antibacterial effect).[9]

Asthma presenting to the on-take medical team will, on the whole, take the form of an acute exacerbation. Most asthmatics will underestimate the severity of their condition since they are so used to living with it. Investigation should include a peak flow, the only objective measure of response to treatment. Pulse oximetry is also mandatory – recent BTS guidelines recommend that arterial blood gases are not performed unless saturations are under 92% (in part to avoid putting asthmatics off returning to hospital in the future). These are guidelines, not tablets of stone, and where there is any doubt as to a patient's condition, an arterial blood gas should be performed.

....

7   Currie *et al.* BMJ (2005) 330: 585–589.

8   Kitch *et al* Drugs & Aging (2000) 17: 385–397.

9   Issacs *et al* MJA (2002) 177: S50–S51.

It is helpful to objectively determine the severity of an exacerbation, since patients may look deceptively well (see the following table). This at least gives the physician an idea as to who should be particularly closely monitored or referred to intensive care. Patients at particular risk include those who misuse drugs, those who have a psychiatric illness, socioeconomic or learning difficulty, who deny their condition or symptoms, or who do not comply with prescribed medication. Patients with brittle asthma, those who have previously been admitted to intensive care or those recently discharged from hospital are also at increased risk.

Severity of acute asthma

Acute severe
PEFR 33–50% predicted or best
Respiratory rate > 25
Heart rate > 110
Inability to complete sentences
Life threatening
PEFR < 33%
SpO_2 < 92% (or PaO_2 < 8 kPa)
$PaCO_2$ 4.6–6.0
Silent chest, feeble respiratory effort
Cyanosis
Bradycardia, dysrhythmia, hypotension
Exhaustion, confusion, coma
Near fatal
$PaCO_2$ > 6.0, or requirement for ventilation with raised pressures

Acute treatment of asthma is second nature to many general physicians. However, evidence now suggests that a change in approach is needed. The first change is oxygen therapy: classically, the asthmatic patient will receive high flow oxygen via a non-rebreathe mask. A recent study has shown that it is better to give low flow oxygen, titrated up to keep oxygen saturations above 92%. A number of asthmatics will start to retain carbon dioxide as they develop hyperinflation and air trapping: limiting the flow of the oxygen minimizes this effect.[10] A second area of evolution relates to β-agonist therapy. This is

[10] Rodrigo *et al.* Chest (2003) 124: 1312–1317.

traditionally delivered by nebulizer, either as a continuous or intermittent treatment. However, there is good evidence to support the use of metered dose inhalers coupled with a spacer. This is as effective, if not more so, due to the duration of time required to inhale the drug (1 min compared to 15 min). One recent review suggested that it might be best to give 4 puffs via a spacer every 10 min.[8] There is much less evidence for the use of anticholinergic agents in acute asthma than for β-agonists. However, ipratropium appears to have a mild bronchodilating effect although it may be more beneficial in some patients than in others. In more severely affected patients, it seems reasonable to add it to the β-agonist regime every 6 h.[11] However, experience suggests that more frequent use may increase retention of secretions, which may make the asthma worse.

Aminophylline has been shown not to improve response and is now not recommended as first-line treatment.[12] It is a drug to consider in a patient not responding to conventional treatment but it is important that it is not allowed to delay onward referral to intensive care. The main problem with theophylline is its side effects, which are more likely to arise when the patient is not monitored and when plasma concentrations are not diligently checked (a minimum of 6 h after starting, then daily).

Magnesium infusion has been included in recent BTS guidelines on the grounds of a multicentred randomized control trial published in 2002.[13] In the study, 254 asthmatic patients with a mean FEV_1 of 22.9% of predicted on arrival in A&E, were randomized to receive magnesium or placebo. During this study, patients were only given β-agonists every half an hour. The mean improvement was to a FEV_1 48.2% predicted compared with 43.5% in the placebo group ($p = 0.045$). There was no change in hospital admission rates. This and subsequent evidence remains far from compelling. Since magnesium is relatively harmless at low doses (adverse effects include flushing and hypotension), it is not unreasonable to give it. However it is crucial that the other drugs such as β-agonists and steroids are not delayed in order to do this. It is also imperative that if the patient does not respond, they are not given further doses of magnesium, which can potentially depress respiratory muscle function and cause confusion and coma.

Steroids must never be forgotten – often the asthmatic who is not responding rapidly has a great deal of airway inflammation and steroids are the lynchpin of treatment. Prednisolone (or IV hydrocortisone) is recommended but it may

11 Phipps et al. Thorax (2003) 58: 81–88.

12 Hart, QJM (2000) 93: 761–765.

13 Silverman et al. Chest (2002) 122: 489–497.

be worth also considering inhaled steroid which has some additional thera-peutic benefit (and also reinforces to the patient the need to take the medica-tion regularly).[14] Any patient developing fatigue or progressive respiratory distress should be discussed with intensive care and ideally looked after there until the attack starts to resolve. When on the intensive care unit, it is impor-tant to avoid intubation if possible. Intubation is associated with a consider-able increase in hyperinflation, risk of pneumothorax and CO_2 retention. Bronchospasm can recur on extubation and any period of intubation increases the risk of pneumonia and sepsis. Non-invasive ventilation (NIV) has been used with modest success in a few small trials with patients manag-ing to avoid intubation. The evidence is not yet clear and NIV for asthma should not be undertaken outside intensive care, where appropriate facilities to intubate rapidly are to hand. Other therapies may become more impor-tant in the management of acute asthma within the next few years such as leukotriene antagonists–some evidence is accumulating to suggest that these may improve outcome in acute attacks.[15]

During an admission, every opportunity should be taken to review a patient's normal asthma control and reinforce good management. The best people to undertake this are often respiratory specialist nurses who can help the patient manage inhaler problems, peak flow plans and other issues. At the very least, the doctors looking after the patient should be able to review inhaler and peak flow technique and check that the patient knows the stage at which to step-up their medication. One should ensure that all patients are discharged with a peak flow meter and diary so that at the clinic, peak flow charts can be reviewed and modi-fication of medications can be informed. Efforts should be made to ascertain the trigger for the exacerbation and to explore any psychological problems, which are also recognized to be associated with poor outcome. It is vital to readdress the issue of smoking and drug use, since both hospitalization rates and intuba-tion rates are significantly higher in patients smoking, or using cannabis or cocaine.[16] All patients who have required admission to hospital as a result of their asthma should be referred to a respiratory specialist for follow up.

Puffers and bloaters

Chronic obstructive pulmonary disease (COPD) affects 3 million people in England and kills 30,000 per year, leading to £800 million in direct healthcare

---

[14] Rodrigo *et al.* Chest (2004) 125: 1081–1102.

[15] Dockhorn *et al.* Thorax (2000) 55: 260–265.

[16] Levine *et al.* Chest (2005) 128: 1951–1957.

costs annually. The UK's mortality rate from respiratory disease (including COPD) is almost double the European average–in parts of the country it outstrips heart disease.[17] Chronic inflammation (and the resulting soup of cytokine mediators) causes destruction of the airways, parenchyma and vasculature, along with increased mucus production. Airway inflammation and the loss of cilia in turn lead to repeated infection, setting up an ongoing cycle. Destruction of lung parenchyma leads to the damage of bronchioles and impaired gas exchange causing hypoxia, pulmonary vasoconstriction, and ultimately cor pulmonale. COPD is strongly linked to smoking; so strongly in fact that unless a patient has a significant history (over 20 pack years), an alternative diagnosis should be sought. Smoking during pregnancy may increase the risk of the foetus subsequently developing COPD in adult life (if they smoke) by priming the immune system.[18]

The diagnosis of COPD should be entertained in any smoker who has cough, shortness of breath and recurrent infections. If the diagnosis is considered, spirometry should be obtained in order to determine a FEV1:FVC ratio. The GOLD guidelines classify COPD according to the severity of the abnormalities on spirometry.[19] Spirometry results should be interpreted with caution, so as not to miss an underlying fibrotic lung condition or an alternative explanation for the patient's symptoms. In particular, chronic infection, bronchiectesis, cystic fibrosis, TB and asthma (all of which can present with recurrent infection, cough and shortness of breath) should be considered.

Often a patient with COPD will present having been told that they have asthma and this can cause confusion in the admissions unit. When a patient presents with an acute exacerbation of COPD, it is extremely important to obtain a baseline daily function (including exercise tolerance and household tasks) so as to set appropriate goals for recovery. It is important to address any change in shortness of breath, sputum quantity or colour, and other systemic symptoms. Throughout the admission, it is worthwhile to continue to address the topic of smoking since this is the only factor likely to influence long-term outcome. Ideally, all patients with COPD should have their spirometry checked during an admission although this is often not feasible. A patient with an oxygen saturation of less than 92% on air should have an arterial blood gas analysed; a $PaO_2 < 6.2$ kPa or a pH < 7.30 suggests a life-threatening episode. A pH < 7.30 has been associated with significantly higher mortality – in one

[17] Chief Medical Officer, Annual Report. Crown copyright, London, 2004

[18] Morgan et al. Am J Respir Crit Care Med (1998) 158: 689–690.

[19] Pauwels et al. Am J Respir Crit Care Med (2001) 163:1256–1276.

study, patients with a pH > 7.30 had a 15% mortality, compared with 27% in those with a pH < 7.30.[20]

When patients present acutely with COPD, it is important to exclude a pneumothorax, malignancy and infection. Pneumothorax is common in patients with emphysema. However, beware of mistaking bullae for pneumothoraces–discussion with a radiologist can avoid a potential disaster! Bacterial infection is more common in COPD than in asthma and can cause further lung destruction, so it is vital to treat early where there is any objective evidence of infection. Right heart failure is also common in patients with severe COPD and the introduction of a small amount of diuretic may improve their symptoms (particularly ankle swelling). Unlike patients with left heart failure, most COPD patients have normal kidneys (although some do of course have widespread cardiovascular disease) and therefore the dose of diuretic required is usually modest. It is important to be on the lookout for malignancy: all too often, chest X-ray abnormalities are overlooked in the heat of the moment and a potentially curable cancer is missed.

There is rarely any place for discussion of long-term oxygen therapy (LTOT) at the time of admission: this decision must be made when a patient is in steady state, not in the throes of an exacerbation. It is helpful in clinic to know the arterial blood gases of a patient during their admission but alone, this will not fulfil oxygen prescription guidelines. To embark upon this route prematurely is not going to make a difference to the patient in the short term and it can be disabling and stigmatizing. If not indicated, LTOT proves extremely costly.

NIV has been the biggest advance in the management of acute COPD in recent years. NIV is a very elegant treatment and has a firm grounding in evidence for patients with a pH < 7.35 or a pCO_2 > 6 kPa.[21] Trials have shown 80–85% success rates, with improvement in pH, reduction in pCO_2, reduction in breathlessness and reduced hospital stay when NIV is used in patients with acute respiratory failure.[22] Patients are not appropriate for NIV if they have previously had a respiratory arrest or have an impaired mental state, if they have cardiovascular instability or if they are at high risk of aspiration. In addition, recent facial or oesophageal surgery, craniofacial trauma or other facial abnormalities are contraindications to NIV. Obesity is a relative contraindication. It is always good to be one step ahead in the management plan, so that if the patient fails non-invasive therapy, it is clear whether they are for full

[20] Plant et al. Lancet (2000) 355: 1931–1935.

[21] Ram et al. Cochrane Database Syst Rev (2004) CD004104.

[22] Lightowler et al. BMJ (2003) 326: 185.

intubation, resuscitation and intensive care. There is very little evidence for NIV for conditions other than COPD outside the intensive care setting, so any patient in whom there is doubt about the diagnosis should be discussed.

Applying NIV is a very simple skill to learn and if available, all doctors should take the opportunity to familiarize themselves with its settings and gain some hands-on experience with a knowledgeable colleague. On occasions, the physician wants to use the machine but there may be no trained nurse available, which can be a cause of considerable frustration. Being able to commence treatment by oneself is extremely satisfying.

Non-invasive ventilators blow air at two pressure levels (inspiratory and expiratory), sometimes called BiPAP – bi-level positive airways pressure. CPAP (continuous positive airways pressure) blows air at a constant pressure and is used for sleep apnoea and cardiac failure: it is not useful in COPD exacerbations. Because there are many different makes and models, it is important to familiarize oneself with the relevant machine and its instruction manual! NIV connects to a mask: this may just fit over the nose, the nose and mouth, or the whole face and is the most crucial part of non-invasive ventilation. Finding a mask that fits the patient is time well spent. The seal around the face is the key to success and an ill-fitting mask will not seal properly. Most masks come with some advice for measuring the patient to ascertain the correct size but this may require a certain amount of experimentation. Once a good fit has been established, the patient should not simply be strapped in and left to it: NIV can be very frightening for patients, especially in the middle of an acute exacerbation with buzzers sounding left, right and centre. Holding the mask on to the patient's face without any straps until they have acclimatized is a good idea—only then should the head straps be employed. The more time spent at the beginning ensuring comfort and gaining trust, the more successful NIV will be.

There is a current vogue for managing patients with exacerbations of COPD at home, partly driven by an effort to reduce bed days. If the patient is acidotic or has consolidation on their CXR, they should generally remain in hospital. Normally, a respiratory outreach team facilitates early discharge. The team usually consists of experienced nurses and physiotherapists who visit patients regularly at home to ensure they are improving. It must be remembered that patients can become very anxious and a home environment is very different from a hospital ward, so there should be no pressure on either the outreach team or the patient to go home earlier than they feel able. NICE has produced guidance on the subject.[23]

....

23 CG012 (February 2004) (www.nice.org.uk)

Any patient who has been admitted to hospital as a result of a COPD exacerbation should probably be followed up in the respiratory clinic, where formal lung function can be assessed. In addition, interventions such as long-acting anticholinergic inhalers, long-acting β-agonist inhalers and referral for surgery (such as lung volume reduction or bullectomy) can be considered. The main route for referral to pulmonary rehabilitation is also through the chest clinic and patients should be assessed for this in their steady state.

Still working out wheeze

Almost invariably, patients are given the label of asthma or COPD when they present with wheeze. One common scenario is that of the patient who presents as an adult with wheeze. Here, occupational history must be explored and it is important to find out about exposure to chemicals or dust, and the relationship of symptoms to time at work and holiday periods. Any suggestion of occupational disease necessitates referral to a physician with expertise in these matters.

The nature of the wheeze can be telling–a monophonic wheeze suggests a single obstructing lesion and should precipitate a CXR and referral for bronchoscopy or a CT scan. A polyphonic wheeze may be due to bronchospasm, as in asthma, but is also often heard in pulmonary oedema: the humble chest X-ray should help distinguish these.

Other symptoms may give clues, such as sputum production–sputum in asthma tends to be yellow or clear: any suggestion of green or brown sputum should alert the physician to the possibility of bronchiectesis, cystic fibrosis (more benign variants can present even in middle-aged adults) or other chronic infection. Churg–Strauss disease is another well-defined cause of late-onset asthma. It is associated with a high eosinophil count and markers of vasculitis, although often the asthma can predate these other aspects. Clearly, it is not practical or cost effective to perform a vasculitic screen on every adult presenting with wheeze but a careful examination should be performed each time the patient is seen and any question of vasculitis should prompt investigation.

Gastro-oesophageal reflux is another common condition that can be mistaken for asthma if the fine print of the history is not ascertained. The patient may present with cough, particularly on lying down, which may be taken to be a diurnal variation. Sometimes chronic aspiration can cause shortness of breath and recurrent infections, or even bronchiectesis. In any patient presenting with a chronic cough, consideration should be given to a 6-week trial of a proton pump inhibitor. The patient should be warned to take the medication even if they feel no immediate change, as the cycle of chronic cough (which is likely to have become habitual) can be difficult to break. Other important causes of chronic cough include post-nasal drip (where sinus X-rays can be very helpful in diagnosis), asthma variants and the use of ACE inhibitors.

Deadly clots

Pulmonary embolism (PE) is a common condition, which on the whole is managed well by general physicians. Studies suggest that the incidence of venous thrombo-embolism is 60–70/100,000 with half of these events occurring in hospitalized patients.[24] Inpatients who develop venous thromboembolism have a mortality estimated at between 6 and 15%.[25] The key to diagnosing PE is thinking of it in the first place. Clinical symptoms and signs can be very subtle. PE presents in many guises and is often a fatal condition when missed. Most doctors are aware of the standard 'risk factors'–recent major surgery, malignancy, immobility, obesity, thrombophilia, family history, pregnancy, oestrogen therapy and smoking. Air travel is particularly topical although it seems likely that any period spent in cramped conditions is risky. Air travel is also associated with alcohol and dehydration, which possibly add to the risk. One recent study demonstrated pro-coagulant changes in the blood of those who had travelled long distances by air (and not in those who had simply taken it very easy on the ground).[26] About 25–50% of all venous thromboembolic events are associated with a thrombotic tendency such as protein C or S deficiency, antiphospholipid syndrome, antithrombin III deficiency or factor V Leidin deficiency.[27] The BTS guidelines recommend performing a thrombophilia screen in patients under 50 years of age or in those with recurrent episodes.

The development of venous thromboembolism is associated with malignancy, particularly when there is no other apparent cause, although the incidence of thromboembolism is such that only a tiny minority of patients subsequently turn out to have cancer. The current recommendation is that a CXR and routine blood tests are performed but that ultrasound and CT are not, due to a very low pick up rate, unless otherwise prompted, following a thorough history and clinical examination.

In diagnosing PE, some hospitals employ scoring systems whereby the patient is categorized into high, intermediate or low probabilities, depending

[24] Heit *et al.* Mayo Clin Proc (2001) 76: 1102–1110.

[25] Heit *et al.* Arch Intern Med (1999) 159: 445–453.

[26] Schreijer *et al.* Lancet (2006) 367: 832–838.

[27] Greaves, Clin Med (2001) 1: 432–435.

on the presence of dyspnoea, pleuritic pain, haemotysis, tachypnoea or a defined risk factor, and the absence of an alternative diagnosis.[28] Such systems allow an estimate of pre-test probability and guide the rational use of further tests.

The D-dimer test is potentially very useful in managing patients with suspected venous thromboembolism. However, it is poorly understood and is often misapplied as a screening test for all-comers on admission. D-dimers carry a high false positive rate, being raised in a multitude of scenarios. The appropriate use of the D-dimer is in the patient where there is a relatively low pre-test probability of PE or DVT (on the basis of a clinical scoring system). If below the defined threshold, thromboembolism is very unlikely to be the diagnosis and no further tests are necessary. In a patient with a high pre-test probability of PE or DVT, a D-dimer should not be requested because the false negative rate in this group of patients is unacceptably high. These patients should go straight to ultrasound, nuclear medicine or CT pulmonary angiogram (CTPA). If a D-dimer has been requested in error, its result can reasonably be ignored. Patients with intermediate pre-test probability pose more of a problem but evidence would suggest that D-dimers are useful in this group as well and they can be managed in the same way as those with low pre-test probability.[29]

Traditionally, patients with a suspected PE were imaged with a ventilation-perfusion (VQ) isotope scan, as opposed to the rather laborious gold standard of the formal pulmonary angiogram. The main problem with VQ is that scans can be difficult to interpret, resulting in reports that may appear a touch non-committal. A normal scan is reassuring and reliably excludes PE (although this is still not universally accepted).[30] However, a high probability scan may not necessarily be caused by PE, depending on co-morbidities (such as COPD). The CTPA has revolutionized the investigation of PE and is now recommended as the primary investigation for the condition. There is good evidence that if a patient has a negative CTPA, further investigation for PE is not warranted.[31] The current issue is that clinical acumen is often being put to one side and a huge number of D-dimer tests are sent inappropriately. Raised levels cause anxiety amongst the medical team and a CTPA is requested to alleviate that. It should be remembered that every scan carries a significant amount of radiation: a standard CTPA delivers 6.7 times more radiation to a woman's

[28] BTS Guidelines, Thorax (2003) 58: 470–484.

[29] Roy *et al.* BMJ (2005) 331: 259–263.

[30] Gray *et al.* Semin Nucl Med (2002) 32: 159–172.

[31] Swenson *et al.* Mayo Clin Proc (2002) 77: 130–138.

breast than a mammogram and this may represent a significant risk in the development of breast cancer in the long-term.[32]

As soon as a diagnosis of PE is seriously entertained, treatment should be started with low molecular weight heparin (LMWH). When the diagnosis is confirmed, warfarin should be commenced and LMWH continued until the INR has been above 2.0 for 2 consecutive days, or for a total of 5 days (whichever is longer). The optimal duration of anticoagulation with warfarin is still unresolved. Ideally, this should be decided for each individual patient based on the risks posed to them by anticoagulation versus the potential benefits. At present there is no good system to aid in this decision-making process. In general, venous thromboembolic disease with an obvious precipitant (which has resolved) requires no more than 6 months of anticoagulation, idiopathic disease (or situations in which the precipitant is persistent) probably requires longer because recurrence rates are high.

Most physicians are aware of the place of thrombolysis in the advanced life support protocol for pulseless electrical activity (PEA) because it may be caused by PE. The difficulty is in assessing its use in other scenarios. A consensus is beginning to form around the use of thrombolysis in 'submassive PE', as defined by haemodynamic indices and importantly, either a firm diagnosis (CTPA) or at least some supportive evidence, such as an echocardiogram showing right ventricular dysfunction or pulmonary artery hypertension.[33]

PLEURAL DISEASE

Pop!

About 18–28/100,000 men and 1.2–6/100,000 women suffer a pneumothorax each year. These cases can be subdivided into primary, where the pneumothorax is spontaneous (perhaps related to the presence of congenital blebs on the lung surface) or secondary, where the patient has underlying chest disease. In all cases of pneumothorax, it is important to review the CXR for signs of underlying lung disease. It may even represent the presentation of conditions as diverse as lymphangioleiomyomatosis (LAM – occurring only in women and associated with pleural effusions and cystic lung), histiocytosis X (associated with cavitations and fibrosis) or AIDS, where the cause is generally pneumocystis.

Pneumothorax commonly presents via the general medical take and despite its apparent simplicity, management carries a number of pitfalls for the unwary.

---

[32] Parker, Am J Roenterol (2005) 185: 1228–1233.

[33] Konstantinides et al. NEJM (2002) 347: 1143–1150

Recent BTS guidelines break down pneumothoraces into those < 2 cm and those > 2 cm. In one analysis, it was asserted that a 2 cm air rim represents a 50% collapse of the lung, although this has been disputed. Unfortunately, any intervention for a pneumothorax considerably increases the risk of intrapleural infection (empyema). In a patient with a primary pneumothorax, where the rim is less than 2 cm and there is no shortness of breath, discharge is appropriate, with instructions to return if symptoms worsen. When the patient is short of breath, or the rim of air is greater then 2 cm, aspiration is recommended. Aspiration should be done aseptically, using a 16–18 gauge cannula in the mid-clavicular line 2nd intercostal space. It is reasonable to attempt aspiration (as opposed to proceeding straight to drainage) on all pneumothoraces, unless there is a suggestion of tension.

Trials show that the success of aspiration depends on the size of the pneumothorax, the age of the patient and the presence of a chronic lung condition.[34] It is advisable to obtain peripheral venous access prior to aspiration and in young patients, administration of 600 mcg atropine should be considered: young people can develop marked vaso-vagal bradycardia in response to pleural irritation and may faint. In patients who refuse aspiration or when the clinician is unsure whether it is indicated, it is reasonable to admit overnight and apply high flow oxygen–this reduces the partial pressure of gas by displacing nitrogen and thereby enhances absorption of gas from the pneumothorax. Many will have been disappointed by the slow response to this technique but it should be remembered that only 1.25–1.8% of the total pneumothorax will resolve in a 24-h period–a lack of progression is a sign of success.[35]

In patients with two failed aspirations or in those with a secondary pneumothorax who have failed one aspiration, a chest drain should be inserted. There is no evidence either way to recommend the type or size of drain and in general, it is better to go for the smallest possible. Exceptions to this rule include patients who have a large air leak or those who have pleural fluid evident, where the diagnosis may be haemo-pneumothorax. Seldinger drains are smaller and easier to insert than the large traditional drain, beloved of the trauma surgeon and hated by patients. If a small bore drain is inserted, then flushing it with 20 ml sterile saline 4 times a day may help to preserve patency. In one study, small drains were associated with a 84–97% success rate. Drains should not be clamped if they are bubbling and if they stop bubbling, it is important to check that the drain is still swinging to ensure it has not become blocked. If a drain is clamped, the patient should be observed closely and not

34 Henry *et al.* Thorax (2003) 58: ii39–ii52.

35 Flint *et al.* Lancet (1984) ii: 687–688, cited in Henry *et al.* Thorax (2003) 58: ii39–ii52.

allowed to leave the ward unsupervised. If a drain stops bubbling for more than 24 h, despite swinging, it should be removed. Any patient who has had a drain in-situ for 48 h and continues to have an air leak should be referred to the respiratory specialists as they will have links with thoracic surgery and specialist knowledge of managing chest drains. Suction should not be attempted until 48 h after chest drain insertion (and therefore usually only under the supervision of a chest physician). If used too early, suction can precipitate re-expansion pulmonary oedema, especially in young patients or in those with a large spontaneous pneumothorax. Pain relief from a chest drain can be achieved by instilling 20–25 ml of 1% lignocaine into the drain at 8-h intervals.[36]

Drain complications are common and the physician should be vigilant: they include infection – 1% of patients with chest drains will develop an empyema as a result of the drain and therefore strict asepsis is required at insertion and with subsequent care. Only nurses well used to their management should care for chest drains, and given the small number inserted in general medical practice, this may require that patients are managed in a dedicated respiratory ward. Other complications include the perforation of organs, which carries an associated mortality. In one series, 3% of chest drains had been placed extra-thoracically and 6% were within the lung parenchyma, when examined with CT.[37] Training in insertion and complete avoidance of any trocar is crucial. In patients where it is unclear whether there is a true pneumothorax or bullous lung disease, a CT scan should be obtained to ensure correct positioning. Surgical emphysema is also a complication, which results from either a mal-positioned, kinked, blocked or clamped drain, where air leaks around the edge of the tube into the subcutaneous tissues. It may also occur in the context of a large air leak where the drain is too small.

If the pneumothorax persists after 5 days, the patient should be discussed with a thoracic surgeon. At this stage there are three options. First, to do nothing more–in one series, 100% of patients with a primary pneumothorax who had a persistent air leak at 7 days had resolved by 14 days; in secondary pneumothorax, 79% of patients had resolved by 14 days. Second, chemical pleurodesis can be considered: talc (the most commonly used) or tetracycline. It should be noted that medical pleurodesis does not reduce the risk of recurrence to nil. Third, the patient can be referred for surgical intervention–either with video-assisted thoracoscopic surgery (VATS), surgical abrasion or surgical instillation of talc (poudage). Unless there are specific contraindications, the evidence suggests that abrasion is the best method. Absolute indications

[36] Sherman *et al.* Chest (1993) 3: 533–536.

[37] Baldt *et al.* Radiology (1995) 195: 539–543.

for referral to the surgeons include a second ipsilateral pneumothorax, a first contra-lateral pneumothorax, bilateral spontaneous persistent air leak at 5–7 days or a spontaneous haemo-pneumothorax.

All patients should be advised not to fly for 6 weeks following complete resolution of a pneumothorax, although the risk of recurrence remains high for a year and some patients will prefer not to fly for this period. In one study, up to 54% of patients had a further pneumothorax, the majority within a year of their primary event.[38] Nor should patients fly for 6 weeks following surgical intervention. All patients should be encouraged to stop smoking as this increases the risk of further pneumothorax. They should also be advised that they should never dive unless they undergo bilateral surgical pleurodesis.

When pneumothorax occurs in a patient with HIV, the most common cause is PCP infection that causes necrotizing alveolitis leading to the replacement of sub-pleural pulmonary parenchyma by thin-walled cysts and pneumatocoeles. A pneumothorax in the presence of PCP has a high mortality and should be treated aggressively. There is a high incidence (40%) of bilateral disease and air leaks tend to be prolonged. Steroids for the treatment of PCP infection may increase the risk of a pneumothorax. Treatment should be early and aggressive, involving referral for surgical intervention as necessary.

In those with cystic fibrosis, a pneumothorax is associated with a median survival of 30 months. This is not a direct effect, rather a reflection on the severity and stage of disease. Treatment is exactly the same as for a secondary pneumothorax but it is also important to commence intravenous antibiotics. If a patient has persistent air leak, it is advisable to try and avoid pleurodesis due to the knock-on implications for lung transplantation. If necessary, local surgical abrasion is acceptable. All patients with cystic fibrosis should be referred to a specialist respiratory physician as soon as possible.

Iatrogenic pneumothorax

Procedure	Risk of iatrogenic pneumothorax (%)[39]
Transthoracic needle aspiration	24
Subclavian central venous line	22
Thoracocentesis	22
Pleural biopsy	8
Positive pressure ventilation	7

[38] Sadikot et al. Thorax (1997) 52: 805–809.

[39] Britten, Injury (1996) 27: 321–322.

Whoops!

Iatrogenic pneumothoraces are common. The table on p289 shows the quoted rates of occurrence. The figure of 22% serves as a reminder that central line insertion, not least subclavian, is not a procedure for the amateur. About 89% of iatrogenic pneumothoraces will resolve with aspiration alone and often the patient can just be watched. In the context of mechanical ventilation or the presence of primary chest pathology, a chest drain is indicated.

A chest full of fluid

Pleural effusions can occur on account of pulmonary disease, pleural disease or extra-pulmonary conditions. Investigation of a unilateral effusion can be challenging. History and examination are naturally prerequisites to investigation: details of previous drug use (such as amiodarone or methotrexate) can give clues on the aetiology. Other medical conditions including cardiac, hepatic or rheumatological disease may be related to a pleural effusion and should be explored. Smoking status and a past or current history of malignancy is important, as is a detailed occupational history (particularly in relation to asbestos exposure). The possibility of a pulmonary embolus (PE) should also be considered: 75% of patients with a pleural effusion secondary to PE will offer a history of chest pain.

Aspiration of pleural fluid is easy to perform and can be very informative. Ideally, 50 ml of fluid should be aspirated, split and sent for microbiology, biochemistry (see below) and cytology. If the fluid is purulent, infection is likely and an intercostal drain should be inserted and antibiotics commenced. If the fluid is not purulent, then a small sample can be put in a heparinized syringe and run through the blood gas analyser for a pH. A pH of less than 7.2 would normally suggest the presence of infection, since the bacteria metabolize glucose within the fluid and decrease the pH through production of carbon dioxide. In this context, an intercostal drain is also indicated. Malignancy can also cause the pH of the fluid to fall but by the time the pH is < 7.2, it is said that the prognosis is very poor. In one study of patients with malignant pleural effusions, a pH of greater than 7.3 conferred a median survival of 9.8 months, compared with 2.1 months in those with pH less than 7.3.[40] A bloodstained effusion can be analysed for the haematocrit (also measured by the blood gas analyser). Significant amounts of blood in the pleural

---

[40] Sahn *et al.* Ann Intern Med (1988) 108: 345–349.

fluid favour malignancy, trauma, cardiac injury syndrome or benign asbestos disease as the cause of the effusion.

Biochemistry of the fluid may help to further determine the aetiology of the effusion. Light's criteria distinguish an exudate from a transudate.[41] If one or more of the criteria are fulfilled, the fluid is an exudate.

Light's criteria for pleural effusions

Pleural fluid protein more than half of serum protein
Pleural fluid LDH divided by serum LDH > 0.6
Pleural fluid LDH more than two-thirds of the upper limits of normal serum LDH

The glucose level of the pleural fluid is also informative; a pleural glucose level of less than 3 mmol/l is found in empyema, rheumatoid disease, lupus, tuberculosis, malignancy and oesophageal rupture. The presence of high amylase suggests acute pancreatitis, pancreatic pseudocyst, oesophageal rupture, pleural malignancy or bizarrely, rupture of an ectopic pregnancy. Occasionally, one can be surprised when tapping an effusion, when the fluid comes out looking like milk. This points to a chylous effusion and it is helpful to send a sample for chylomicron and cholesterol biochemistry. A chylous effusion is suggestive of a thoracic duct injury or occasionally, lymphangioleiomatosis (LAM).

Cytological examination of pleural fluid can be extremely useful. Many malignancies metastasize to the pleura or lung and may be otherwise undetected. A number of studies have suggested that cytology has a diagnostic sensitivity of between 40 and 87% but there is little additional benefit to be had from a blind pleural biopsy.[42]

In the context of an un-diagnosed unilateral pleural effusion, it is extremely important not to aspirate the effusion to dryness. If the patient is particularly symptomatic, aspiration of up to a litre of fluid may improve symptoms. However, bear in mind that a pleural effusion associated with a PE may result in a patient disproportionately dyspnoeic for the size of the effusion. If, despite biochemical and cytological analysis, the diagnosis remains in doubt, the most likely cause is malignancy. Tumours can be scattered around the pleural surface, with areas of sparing. If cytology is not diagnostic, the most sensitive tests to perform are either a CT-guided pleural biopsy or a thoracoscopy. Both tests are available in specialist centres but perhaps not elsewhere. A non CT-guided

---

[41] Light *et al*. Ann Intern Med (1972) 77: 507–513.

[42] Maskell, Thorax (2003) 58: ii8–ii17.

Abram's needle biopsy adds little to the investigation of a malignant pleural effusion. In one study, the yield compared to cytology alone, increased by only 7% (to 27% in that series).[43] Blind Abram's biopsies are, however, frequently positive in the context of a tuberculous effusion and are worthwhile if a patient presents with an undiagnosed pleural effusion from an area of high tuberculosis prevalence. In the context of tuberculosis, the combination of an Abram's biopsy, smear culture and histology has a diagnostic yield of 80–90%.[40] Abram's biopsies carry a significant risk, including pain, pneumothorax, vaso-vagal reaction, haemorrhage and fever. It is therefore important that the operator has had experience in the technique. In the investigation of pleural disease in the context of a pleural effusion, blind Abram's biopsy, CT-guided biopsy and thoracoscopy all require the presence of pleural fluid, so aspirating an effusion to dryness is a false economy.

Mesothelioma is a primary pleural malignancy presenting almost exclusively in patients who have worked with asbestos. Many patients will present with a unilateral pleural effusion. It is vital to mark the area from where fluid has been aspirated, as in up to 40% of cases, mesothelioma will grow along the needle track. This can cause significant pain and disfigurement to the patient. Radiotherapy within 6 weeks of aspiration can significantly reduce the risk of this occurring. India ink is one way to mark the area but ensuring that the dressing is not removed before the patient sees a chest physician is another.

Despite best efforts, the cause of a pleural effusion may remain in doubt. Up to 15% of effusions fall into this category. Here, it is important to try to exclude tuberculosis and PE. Both of these conditions are treatable but potentially fatal if missed. Even if a positive culture or Gram stain is not obtained, the combination of an exudative pleural effusion and a positive tuberculin skin test is reasonable to provoke a course of anti-tuberculosis therapy. However, once the investigations have gone this far, the patient should be under the care of a chest physician who can consider the rare conditions and monitor the effusion.

Muck in the chest

Any patient with a pleural effusion has pleural infection until proven otherwise. Approximately half of pneumonia admissions will be associated with the presence of a pleural effusion. The majority of these will be simple 'parapneumonic' effusions. In some situations, the fluid may show features of infection without being frankly purulent in which case it is termed a complicated parapneumonic effusion. Once the pleural fluid becomes purulent, it is termed

---

[43] Prakash *et al.* Mayo Clin Proc (1985) 60: 158–164.

an empyema. In either case, antibiotics will not penetrate the fluid adequately and it must be drained to treat the patient properly. Antibiotic therapy depends of course upon the context, local sensitivities (microbial) and practices.

Until recently, most respiratory physicians believed in intermittently administering streptokinase via the chest drain for 72 h. It was thought that this helped to break down loculations and resolve effusions more quickly and successfully. A recent multi-centre randomized controlled trial has proven that in fact, there is no benefit to its administration.[44] Studies are underway into alternative strategies but it will be some years before these yield results and until then, patients should be treated with antibiotics and a chest drain alone.

Mesothelioma – a growing problem

Mesothelioma is malignancy of the pleural surface, which carries a dire prognosis of between 6 and 18 months. It frequently evades diagnosis for many months. Although research continues, at present the only chance of curing this terrible malignancy is to diagnose it early so that the patient can have radical surgery. It is likely that chemotherapy, if it works at all, will only have an impact in early stages of the disease, hence timely diagnosis will become increasingly important. Mesothelioma is strongly associated with exposure to asbestos with a dose-dependent relationship (70% of cases have been exposed). 8% of all asbestos workers will die of respiratory failure secondary to asbestos and their lifetime risk of developing mesothelioma is thought to be 8–13%. There is a considerable time delay between exposure and the development of mesothelioma which occurs up to 40 years later. The peak of use of asbestos was in the 1960s and 1970s and hence new cases remain on an upward trajectory, with the peak expected in 2020 when deaths in the UK are likely to number 2700 to 3000 per year.

Most commonly, patients with mesothelioma present with increasing shortness of breath or chest pain. They may also present with an asymptomatic pleural effusion, dysphagia, hoarseness, nerve compression, brachial plexopathy, Horner's syndrome or superior vena caval obstruction. Mesothelioma can cause paraneoplastic syndromes such as disseminated intravascular coagulopathy, migratory thrombophlebitis, haemolytic anaemia, hypoglycaemia or hypercalcaemia. Mesothelioma rarely metastasizes outside the chest cavity but this is not unknown. Examination of the patient may reveal a pleural effusion, reduced lung expansion or dullness to percussion (caused by pleural thickening). Typically the pleural effusion is unilateral but 5% of mesotheliomas

---

[44] Maskell *et al.* NEJM (2005) 352: 865–874.

are bilateral.[45] In any patient with chest pain and a unilateral pleural effusion, the diagnosis of mesothelioma should be considered. Very often, the treatment of mesothelioma is palliative and the chest services will have strong links with the palliative care team to ensure appropriate care for all these patients.

LUNG CANCER

Lung cancer is the commonest cause of death from cancer in the world and each year 38,000 new cases are diagnosed in the UK.[46] At present, 1 in 13 men and 1 in 20 women develop lung cancer. Smoking is the main causative factor, linked to 85% of cases. Lung cancer is rare in patients younger than 40. A large part of the service provided by chest physicians is concerned with the diagnosis of lung cancer and in the UK, government targets now ensure that all patients referred by their family doctor with suspected lung cancer are seen within 2 weeks. These targets do not cover intra-hospital referrals and so the referring hospital physician must take great care in the way a referral is made to ensure timely investigation. The key to treatment of lung cancer is early diagnosis. A patient who has an operable lung tumour has a 45% 2-year survival (35% at 5 years) but less than 1 in 5 patients are operable and the mean survival of all newly diagnosed patients with lung cancer hovers around 6 months (10% at 2 years).

Persuading a patient to stop smoking will significantly reduce the risk of lung cancer but not for some years. Currently, half of all lung cancer is diagnosed in ex-smokers. Other risk factors include passive smoking (up to 2% of all lung cancers in the US are thought to be caused by passive smoking); radon is also linked with lung cancer (additive to smoking) and people who live in houses built on granite are particularly at risk of this effect. Occupational exposures such as asbestos, silicon and coal dust will increase the risk of lung cancer. Lung fibrosis, of whatever cause, will also heighten the risk in an individual–up to 15% of patients with fibrosis will develop lung cancer.

About 15% of new diagnoses present on the acute medical take, half present via primary care, leaving 35% to present sub-acutely (in clinic or via other specialties). Most general physicians are well aware of the myriad of different ways in which lung cancer can declare itself. Squamous cell lung carcinoma is the commonest form, accounting for up to 45% of all tumours within the lung. Metastases are late and tend to occur in large airways. Adenocarcinoma (15%) is often more peripheral and is much less strongly correlated with smoking than

---

[45] Sterman *et al.* Up to date (2004) (www.uptodate.com)

[46] www.cancerresearchuk.org/cancerstats/

the other types of lung cancer. It is important to ensure that adenocarcinoma within the lung is not metastatic from elsewhere and the histopathologist may be able to help through immunostaining. Small cell carcinoma is the most aggressive tumour and accounts for 20% of all lung cancers. Specific catches, which may cause a case of lung cancer to be missed, include the non-resolving pneumonia. Any patient who has a significant smoking history is considered high risk and if they have presented on the acute take with symptoms of a chest infection, they should be reviewed at 4–6 weeks. A repeat CXR should be done at this stage and if either the CXR has not resolved or symptoms persist despite antibiotics, the patient should be referred for review by the chest team. It is important to remember that chest X-rays are not all-seeing and a tumour is not always visible, hiding behind patches of consolidation, ribs or the mediastinum. All chest X-rays should be reviewed by the requesting physician and any abnormality such as collapse, consolidation, effusion, lymphadenopathy or an abnormal shadow should be acted upon. Formal radiological reports may not be available on the post-take ward round and in a number of cases, reports have been mislaid, leading to missed diagnoses, patient misery and justified medicolegal action. High patient turnover and a lack of continuity of care from junior staff is unlikely to go a long way in Court.

The pulmonary nodule

A nodule seen on a chest X-ray or CT scan may pose diagnostic difficulties. A CT can never offer certainty as to the composition of a nodule and nodules may be too small or positioned such that bronchoscopy or transcutaneous needle biopsy is not inviting. Do these nodules represent early lung cancer or simply an area of fibrosis, consolidation or rheumatoid lung disease? A nodule which has not changed on imaging for more than 2 years is unlikely to be lung cancer and examination of previous chest X-rays and reports is helpful. However, other than in this unusual circumstance, all cases of lung nodule should be referred to the chest physician to be investigated and followed up. Commonly, an attempt at biopsy will be made and if this fails, a repeat CT scan will be considered.[47]

In the context of suspected lung cancer, it is inappropriate to send a patient home without arranging investigation and follow-up. If any delay in referral is anticipated, it may be helpful to request a CT chest. However if this is done, it is important to ask for a staging CT chest that includes the upper abdomen. Many chest physicians like to have a CT prior to bronchoscopy to facilitate

[47] Ost *et al.* NEJM (2003) 348: 2535–2542.

navigation and targeting of the most appropriate areas of the lung. When a diagnosis is not clear-cut, the multidisciplinary team will discuss further investigation: transthoracic biopsy may be useful or alternatively, in a patient with a central tumour, a limited surgical procedure (such as mediastinoscopy) may be suggested.

PET (positron emission) scanning is a relatively new investigation, useful in the staging of lung cancer. Radiolabelled glucose molecules (^{18}FDG) are taken up in areas of high cellular metabolism due to the action of the enzyme GLUT1, found in high levels in malignant cells. The ^{18}FDG undergoes decay, emitting photons that can be detected radiologically, producing a 'map' of the tumour. Small nodules, metastatic deposits and involved lymph nodes can be detected. PET scanning allows accurate staging, which should improve assessment of appropriateness for surgery. PET is more specific than CT (75% versus 66%) and more sensitive (91% versus 86%) at detecting metastases, particularly in lymph nodes and outside the thorax.[48] It is very useful in investigating enlarged mediastinal lymph nodes. In some areas of the UK, combined CT–PET scanners exist and can do the two scans simultaneously, which increases the sensitivity and specificity still further.

One of the responsibilities of the multidisciplinary team is to accurately stage the tumour and taking this together with a patient's performance status, decide upon the most appropriate treatment. Performance status determines a patient's ability to withstand the trauma of chemo- or radiotherapy and therefore, its appropriateness. It is not helpful to give assessments of life expectancy or proposed treatment plans at initial diagnosis. It is better to wait until a specific diagnosis has been made, the tumour has been staged and the treatment plan discussed at a lung cancer multidisciplinary meeting.

Screening for lung cancer

There has been much discussion over whether, in the light of such a dire prognosis and the knowledge that early operative intervention is potentially curative, smokers and ex-smokers should be screened for early lung cancer nodules. In screening pilots, 55–85% of cancers detected on a baseline scan (and 60–100% on subsequent scans) are stage 1 cancers, compared with only 16% presenting in the usual way.[49] Since stage 1 lung cancer carries a 60% cure rate, this has led to considerable interest in screening. Screening methods currently under investigation include CXR, CT scanning and sputum cytology.

---

[48] Pieterman *et al.* NEJM (2000) 343: 254–261.

[49] Mulshine *et al.* NEJM (2005) 352: 26.

CT scanning was considered unsuccessful following early trials although there has been much criticism on the way these studies were conducted. Two recent trials have proved more promising. One study performed in Japan with 15,342 patients showed that of those lung cancers detected, 78% were stage 1. The 5-year survival rate in cases detected by a chest radiograph was 49%, which improved to 84% on those detected by CT scan.[50] More recently the ELCAP trial has proved even more promising: in this study, people aged over 60 years who had a 10 or more pack year smoking history were screened using low dose CT scanning. If the patient had between 1 and 6 non-calcified nodules, they went on to have a normal CT and HRCT through the nodules. Repeat HRCT was done at 3, 6, 12 and 24 months. When a nodule reached 6–10mm, a biopsy was performed. A nodule > 11mm received standard care. 26,577 patients were initially studied with follow-up screening of 19,555.[51] A large proportion of patients had non-malignant nodules detected on their scans but 350 lung cancers were identified, of which 82% were stage 1. The survival for patients who had lung cancer detected was 95% at a median follow up of 40 months. One of the main concerns over these trials is a significant lead-time bias, as tumour doubling takes a fair period of time. In addition, we know that a proportion of apparently stage 1 lung cancers will have occult bone metastases at presentation. Furthermore, the costs and risks of screening patients in terms of radiation exposure and the anxiety generated are real. Randomized controlled trials are now underway involving the use of PET, which may improve the detection of carcinoma through screening, and these results are eagerly anticipated.

PULMONARY INFECTION

Community acquired pneumonia

Pneumonia is common with a reported annual incidence of between 5 and 11 cases per 1000 adults. Approximately 22–42% of patients with pneumonia require hospitalization in the United Kingdom and 5–10% of these admissions require intensive care. Mortality rates are 5–12% and higher in certain groups, such as the elderly and those with coexisting disease.[52] Stratification of risk is of key importance when considering a patient with pneumonia. This allows appropriate antibiotic choice and focuses the mind on those who are most unwell.

---

[50] Sone *et al.* Lancet (1998) 351: 1242–1245.

[51] ELCAP Investigators, Clin Imaging (2004) 28: 317 –321.

[52] BTS Pneumonia Guidelines, Thorax (2001) 56: iv1–iv64.

The BTS guidelines advocate the use of the CURB65 score.[53] A patient scores a point for each criterion fulfilled, as illustrated below:

C	Confusion	AMTS of 8 or less
U	Urea	> 7 mmol
R	Respiratory rate	> 30 breaths per minute
B	Blood pressure	Diastolic < 60 mm Hg or Systolic < 90 mm Hg
65	Age	> 65 years

The patient's score correlates with their intensive care requirement and mortality.

Course of pneumonia by CURB65 score

CURB65 Score	Risk of mortality or need for ICU(%)	Appropriate location for care
0	1	Probably home
1	3	
2	13	Probably hospital
3	17	Consider intensive care unit
4	42	
5	57	

Hypoxia (oxygen saturations of 92% or a pO_2 below 8 kPa) and multi-lobar involvement are other additional risk factors to those outlined in the CURB65 score. The physician should carefully weigh up the individual patient's risk factors in deciding where the patient should be best treated and what antibiotics they should be given.

Patients with severe pneumonia (CURB65 score of 2 or more) require careful investigation including (in addition to routine tests) blood cultures, urinary legionella antigen, pneumococcal antibodies and acute atypical serology. In addition, these patients should be commenced on intravenous antibiotics and regularly reviewed. All patients remaining in hospital should be considered for oxygen and IV fluids. CRP should be monitored and will have fallen by 50% (from its peak) at day 4, if the patient is responding.

[53] Lim *et al.* Thorax (2003) 58: 377–382.

Often textbooks suggest that the cause of pneumonia may be determined by the CXR changes. For example, the presence of upper lobe changes suggests *Klebsiella pneumoniae* and cavitations favour *Staphylococcus aureus* infection. In fact, the literature suggests that although these are classic features, they are neither specific nor sensitive and there are no radiographic features that allow sufficiently accurate prediction of the pathogen to guide antibiotic therapy. Chest X-ray changes tend to lag behind clinical improvement and it is often said that the CXR should have resolved by 6–8 weeks. In one study, 51% of cases had resolved by 2 weeks and 73% by 6 weeks, with slower clearance in smokers, the elderly, and those with multilobar involvement.[54] BTS guidelines now suggest that a repeat CXR during the patient's admission is not indicated unless there is a failure to improve. Treatment for severe pneumonia should include antibiotics for 10 days, extending to 14–21 days when *Legionella*, Gram-negative *Enterobacter* or *Staphylococcus* is isolated. All patients who have had pneumonia should be reviewed at 6–8 weeks. At this time, all patients who have risk factors for malignancy (including age over 50 years or smoking) should have a repeat chest X-ray. In addition, any patient who has persistent signs or symptoms should also have a repeat CXR. Patients with persisting changes should be referred for consideration of CT scan and/or bronchoscopy.

Several conditions should prompt an early inpatient referral to the chest team: multi-lobar pneumonia is uncommon in a normal pneumonic process but can be associated with *Streptococcus pneumoniae*. The involvement of more than one lobe may suggest other pathology, such as broncho-alveolar cell carcinoma, tuberculosis, severe atypical pneumonia or cryptogenic organizing pneumonitis (COP). These conditions require specialist investigation and management. The other time a chest opinion should be sought is when the patient's pneumonia is failing to resolve. This may be for many reasons, such as a resistant or atypical organism, or the development of an empyema or abscess. Aspiration of fluid, with or without the use of ultrasound, is likely to be helpful.

CYSTIC FIBROSIS

Cystic fibrosis is not something that frequently concerns the general physician on the acute take, as patients tend to be very well engaged with their specialist service. The most common reason for a patient with cystic fibrosis to present to the general take is infection. It is important to understand the spectrum of

54 Mittl *et al.* Am J Respir Crit Care Med (1994) 149: 630–635.

infections that can affect such patients, as they require a rather different approach with regard to antibiotic treatment. Cystic fibrosis occurs when the gene coding for the chloride channel in the cystic fibrosis transmembrane conductance regulator mutates. Approximately 1 in 25 people carry a mutation. Clinical cystic fibrosis affects those who are homozygous, equating to approximately 1 in 2500. The abnormality in the chloride channel leads to inadequacy of salt and water transport across the cell membrane and causes thick secretions in the lungs. Consequently, the patient is at high risk of infection due to impairment of clearance of microorganisms. Chronic infection leads to bronchial wall damage and bronchiectesis.

Over the past few years, significant changes in the way that patients with cystic fibrosis are managed has led to a considerable improvement in median survival. In particular, changes in diet (including a high fat, high calorie approach to nutrition) have been important. A baby born in 1990 with cystic fibrosis had an expected survival of at least 40 years. Subsequently, what was previously regarded as a paediatric illness has now encroached on the adult population. Most of the problems that patients with cystic fibrosis encounter are related to respiratory infections. Infections can manifest in a rather different way to those in patients with healthy lungs. Presenting features may include deterioration in exercise tolerance, changing sputum colour or haemoptysis. In addition, patients are prone to pneumothoraces and may present with sudden onset of severe shortness of breath.

All patients with cystic fibrosis presenting on the acute take must have a chest X-ray to exclude this problem. Oxygen saturations and if possible spirometry should also be performed. All patients with cystic fibrosis will have regular sputum testing. If the patient presents in their own hospital, then it is important to review the latest microbiology results. Common infecting organisms include *Staphylococcus aureus*, *Pseudomonas aeruginosa* and *Haemophilus influenzae*. In addition, patients are at risk of *Mycobacteria pneumoniae* and viral infections. Often these organisms chronically colonize and patients may need long-term prophylactic antibiotics. In an acute exacerbation, it is extremely important to send a sputum sample prior to commencing any antibiotics. If it is not possible to consult the chest team prior to starting, then a combination covering Pseudomonas, such as meropenem plus gentamicin, or tazocin plus gentamicin should be given. In addition, the patient must be adequately nourished and receive regular intensive physiotherapy. Pneumothorax in a patient with cystic fibrosis is common, particularly in men, and is associated with a poorer prognosis. If the pneumothorax is extremely small, it may be managed conservatively, but a larger pneumothorax requires insertion of an intercostal drain. Often, expansion of the lung is difficult and the patient may require suction. As previously alluded to, it is extremely important to avoid any temptation to pleurodese.

A patient with cystic fibrosis may also present on the acute take with haemoptysis, when inflammation from chronic infection and persistent coughing can cause rupture of a vessel. Here, the primary consideration should be to treat underlying infection. Clearly, other factors may be contributing to the bleeding problem such as a low platelet count (from infection or drugs) and the use of non-steroidal anti-inflammatory drugs. There have been reports demonstrating success in using tranexamic acid for persisting symptoms.[55] Occasionally haemoptysis can be caused by erosion of a bronchial artery. In this case, blood loss of 250 ml or more can occur in 24 h. On the whole bronchoscopy is not particularly helpful in resolving severe bleeding, since it is technically difficult. The life-saving intervention in this case is basic resuscitation and referral for angiography and embolization of the vessel. If this is unsuccessful, the patient should be referred to the surgeons for ligation.

OTHER RESPIRATORY PROBLEMS

Diving low

Diving is a popular pastime, but one with potentially serious implications for patients with respiratory disease. An average of 12 deaths occur every year in the UK as a result of diving with a further 100 cases of serious decompression illness.[56] When a diver descends, pressure increases by 1 bar (100 kPa) every 10 m, with a proportional increase in partial pressure of gases. Inert gas (nitrogen) dissolves more easily into tissues at depth and may form bubbles within the tissues on ascent, leading to decompression illness. In addition, gas within a cavity is compressed on descent and re-expands on ascent. This can cause barotrauma unless, as a diver ascends, he breathes out to allow expanding gas to escape from the lungs. Gas can track to the mediastinum or retroperitoneum, or cause gas embolism if within the pulmonary circulation. In addition to barotrauma and decompression problems, divers may suffer anxiety, panic, physical injury and equipment failure leading to hypoxia, hyperoxia or gas poisoning. Divers in general have large lung volumes with an increase in vital capacity. They tend to have reduced expiratory flow rates at low lung volumes which may represent small airways disease. The lung volume tends to

---

55 Graff, Respiration (2001) 68: 91–94.

56 Wilmshurst, BMJ (1998) 317: 996–999.

decrease at an accelerated rate with age.[57] The most common scenario in which diving is an issue is in the case of a pneumothorax. Guidelines are very clear: anyone who has had a spontaneous pneumothorax should not dive again unless they have undergone a bilateral surgical pleurectomy (failure rate < 0.5%) and have had normal lung function tests and CT chest post operatively. This does not apply to the individual who has had a traumatic pneumothorax, as long as the injury has healed and lung function tests and CT scan are normal.

Patients with lung bullae are also excluded from diving. Asthma is not an absolute contraindication but extreme caution must be taken in advising patients – any evidence of cold, exercise or emotion-induced asthma and the patient should be cautioned against diving. In addition, those with acute symptomatic asthma (having had recourse to use a bronchodilator in the previous 48 h) or those with abnormal spirometry, should also refrain.

Flying high

Aircraft cabins are pressurized to 8000 ft, which gives an equivalent oxygen concentration of 15.1%. The PaO_2 experienced by a healthy person will be dependent on minute volume and age but generally falls to between 7.0 and 8.5 kPa (saturations 85–91%).[58] Hence patients with underlying respiratory problems will experience potentially troublesome hypoxia during a flight. Regardless of cause, a resting oxygen saturation of less than 95% or an FEV_1 of less than 50% puts patients at risk of developing hypoxia on the plane. These patients should probably undergo an investigation such as a hypoxic challenge or an exercise test, which can be arranged through the lung function laboratory. In some centres, the practice is to recommend that if the patient can walk the distance from the airport to the plane, they should be safe to fly! Although this may sound pragmatic, it is not validated: indeed, nor is exercise testing itself, although it is recognized by a number of airlines. In general, a patient with oxygen saturations of less than 92% on air should have supplemental in-flight oxygen.

As alluded to earlier, air travel is strongly linked with an increased risk of PE due to a combination of dehydration, poor mobility, venous stasis and possible alcohol ingestion. One study suggested that up to 10% of people travelling on aircraft will have sub-clinical DVTs.[59] No data are yet available to recommend the use of aspirin, or indeed to quantify the health merits of upgrading

57   BTS Guidelines, Thorax (2003) 58: 3–13.

58   Coker et al. Thorax (2002) 57: 289–304.

59   Scurr et al. Lancet (2001) 357: 1485–1489.

or avoiding alcohol, although there is some evidence for the use of graduated compression stockings (TEDS). Patients who have a high risk of embolism should be considered for low molecular weight heparin for the duration of their journey. Patients with a moderate risk of PE may wish to consider aspirin in addition to TEDS. Patients who have had a thrombo-embolism should be carefully assessed before being allowed to fly again. As a general rule a resting oxygen saturation of 95% or more should be safe for travel and if the patient is on anticoagulation, the risk of further embolism is minimal.

Infections are a further issue when considering aircraft flight. In particular, communicable diseases such as tuberculosis are a concern in the closed environment of the aircraft. Currently, however, the World Health Organization advises that the risk of infection with TB on aircraft is no greater than the risk when travelling by rail or bus. Current recommendations are that the patient should have been rendered non-infectious prior to travel. Three negative smears on separate days or a negative culture suggest a very low risk but in practice, if a patient has been on full anti-tuberculosis treatment for 2 weeks, they are generally considered non-infectious.

Pregnancy and the lung

Maternal deaths are recorded on an ongoing basis in the UK and the collated results are published every 3 years.[60] In 2000–02, 30 women died from venous thromboembolism around the time of their pregnancy. Although this is a marked improvement on the figure of 138 deaths for the period 1952–54, many of these deaths are preventable. It is common for the medical team to be asked to review a woman who has become breathless while pregnant. A number of diagnoses should be considered but first and foremost is PE. If suspected, PE must be excluded due to the substantial mortality that it carries, not just for the mother but also the baby. As soon as a PE is considered or diagnosed, the woman should be treated with IV heparin or low molecular weight heparin (typically increasing the dose to the acute coronary syndrome regime, on the basis of an increased glomerular filtration rate). Liaison with the obstetricians is vital. Pregnant women, with appropriate shielding, should be investigated and scanned. D-dimer is not validated in this situation. Women in the UK die from pulmonary emboli in pregnancy at a rate of more than one a month, and misplaced worries over modest amounts of radiation are in part to blame.

Pregnancy causes a number of physiological changes within the mother which affect the lungs. As the foetus grows, diaphragmatic descent is impaired

[60] www.cemach.org.uk

and the woman is less able to expand the lungs. It seems reasonable that pregnant women may be more at risk of bacterial lung infection but in fact, the majority tend to be viral and self-limiting.

Sleep

Sleep medicine has grown in standing over the years. Making the diagnosis of sleep apnoea is enormously satisfying as the physician can bring about a significant improvement in a patient's quality of life with a single intervention. The challenge in diagnosis is that symptoms are often indolent and progress over many years, so the patient may think that those symptoms are 'normal'. All patients should be asked about their sleep patterns—key questions concern snoring, witnessed episodes of apnoea and inappropriate sleeping during the day. If the answers are suggestive of sleep apnoea, an Epworth score should be carried out (see table below). A score of 10 or more makes the diagnosis very likely. Examination should focus on baseline oxygen saturations, dentition, jaw alignment and tonsillar size. Patients with sleep apnoea often tend to be obese or have craniofacial abnormalities. In addition, signs of hypothyroidism should be sought (and biochemistry sent). Any patient with very large tonsils should be referred to an ENT surgeon for tonsillectomy as this can be curative. It may be worth referring to the local sleep service simultaneously, as waiting times can be lengthy. All of the above findings should be documented in the referral letter.

Epworth Sleepiness Scale

Situation	Chance of dozing
Sitting and reading	
Watching television	
Sitting inactive in a public place (such as in the theatre)	
As a passenger in a car for an hour without a break	
Lying down to rest in the afternoon when circumstances permit	
Sitting and talking to someone	
Sitting quietly after a lunch without alcohol	
In a car, while stationary for a few minutes in the traffic	
Chance of dozing: 0 – never; 1 – slight; 2 – moderate; 3 – high.	

It is important to advise patients with possible sleep apnoea regarding driving. The DVLA states that all patients with 'sleep apnoea, narcolepsy/cataplexy or any other condition which causes excessive daytime/awake time sleepiness' should notify their condition.[61] Driving must cease until control of symptoms is obtained. For those holding a group 2 licence, specialist follow up and annual licence renewal is required. In practice, anybody who is sleep deprived, for whatever reason (shift worker or party animal), is at increased risk of motor vehicle accidents. Sleep apnoea is a common condition and may frequently be seen on an acute take as an incidental finding. Having advised a patient about not driving, referral should be quick (particularly if the patient's livelihood depends upon their ability to drive). Many sleep units will prioritize HGV drivers, or other patients who drive for a living, so it is important to stress this issue in the referral.

Dietary advice is often an important part of therapy for sleep apnoea: weight loss can be extremely difficult in a patient who has sleep apnoea on account of fatigue but it is important to motivate the patient early so that as soon as treatment is initiated, they attend to losing weight. This can dramatically reduce the need for ongoing therapy. Once a patient is referred to a specialist they will initially attend for some form of sleep study. This may be conducted at home with portable equipment or it may necessitate an overnight stay in a sleep laboratory. If sleep apnoea is confirmed on the study, the patient will be prescribed CPAP therapy–air blown at constant positive pressure via a nasal mask in order to maintain the patency of the upper airway and prevent closure during sleep.

It is logical to treat sleep apnoea in symptomatic patients, as the very disabling symptoms are likely to fully resolve. In recent years, debate has raged as to whether treatment is appropriate only on the grounds of symptomatic relief or whether it may in fact confer a mortality benefit. The argument goes that frequent awakening (in response to apnoea) is accompanied by reflex brain stem arousal, catecholamine release and a profound temporary increase in blood pressure. Some authorities feel that such a response is bound to be detrimental in terms of cardiovascular morbidity and a recent study looking at the mortality of those with untreated sleep apnoea compared to treated controls appeared to decisively support this.[62] However, others point to the fundamental flaws of cohort studies and the powerful 'healthy adopter' effect (those who do not use CPAP will be different in many ways from those who do). The small number of randomized controlled trials (using sham versus real CPAP) show that blood pressure reductions are modest and importantly, only occur in those with symptoms of sleep apnoea.[63] It may be that any excess

[61] www.dvla.gov.uk

[62] Marin *et al.* Lancet (2005) 365: 1046–1053.

[63] Pepperell *et al.* Lancet (2002) 359: 204–210.

mortality in those with sleep apnoea is actually due to their excess neck circumference, regarded by some as a better measure than BMI or waist-to-hip ratio, when considering the metabolic syndrome. Sleep apnoea may simply be an almighty confounder. The jury is out.

Other treatments, which have been used for sleep apnoea and snoring include uvulopharyngopalatoplasty–an operation offered by ENT surgeons. It is best not to advise a patient to go down this path until a sleep study has been conducted. The operation is, by all accounts, as painful as it sounds, it may not improve symptoms and it may make CPAP therapy more difficult. Patients should be advised to minimize their use of alcohol and benzodiazepines as both will make sleep apnoea worse.

PULMONARY FIBROSIS

The finding of fibrosis on a chest X ray or its appearance as a chance finding on a CT scan fills most physicians with a degree of trepidation. Like many other conditions that have been incompletely understood over the years, pulmonary fibrosis has had its fair share of re-classifications and re-definitions, all of which run the risk of generating confusion. The table below shows the current system for the classification of fibrosis.[64] Idiopathic diffuse parenchymal lung diseases (DPLD) were formerly known as cryptogenic fibrosing alveolitis (CFA).

Classification of diffuse parenchymal lung disease (DPLD)

DPLD of known cause	Granulomatous DPLD	Idiopathic DPLD	Others
Rheumatoid arthritis	Sarcoidosis	Usual interstitial pneumonia (UIP)	Langerhans histiocytosis
Asbestosis		Non-specific interstitial pneumonia (NSIP)	Lymphangioleiomyomatosis
Methotrexate lung		Cryptogenic organising pneumonia (COP)	

The rationale for the re-classification is to try and separate out those patients who have a better response to steroids or immunosuppression.

In reality, patients presenting on the acute take with fibrosis prominent on CXR or CT have normally decompensated as a result of infection. It is important to

---

64 Martinez, Proc Am thoracic Soc (2006) 3: 81–95.

treat such decompensation promptly with antibiotics. Steroids are unlikely to make a significant difference in the acute stages and should be avoided until a firm diagnosis has been made. Patients with a new finding of fibrosis should be referred to the chest team for consideration of lung function testing, HRCT scan and biopsy (either by bronchoscopy, VATS or an open approach). Patients treated for known fibrosis may present on an acute take with deterioration and in this circumstance, consideration should be made of unusual organisms. Fungal infections, including *Pneumocystis carinii* (now known by some micro-biological connoisseurs as *Pneumocystis jiroveci* after a Czech pathologist), are more common when a patient is immunosupressed by their medications. Sputum sampling is important, preferably prior to starting antibiotics, although treatment for PCP with septrin and steroids should not be unduly delayed.

Chapter 13

Kate Scatchard, David Church and Ed Gilby

ONCOLOGY

INTRODUCTION

In the UK, 1 in 3 people develop cancer during their lifetime, and malignancy is the cause of 1 in 4 deaths. Nearly all clinical disciplines in medicine are involved in some way in either the diagnosis or management of cancer patients, and while the last few decades have seen tremendous advances in the treatments available in the UK, there has been even greater change and progress in the delivery of cancer care.

The rapid pace of scientific and clinical research in the field of cancer has made it increasingly difficult for the generalist to keep up with changes in oncological practice over recent years. This may lead to problems for the harassed on-call physician. It is always embarrassing when the patient asks whether they should continue to take a drug that one has never heard of; and the vexed decision as to whether cardiopulmonary resuscitation is appropriate for a patient is rendered even more so if one does not have a clue as to the prognosis. Not every centre has a friendly oncologist who can be called upon for advice. Here, we aim to give a snapshot of this rapidly changing field for some of the commonest tumours in the West and to highlight a few specific scenarios in cancer medicine, of which clinicians should remain mindful.

The UK Government appointed a 'cancer tsar' to lead developments in cancer care, who established a Cancer Collaborative in 1999. The results of wide-ranging consultation and discussion were then crystallized into the National Cancer Plan, which outlines a number of targets (such as the 2-week wait for a first appointment following first referral from primary care).[1] Diagnostic investigations

---

[1] Department of Health, the NHS Cancer Plan: a plan for investment, a plan for reform (2000) (www.dh.gov.uk).

should reach a conclusion within 31 days, and treatment should start in all cases within 62 days. Many protest about the wisdom of a 'target culture' and in some trusts, seemingly perverse systems may be in operation: the lower level of priority often attached to intra-hospital referrals being one such example. It is doubtless, however, that the average patient receives a more timely and comprehensive service than a decade ago. This is not to say that some patients do not continue to experience many weeks of delay, particularly if the nature of their illness is not properly recognized.

It is now uniform practice for all newly diagnosed cancer cases to be discussed at a multidisciplinary meeting with the presentation of pathology (from a biopsy or operative specimen), review of cross-sectional imaging and a thorough discussion of the management options. Such meetings are well established for the commoner malignancies but a little more challenging for rarer diseases (such as sarcomas, germ cell tumours and melanoma) when regional discussion may be more appropriate. To state simply that 'there is a multidisciplinary meeting' is not of course to guarantee the quality and value of the deliberations that take place there.

Opinions vary considerably on this wholesale redesign of cancer services. It has been shown for breast and bowel cancer, for example, that early diagnosis clearly results in better prognosis and survival. It is less clear that a 2-week referral deadline is as relevant for a more indolent case of prostatic cancer. In many units, patients with suspected breast cancer, having discovered a lump in the breast and been referred by their general practitioner, are seen at their initial consultation by a breast surgeon, undergo imaging and a biopsy procedure all in the same visit. A patient presenting with microcytic anaemia, on the other hand, gives rise to a suspicion of bowel cancer and may require upper gastrointestinal endoscopy coupled with colonoscopy or appropriate radiological imaging such as a barium enema, a CT scan of the colon or indeed the more complex double-contrast CT pneumocolon (10% of those with an apparent cause identified on upper gastrointestinal endoscopy will have a coexisting large bowel diagnosis). The complexity of investigations and the increasing number of hospital departments involved make the 'one-stop shop' a more challenging endeavour.

The use of CT, MRI and PET scanning has increased markedly in the last decade, putting huge burdens on radiology services. Advances in endoscopic and laparoscopic techniques, backed up by CT-guided biopsy procedures, have meant that in more than 95% of cancer cases, a histological confirmation can be obtained, and major surgery is, thankfully, now largely confined to patients where the procedure will constitute definitive treatment. One such example is planned surgery for oesophageal tumours following neo-adjuvant chemotherapy to cause shrinkage. Oesophageal cancers can now be assessed with remarkable precision using endoscopic ultrasound, predicting the stage of the primary tumour and the extent of lymph node involvement with an accuracy approaching 85%.[2] The scale of the surgical undertaking is such that avoiding inappropriate procedures is a very sound goal.

Not only has the number of biopsy specimens obtained from suspected cancer patients grown, but the immunohistochemical techniques available to pathologists has allowed them to make a confident statement about the likely tissue of origin in more than 80% of cancers.[3] In some cases, the finding of binding sites or hormone receptors can predict responsiveness to drug or hormone therapy. For example, the demonstration of C-KIT receptors in GIST (gastrointestinal stromal tumours) predicts their excellent response to imatinib, which inhibits the growth factor driving the tumour. Unfortunately, this treatment, virtually devoid of side effects, is usually followed by resistance and tumour recurrence after a year or two, but the initial relief for such patients is immense.

When it comes to the choice of active treatment for the accurately diagnosed and staged case, a good deal of uniformity has been achieved in most centres, and local networks of hospitals agree on a portfolio of protocols for management. Understandably, the introduction of new agents such as the monoclonal antibodies trastuzumab (Herceptin) and cetuximab (Erbitux) – targeting the growth factor receptors HER2 and EGFR respectively – and bevacizumab (Avastin) – targeting a ligand responsible for angiogenesis – is expensive and requires thorough testing in clinical trials. To this end, all oncologists are actively engaged in submitting as many patients as possible to clinical trials, and a number of national centres are developing units specifically concentrating on phase I (dose finding) and phase II (initial cancer activity) studies of new agents. The evidence base for all treatments offered these days is one of solid clinical trial evidence.

Chemotherapy drugs tend to be extremely expensive, especially when first marketed, and all have toxic side effects to a greater or lesser degree. Experience with combination regimens used in maximally tolerated doses during the 1970s and 1980s led to the realization that a balance needs to be struck between the probable benefits and probable toxic burden if valuable resources are to be best used.

---

2 Heeven et al. Endoscopy (2004) 36: 966–971.

3 Lagendijk et al. Human Pathology (1998) 29: 491–497.

Given finite resources, health economics and the concept of the 'quality-adjusted life year' (QALY) have become increasingly important. In recent times, the decision on choice of drugs and regimens has increasingly been made at the national level by NICE on the basis of cost per QALY gained, and many commissioners will only finance prescriptions made in accordance with NICE guidelines. It remains the oncologist's job to decide with the patient when to continue or stop therapy.

THE BIG THREE

There are three giants in the cancer world, each presenting between 30,000 and 40,000 new cases a year in the UK: breast, lung and bowel.[4]

Breast cancer

Early-stage breast cancer is a disease confined to the breast or regional lymph nodes. Its prognosis depends on a variety of factors, including (most importantly) the presence or absence of nodal involvement, hormone receptor positivity, HER2 status, tumour grade and size, and whether the tumour has invaded vascular spaces. It is an extremely heterogeneous malignancy, with huge variability in prognosis between different tumours; while a post-menopausal woman with a small oestrogen-receptor-positive tumour with no involved nodes may have a greater than 90% chance of being alive at 10 years following treatment; a 30-year old with a large, heavily node-positive cancer that is oestrogen receptor negative may have only a 50% chance of long-term survival after surgery, even with state-of-the-art therapy. The overall 5-year, age-standardized relative survival for women with breast cancer, diagnosed between 1996 and 1999 in England and Wales, was 77%.[4]

The oncological management of early breast cancer is tailored according to these risk factors, as well as the patient's general health and choice. Typically, it comprises varying combinations of chemotherapy, hormone therapy (for the two-thirds of women whose tumour is oestrogen receptor positive) and radiotherapy. Other treatments such as adjuvant trastuzumab (Herceptin) are becoming an integral part of care in selected patients.

Chemotherapy may be given before surgery (neoadjuvant therapy) or subsequently (adjuvant therapy). The improvements in survival it provides are well proven in numerous trials and meta-analyses such as the pivotal Early Breast Cancer Trialists Collaborative Group (EBCTCG) overviews.[5] The current

---

[4] www.canceresearchuk.org/cancerstats/

[5] Early Breast Cancer Trialists Collaborative Group, Lancet (2005) 365:1687–1717.

standard of care in the UK is four to eight cycles of an anthracycline-based regimen, which reduces the annual risk of death by about two-fifths in women under 50 and by a fifth in women aged 50–69 years. This relative risk reduction is generally constant across different prognostic groups, although the absolute benefit of chemotherapy depends on the initial risk of relapse. Thus, while all oncologists would recommend adjuvant chemotherapy to a 35-year old with an aggressive tumour and involved nodes, only a card-carrying chemophile would do so to a 69-year old with a 1-cm, hormone-receptor-positive, node–negative cancer. Taxanes, newer drugs derived from yew tree bark, provide a small but definite additional reduction in the risk of relapse when added to anthracycline-containing regimens, but at present are not widely used in this context in the UK. An aim of much current research is the discovery of molecular markers predictive of relapse, in order to target chemotherapy at those who require it, while sparing those who do not from the needless associated toxicity.

The role of hormonal manipulation in breast cancer treatment has been recognized for over 100 years since George Beatson removed the ovaries of women with the disease and observed tumour regression. Tamoxifen binds the oestrogen receptor in place of oestrogen and suppresses cell growth. We now know that 5 years of adjuvant tamoxifen for women with oestrogen-receptor-positive tumours reduces the risk of recurrence by a half and the risk of death by a third, making this one of the most effective interventions an oncologist can make.[5] Aromatase inhibitors, the (not so) new kids on the block, work by preventing peripheral conversion of adrenal steroids to oestrone and oestradiol, thus depriving post-menopausal women of their major source of oestrogens. Whether they should replace tamoxifen as the standard of care for the adjuvant treatment of post-menopausal women with breast cancer is a matter of intense current debate. Proponents cite the 3–4% absolute risk reduction in disease recurrence demonstrated in the large ATAC trial and the improved side-effect profile of the drugs (no increase in endometrial cancer compared with tamoxifen).[6] Detractors cite both the lack of survival advantage in the study at present, the significantly increased cost of the drugs and the increased risk of osteoporosis. A pragmatist might speculate that selected use of these drugs in subgroups of women most likely to benefit may be the optimum approach, but controversy remains.

Another development that has provoked enormous controversy in the UK is the use of trastuzumab (Herceptin) for both early-stage and advanced

---

[6] Howell *et al.* Lancet (2005) 365: 60–62.

breast cancer. Growth factor receptors are found on the surface of many cells, and, unsurprisingly, given their name, mediate progrowth and prosurvival signalling. Around two decades ago, it was demonstrated that about a quarter of breast tumours have increased amounts of a growth factor receptor known as HER2 (or c-erbB2) on their surfaces, and that this was associated with a more aggressive disease course and poorer prognosis. A humanized monoclonal antibody was developed to the HER2 receptor, and progressed rapidly through clinical trials. As with oestrogen receptor status and tamoxifen therapy, trastuzumab only works in tumours that overexpress HER2; but it most certainly does work. A pivotal phase III trial demonstrated a 5-month survival improvement for women with HER2-positive metastatic breast cancer who received a trastuzumab/chemotherapy combination compared to chemotherapy alone, and several recent trials have shown similarly striking results in the adjuvant setting. The addition of trastuzumab to standard adjuvant treatment produces a 50% relative reduction in the risk of relapse.[7, 8, 9] In the HERA study of over 5000 women, 77.4% of women who received standard therapy were alive and free of disease after 2 years, compared to 85.8% of women who had standard therapy plus trastuzumab.

Adjuvant use of the drug has now been advocated in the UK, albeit via a political process bypassing the niceties of licence requirements and the government's own advisory body, NICE! A side effect we will see more frequently is cardiotoxicity, specifically a fall in left ventricular ejection fraction. NYHA class III or IV heart failure occurred in 4% of treated patients in one study. Current recommendations are that echocardiography should be performed every 3 months while patients are on trastuzumab, with discontinuation of the drug if a significant drop in LVEF is noted. The cost effectiveness of adjuvant trastuzumab is uncertain. The high acquisition cost of the drug and the lack of long-term outcome data mean that at present the costs per QALY are likely to be extremely high. Things may change if and when overall survival data are available and the benefits can be modelled over a more meaningful time period.

Radiotherapy has been a mainstay of breast cancer treatment for over 50 years. In women who have had a lumpectomy, treatment of the breast reduces the risk of local disease relapse from around a third to less than 1 in 20. It is also used to treat the chest wall and/or draining lymph nodes in women

[7] Slamon *et al.* NEJM (2001) 344: 783–792.

[8] Piccart-Gebhart *et al.* NEJM (2005) 353: 1659–1672.

[9] Romond *et al.* NEJM (2005) 353: 1673–1684.

with high-risk tumours. For a long time, a survival advantage from radiotherapy was never demonstrated, probably due to excess cardiac deaths from inadvertent irradiation of the left anterior descending artery. However, with modern planning techniques and newer machines, it appears that the absolute improvement in survival it affords is between 2 and 5%. Current research is aimed at maintaining such outcomes, while minimizing toxicities.

In all but a tiny minority of women (in whom surgical resection of a metastasis may be undertaken), the presence of distant metastases from breast cancer indicates incurable disease. The commonest sites of breast cancer metastases are bone, lung, liver and brain.

Two subgroups of patients with disseminated disease are worthy of special discussion. First, patients with bone metastases, in whom treatment must be tailored to minimize skeletal complications such as fracture, pain and spinal cord compression. While systemic antineoplastic therapy may help achieve this aim, further benefit is provided by the use of bisphosphonates, agents proven to decrease the rate of skeletal complications in such women through inhibition of osteoclast activity. Palliative radiotherapy for painful secondaries improves symptoms in a sizeable majority of these women and contributes significantly to the workload of clinical oncologists. Management of spinal cord compression and hypercalcaemia, both common complications of bone metastases, are discussed later. Second, in patients with HER2-positive metastatic disease, who often have a dramatic clinical response to chemotherapy combined with trastuzumab, elimination of all radiological evidence of disease is not uncommon. In such patients, trastuzumab is continued as monotherapy for as long as the disease is responding, and control of disease for some years, even after diagnosis of brain metastases, is well documented.[10]

The systemic management of metastatic breast cancer includes hormone therapy in patients with hormone-receptor positive disease, chemotherapy, and the increasing use of novel agents. Breast cancer is arguably the disease in which the therapeutic armamentarium is largest, and it is not unusual to see a woman receiving fourth- or fifth-line chemotherapy for metastatic disease. Prognosis depends on the sites of metastases, and it should be remembered that although the median survival of women with visceral secondaries in general remains less than 24 months, patients with soft-tissue or bone metastases may live considerably longer, and it is by no means unheard for a woman with bone-only metastases to live for over a decade.

....

[10] Kirsch et al. J Clin Oncol (2005) 23: 2114–2116.

With the plethora of active agents available, breast cancer increasingly represents the paradigm of metastatic malignancy as a chronic disease, often with a prognosis comparable to nonmalignant conditions. It is vital that generalists be aware of this when considering how aggressively to treat a woman with metastatic breast cancer who has a concurrent acute, reversible condition.

Lung cancer

As any medical student who has been within a mile of a textbook knows, lung cancer is divided into small-cell lung cancer (SCLC), accounting for approximately 15% of the total, and non-small-cell lung cancer (NSCLC) histologies. Both are bad news. In the UK in the year 2002, 37,699 people were diagnosed with lung cancer and 33,602 people died from the disease, with only 6% of patients alive after 5 years.[11]

SCLC is an aggressive tumour that is normally fatal within 3 months if left untreated, and one in which there has been frustratingly little progress in treatment over recent years. For the third of patients who have limited-stage disease (loosely defined as disease confined to one hemithorax) at presentation, the standard of care is a combination of platinum-based chemotherapy and radiotherapy to the primary tumour, best delivered concurrently if the patient is fit enough.[12] Thus treated, between 1 in 10 and 1 in 3 patients can expect to be long-term survivors.[13] SCLC has a predilection for CNS spread, and the fact that over half of patients with limited-stage disease relapse with brain metastases led to the use of prophylactic cranial irradiation for patients whose local disease responds to treatment.[14] Patients with extensive-stage disease (distant metastases) are incurable, although chemotherapy may extend life to a median of 7–11 months.[15]

NSCLC has a similarly dismal prognosis. Often advanced at the time of presentation, disease is seldom resectable, and most patients who undergo surgery relapse and die within 5 years. Recent efforts have been directed at avoiding unnecessary thoracotomy in patients with occult metastatic disease, at improving outcomes for those who undergo resection with adjuvant therapy and at the use of new agents in the palliative setting. Positron emission tomography (PET) scanning uses a radioactively-labelled glucose tracer, 18-flurodeoxyglucose (FDG),

[11] www.cancerresearchuk.org/cancerstats/

[12] Fried *et al.* J Clin Oncol (2004) 22: 4837–4845.

[13] Turrisi *et al.* NEJM (1999) 340: 265–271.

[14] Auperin *et al.* NEJM (1999) 341: 476–480.

[15] Albain *et al.* J Clin Oncol (1990) 8: 1563–1574.

which is taken up preferentially by metabolically active tissues (such as malignant cells). Although still finding its place in the imaging arsenal, one area in which there is consensus of benefit is in the work-up of NSCLC patients being considered for surgical resection. Several studies have demonstrated that FDG–PET is superior to CT for accurate staging of both extrathoracic metastases and mediastinal nodal involvement. An analysis of 53 studies evaluating its use in staging showed a sensitivity and specificity for FDG–PET of 79 and 91%, respectively, compared to 60 and 77% for CT.[16] Another study revealed that a third of patients with NSCLC being worked-up for surgery were 'upstaged' by FDG–PET when compared with CT.[17] Current NICE guidelines recommend that all patients being considered for surgery should have FDG–PET as part of their work-up.[18]

Another recent change in practice in the management of NSCLC is the use of adjuvant chemotherapy following resection of early-stage disease. Although initially a number of trials demonstrated no benefit for this approach, when a meta-analysis of cisplatin-based regimens in 1995 showed a 13% relative risk reduction in risk of death, the issue was revisited.[19] The Adjuvant Lung Project Italy (ALPI) randomized 1209 patients with completely resected stage I to III disease to chemotherapy or observation. At median follow up of 64.5 months, there was no difference in overall survival between groups.[20] The International Adjuvant Lung Trial (IALT) randomized 1867 patients (stages I–III) after surgery to cisplatin-based chemotherapy or observation. In the chemotherapy group, 5-year survival rates were 44.5%, and 40.4% in the control group.[21] A more striking result was obtained by the National Cancer Institute of Canada, which randomized 482 patients with resected stage IB and selected stage II patients to a more modern cisplatin combination or observation, and demonstrated 5-year overall survival rates of 69 and 54%, respectively ($p = 0.012$).[22] Similar results were obtained in a trial conducted by the Cancer and Leukaemia Group B (CALGB), which showed a 12% absolute improvement in survival at 4 years for treated patients ($p = 0.028$).[23] The overall

[16] Gambhir et al. J Nucl Med (2001) 42: S1–S92.

[17] Hicks et al. J Nucl Med (2001) 42: 1956–1604.

[18] CG024 (February 2005) (www.nice.org.uk)

[19] NSCLC Collaborative Group, BMJ (1999) 311: 899–909.

[20] Scagliotti et al. J Nat Cancer Institute (2003) 95: 1453–1461.

[21] Arrigada et al. NEJM (2004) 350: 351–360.

[22] Winton et al. NEJM (2005) 352: 2589–2597.

[23] Strauss et al. J Clin Oncol (2004) 22: 621.

conclusion of most oncologists is that adjuvant chemotherapy for fit patients after resection of NSCLC produces a 5–15% absolute improvement in 5 year survival.

Although adjuvant chemotherapy will hopefully mean that fewer patients relapse in the future, at present all too many patients with NSCLC develop distant metastases, associated with a median survival of under 12 months. Though traditional forms of palliative chemotherapy for fit patients in this situation are proven to improve symptoms and extend survival, recent efforts to improve outcomes have focused on the use of new agents. The epidermal growth factor receptor (EGFR), a member of the same family as HER2, mediates prosurvival and progrowth signals and is overexpressed in most cases of NSCLC. Gefitinib and erlotinib are both orally administered, well-tolerated agents that inhibit EGFR, and their efficacy in the metastatic setting has been examined in several large studies. Unfortunately, the largest to date, which randomized 1692 patients with progressive disease after chemotherapy to gefitinib or placebo, failed to show any survival improvement.[24] However, the story does not end here, as a search for tumour-specific factors predictive of response was undertaken and demonstrated that the vast majority of patients who have a dramatic response to EGFR inhibitors have mutations in EGFR in their tumours (a group making up approximately 13% of the wider patient population). Such mutations are found most commonly in women with adenocarcinoma who are lifelong nonsmokers.[25] So, it seems oncologists need to be a little smarter in targeting the drug to the patients most likely to benefit, an approach currently being investigated in various trials testing mutation status prospectively. It is plausible that numerous drugs have been prematurely binned on the basis of a poor showing in heterogeneously populated trials, when they may be both efficacious and less toxic in a molecularly defined subgroup.

Colorectal cancer

The oncological treatment of colorectal cancer (CRC) has recently changed from something of a 'Cinderella area' to one of the most exciting parts of cancer medicine. In summary, curative treatment of CRC requires surgical resection of tumour, the likelihood of cure depending on how far through the bowel wall the cancer has invaded, whether it has spread to draining lymph nodes or, worse still, further afield. Adjuvant chemotherapy, as with breast and

---

[24] Thatcher *et al.* Lancet (2005) 366: 1527–1537.

[25] Paez *et al.* Science (2004) 304: 1497–1500.

now lung cancer, is standard care in fit patients and gives a 5–10% absolute improvement in overall cure after surgery. Until recently, the presence of liver metastases was regarded as terminal.

However, this has changed over recent years. Patients who relapse with liver metastases without extrahepatic disease have a 30–40% chance of 5-year survival if the tumours are surgically resected.[26] If the metastases are not initially amenable to surgery, thanks to new drugs, chemotherapy renders them resectable in around 10–20% of cases. Oncologists have had to raise their game in assessing these patients to make sure they are not denied potentially life-saving treatment. For the generalist, it is vital that the patient on the admissions ward, with liver metastases 2 years out from his bowel-cancer operation, is not written off as terminal but rather referred to the appropriate multidisciplinary team.

The most interesting developments in CRC have come in the treatment of metastatic disease, where the increasing availability of effective new drugs has produced dramatic results. Until recently, metastatic CRC was largely treated with one chemotherapeutic drug, 5-fluorouracil (5-FU), which gives an 4-month advantage over the 6-month median survival expected in such patients with supportive care alone.[27] In the 1990s, the addition of irinotecan to the chemotherapeutic options provided an additional 3-month survival benefit, and more recently the use of oxaliplatin, a platinum compound, has further extended median survival to 19 months in one large trial.[28,29] However, the greatest excitement has been generated by a nonchemotherapeutic agent, bevacizimab (Avastin). This is a monoclonal antibody against vascular endothelial growth factor (VEGF), a key player in tumour blood vessel supply and, consequently, growth. Combined with 5-FU and irinotecan chemotherapy, bevacizumab produces a further 5-month survival improvement over the same chemotherapy alone, and takes median survival beyond the 20-month mark.[30] This agent does have toxicities that may be relevant to the generalist with an increase in hypertension and thromboembolic events that are likely be seen more often as it becomes more widely used. Currently, investigators and pharmaceutical companies are falling over themselves to test these drugs

26 Hughes *et al.* Surgery (1986) 100: 278–284.

27 Simmonds. BMJ (2000) 321: 531–535.

28 Saltz *et al.* NEJM (2000) 343: 905–914.

29 Goldberg *et al.* J Clin Oncol (2004) 22: 23–30.

30 Hurwitz *et al.* NEJM (2004) 350: 2335–2342.

in the adjuvant setting, with encouraging results in the case of oxaliplatin.[31] However, as with trastuzumab, the huge cost of these drugs, particularly bevacizumab, is raising questions for funders and providers of health care. There has been much discussion in recent years around the prevention of CRC through screening. This is discussed further in Chapter Eleven.

SIGNIFICANT OTHERS

Ovarian cancer

Ovarian cancer, of which there were 6959 new cases in 2002, has long been known to be responsive to chemotherapy. In the early days, alkylating agents such as melphalan and cyclophosphamide were the first choices. The introduction of cisplatin and, later, carboplatin in the 1980s produced response rates as high as 60% in combination with cyclophosphamide and were hailed as a breakthrough. Carboplatin has now been the first-line drug for more than two decades, but the introduction of paclitaxel (Taxol) in the early 1990s altered the scene dramatically. Paclitaxel was discovered during a wide biological screening programme of natural sources carried out in the 1960s by the National Cancer Institute in the US and was derived from an extract of the bark of the Pacific Yew Tree, *Taxus brevifola*.[32] This slow-growing, protected species produced such a low yield that it would have meant the felling of six 100-year-old trees to produce enough drug for 1 patient. Fortunately a more abundant and sustainable European species also produces the parent molecule. Needless to say, paclitaxel was, and still is, expensive by comparison with predecessor drugs. In early clinical trials of paclitaxel, interim analysis of disease-free survival suggested that when it was included in a combination therapy, the patient might enjoy a full year extra free of disease. NICE advised in 2000 that paclitaxel, in combination with carboplatin, should be the first line of chemotherapy. It was therefore a surprise to many when the large multinational ICON3 trial showed no difference in outcome between the paclitaxel/carboplatin combination, single-agent carboplatin and the old-fashioned CAP regime (cyclophosphamide, doxorubicin and cisplatin).[33] NICE revised its recommendation to single-agent carboplatin as a reasonable first-line treatment, and that is now standard practice.[34] Champions of expensive novel compounds beware!

---

[31] Andre *et al*. NEJM (2004) 350: 2343–2351.

[32] Schellens *et al*. *Cancer Clinical Pharmacology*. OUP, Oxford, 2005.

[33] ICON3 Investigators, Lancet (2002) 360: 505–515.

[34] TA055 (January 2003) (www.nice.org.uk)

Unfortunately, despite response rates of 60–70% to first-line treatment, between half and three-quarters of patients relapse within 2 years. Virtually none of them survives in the long run but use of second and subsequent treatments can be very rewarding, inducing further remission and prolonging survival. Patients with a complete first remission and those with a long tumour-free interval are most likely to benefit. Seven drugs are licensed for second-line treatment in ovarian cancer, and many patients receive a majority of these before active treatment gives way to palliative support.

Future developments include the addition of gemcitabine to the list of seven drugs following recent demonstration of its activity, but of greater interest are two different lines of research. The first is the attempt to assess response of ovarian cancer at an early stage in the hope of increasing the intensity of chemotherapy in those with the best response. One study recently showed that PET scanning the abdomen before and after one cycle of chemotherapy can select responding patients who had better survival.[35] This deserves a proper randomized trial. Second, interest has increased in the use of intraperitoneal chemotherapy for this disease, which so often stays confined to the abdomen. A Cochrane review has been published describing a meta-analysis of eight trials involving nearly 2000 patients, concluding that there is a significant survival advantage to including intraperitoneal therapy in first-line treatment.[36] The introduction of cisplatin or carboplatin via a catheter placed either at the time of surgery or by careful direct positioning can be used to introduce high concentrations of drug. In some studies, the drug has been heated above body temperature: side effects, particularly pain, are more common, and only 42% of patients completed the planned treatments.[37] They did, however, show a disease-free survival of 23.8 months compared with 18.3 months. The big question is "will they have a better long-term survival or will we just be repeating the paclitaxel story?" The Cochrane review suggests that some lives may be saved if we adopt this new approach.

Prostate cancer

Prostate cancer is the commonest malignancy in men in the UK, and the incidence is likely to rise with the increasing use of serum-prostate-specific antigen (PSA) to 'screen' asymptomatic men.[38] In the US, where the measurement of PSA became

[35] Avril *et al.* J Clin Oncol (2005) 23: 7385–7387.

[36] Jaaback, Cochrane Database Syst Rev (2006) Issue 1.

[37] Armstrong *et al.* NEJM (2006) 354: 34–43.

[38] www.cancerresearchuk.org/cancerstats/

widespread in the late 1980s, the incidence of diagnosed prostate cancer dramatically increased.[39] As with breast cancer, carcinoma of the prostate is a hugely heterogeneous malignancy, and acceptable treatment options range from watchful waiting to radical treatment with neoadjuvant and adjuvant therapy. With PSA screening, over-treatment may be a significant issue, particularly in older men.[40] The key aim of management is therefore to administer appropriate therapy to those who require it, rather than therapy *per se*.

The workup of the patient with suspected prostate cancer includes biopsy to obtain histological confirmation in almost all cases (patients with grossly elevated PSA and clear evidence of metastatic disease may occasionally be treated on clinical grounds alone). Further investigations may include MR of the prostate and pelvic lymph nodes, together with isotope bone scan. The chances of an asymptomatic individual with prostate cancer developing clinically relevant manifestations of disease are related to a combination of the biology of the tumour and the life expectancy of the patient, and these should both be taken into account when planning investigations and treatment. National US guidelines recommend that patients with life expectancy of less than 5 years diagnosed with prostate cancer may be observed without further investigations unless adverse risk factors are present.[41] In the UK, there is a general consensus that radical treatment is appropriate only for patients with a life expectancy of more than 10 years. The tumour features most relevant to outcome include the anatomical stage of disease, Gleason score (a measure of the degree of differentiation of tumour) and level of serum PSA. It should of course be remembered that there is an anaplastic variant of prostate cancer, where the malignant cells are less capable of pouring out PSA: therefore, PSA levels may be normal despite advanced malignant disease.[42]

Although a gross oversimplification of an extensive literature, an attempt follows to summarize the different management options for fit patients with localized disease.

Active surveillance is acceptable for low-risk patients with indolent disease (typically PSA doubling time of > 3 years). This strategy requires regular PSA measurements and periodic repeat biopsies of the prostate, with a view to radical intervention if required.[43]

[39] Jemal *et al.* CA Cancer J Clin (2005) 55: 10–30.

[40] Cooperberg *et al.* J Clin Oncol (2005) 23: 8146–8151.

[41] National comprehensive cancer network practice guidelines (2005) (www.nccn.org)

[42] Schwartz *et al.* Radiology (1998) 208: 735–738.

[43] Klotz, J Clin Oncol (2005) 23: 8165–8169.

Radical prostatectomy can be appropriate as radical treatment of patients with low- or intermediate-risk disease. Patients with high-risk disease treated with radical prostatectomy have a modest progression-free survival of 28–36% and are, therefore, often considered for alternative therapies.[44] Patients with very-high-risk disease (tumour spread to seminal vesicles, adjacent organs or pelvic lymph nodes) are not surgical candidates.

Prostate brachytherapy involves the implantation of radioactive seeds within the prostate to deliver a highly focused dose of radiation. This treatment is acceptable only for low-risk patients if used as the sole treatment, but can be combined with external beam radiotherapy for higher risk groups. External beam radiotherapy is acceptable for all stages of disease, though it is now combined with a hormone therapy for 3 months beforehand and up to 2 years later for high-risk tumours, in a strategy that improves outcome.[45] Hormone therapy alone is appropriate for patients with very-high-risk disease, where the principal risk of relapse is at distant sites.

The choice between the radical treatment options cannot be said to be particularly evidence based, as trials comparing modalities are somewhat lacking. The most recent example of this is the widespread adoption of brachytherapy without randomized evidence to support its use. However, observational studies suggest comparable efficacy of the three treatments for low-risk disease.

At diagnosis, many patients with prostate cancer have distant metastases, most often in the bone. Treatment in this context is palliative with the aim of extending life and minimizing symptoms. Hormone therapy works on the principle that the vast majority of prostatic carcinomas express the androgen receptor, and their growth is dependent on testosterone levels (hence the traditional therapy of castration). Nowadays, management is thankfully pharmacological: luteinizing-hormone-releasing hormone (LHRH) agonists are the most commonly used agents. Following a tumour flare (which must be covered with an antiandrogen), these cause down-regulation of the LHRH receptor with consequent decrease in LH and, thus, testosterone levels. The duration of disease response achieved with LHRH agonists is typically 12–18 months. Hormone-resistant prostate cancer (HRPC) is defined as disease progression in the context of 'castrate' levels of serum testosterone, and is a condition with a poor prognosis and a median survival of less than a year.

---

44 Lau *et al.* J Urol (2002) 167: 117–122.
45 Bolla *et al.* NEJM (1997) 337: 295–300.

Further options for management include antiandrogen therapy, oestrogens and low-dose steroids. A recent development is the widespread use of cytotoxic chemotherapy for HRPC. While it was previously thought that this disease was chemoresistant, two recent phase III randomized trials have demonstrated that docetaxel-based chemotherapy produces a survival benefit of approximately 3 months when compared with mitoxantrone and prednisolone therapy, the previous standard of care.[46,47] It should be noted that LHRH agonists are normally continued in HRPC as there is evidence that the androgen receptor on carcinoma cells remains active. Bisphosphonates reduce osteoclast activity, important despite the fact that bone metastases in prostate cancer are frequently osteoblastic radiologically. When used in patients with HRPC and skeletal metastases, zolendronate significantly decreases skeletal complications.[48] Nonetheless, prostate cancer is one of the commonest causes of spinal cord compression.

Current research themes around prostate cancer include improving the accuracy of radiotherapy using intensity-modulated radiotherapy, incorporating active cytotoxics (such as docetaxel) into treatment of early-stage disease and identifying new molecular targets amenable to drugs (such as monoclonal antibodies and small-molecule tyrosine kinase inhibitors).

Carcinoma of unknown origin

Metastatic carcinoma of unknown primary accounts for 3% of all cancer diagnoses and regularly causes a conundrum for general physicians. Such patients have a poor prognosis (3-to-4-month median survival) and, therefore, it is vital to quickly establish a diagnosis of malignancy by biopsy of an involved site in order that appropriate treatment can be initiated, rather than organizing a protracted hunt for a silent primary. With improvements in immunohistochemistry, the origin of many poorly differentiated tumours can be identified by the pattern of staining, allowing organ-specific chemotherapy to be initiated. This is particularly important for potential breast and prostate cancers as successful hormone manipulation will improve survival, and also in ovarian cancer where aggressive surgical debulking prolongs life.

46 Petrylak *et al.* NEJM (2004) 351: 1513–1520.

47 Tannock *et al.* NEJM (2004) 351: 1502–1512.

48 Saad *et al.* J Natl Cancer Inst (2002) 94: 1458–1468.

For all other types of carcinoma, finding the culprit organ is less important as the prognosis of aggressive poorly differentiated tumours is poor, irrespective of the site of origin. For these patients, combination chemotherapy (such as cisplatin with 5-FU or etoposide, leucovorin and 5-FU) is used to cover most possibilities, giving a response rate of 10–40% and a median survival of approximately 6 months.

The aim of investigation in this context is, therefore, to identify the extent of disease and possible biopsy sites. History taking should concentrate on which system merits further scrutiny: constitutional symptoms are common and the rate of deterioration is usually rapid.

Physical examination should focus on the head and neck, peripheral lymph nodes, breasts, pelvis and rectum. The sensitivity and specificity of most tumour markers are too low to be useful in a diagnostic trawl but PSA, CA-125, AFP and β-HCG are worthwhile. The CT scanner tends to be the next port of call and often guides biopsy. Mammography is particularly useful in women with isolated axillary lymphadenopathy, as 40–60% will have an occult breast primary. PET scanning may help identify biopsy sites and disease extent but will not usually find a primary that evaded identification by other means. Upper-GI endoscopy, colonoscopy and bronchoscopy should not be done routinely in the work-up of unknown primaries, unless the patient has specific symptoms raising suspicions of a primary in one of these sites.

MANAGEMENT OF ONCOLOGICAL EMERGENCIES

Although it is important to remember that cancer patients can experience illnesses unrelated to their malignancy, most of the time an acute admission is likely to be precipitated by either the cancer or its treatment. Some of the scenarios that follow are also addressed in Chapter Fifteen.

Neutropenia

Febrile neutropenia is the commonest reason for admission in cancer patients receiving treatment and tends to occur approximately 10–14 days after a dose of chemotherapy. Its frequency is directly proportional to the severity and duration of the neutropenia. The causative organism is identified in less than half of all episodes. Those at highest risk in terms of occurrence and outcome can be identified by virtue of their disease, chemotherapy regimen and clinical state.

Management of febrile neutropenia

Risk group	Patient characteristics	Treatment option
HIGH	• Severe (< 0.1) prolonged (> 14 days) neutropenia • Haematological cancer • Bone marrow stem cell transplant • Significant comorbidity • Haemodynamically unstable	Broad-spectrum intravenous antibiotics for duration of febrile episode
MEDIUM	• Solid cancer receiving intensive chemotherapy (including stem cell transplant) • Expected neutropenia for 7–14 days • No comorbidities • Haemodynamically stable	Initial inpatient iv antibiotics, then discharge with oral antibiotics
LOW	• Solid cancer receiving conventional chemotherapy • Expected neutropenia <7 days • Haemodynamically stable • Fever of unknown origin/simple infection	Outpatient oral antibiotics

Risk stratification can also be used to identify those patients who do not require a prolonged hospital admission (particularly as hospitals are increasingly seen, both in perception and reality, as a hotbed of potential infection rather than a place of safety). Instead, they can either receive a short course of intravenous antibiotics (24–48 h) and then be discharged on oral therapy, or indeed receive oral antibiotics from the outset, often with a combination of ciprofloxacin and co-amoxiclav.

Due to the lack of a functional immune system, the source of infection is usually unclear or disseminated but it is still worth reviewing device sites, the respiratory system, sinuses and oropharynx (particularly for fungi), and gastrointestinal tract (although digital rectal examination should not be performed here, as it may produce transient bacteraemia). Investigation includes a full blood count, peripheral and line cultures, MSU and CXR. Once cultures have been taken, empirical broad-spectrum antibiotics (such as a third-generation cephalosporin ± gentamicin) should be started immediately with the aim of providing cover for both Gram-positive and Gram-negative organisms. Frequently, severely neutropenic patients remain pyrexial until the WBC recovers and, therefore, timing of any changes in antibiotic cover is important, so as to not run out of options. Generally, antibiotics should only be changed if the patient remains clinically unwell after a minimum 48 h of a regimen unless the microbiology is instructive. Second-line regimens typically focus on covering resistant Gram-positives, particularly staphylococci, with the inclusion of vancomycin. Once a switch to third line is being considered, amphotericin is often used, as the risk of fungal infection at this stage is high. Antibiotics do not need to be continued for the whole duration of neutropenia if the patient has received a minimum of 7 days treatment, is no longer febrile and has intact mucous membranes and skin.

Hypercalcaemia

Hypercalcaemia occurs in 10% of cancer patients, usually during the terminal phases. It is commonest in those with squamous cell lung cancer, breast cancer and multiple myeloma, where osteolytic bony metastases stimulate osteoclasts to release calcium. It is also commonplace in prostate cancer. However, raised calcium can be present in the absence of bone metastases due to PTH-related peptide or abnormalities in vitamin D metabolism (T-cell acute lymphocytic leukaemia, Hodgkin's disease). Pseudo-hypercalcaemia can be produced by the binding of calcium to nonalbumin proteins present in high concentrations in the blood.

Patients may be symptomatic with the full house of 'stones, abdominal groans and psychiatric moans'. The best way to normalize calcium is to treat the underlying disease but as this is frequently not possible in end-stage patients, short-term control can be achieved via generous intravenous rehydration followed by a bisphosphonate infusion. Calcium should fall to normal levels within 2–3 days, and prognosis is particularly poor if this does not occur. Alternative measures include furosemide, steroids (particularly in myeloma, lymphoma and breast cancer) or calcitonin.

Superior vena cava obstruction (SVCO)

About 95% of superior vena cava obstruction (SVCO) is due to underlying malignancy, particularly cancer of the lung (accounting for 85% of cases), lymphoma (10%) or mediastinal metastases.[49] The onset is usually insidious over several weeks, and patients present with a combination of facial oedema, shortness of breath, cough, headache, upper-body cyanosis with dilated peripheral veins and blackouts, all exacerbated by position.

As SVCO is unlikely to be immediately fatal, it is important to establish the underlying diagnosis first with imaging and biopsy, remembering that prior use of steroids may prevent a lymphoma from being identified. Treatment varies with diagnosis as highly chemosensitive tumours such as small-cell lung cancer and lymphoma can respond rapidly to systemic chemotherapy.

---

[49] www.ncicancerweb.ncl.ac.uk/cancernet

In other cancers, high-dose dexamethasone and radiotherapy are more appropriate. SVC stenting is also useful, particularly in patients with recurrent SVCO following radiotherapy.

Spinal cord compression

Spinal cord compression occurs in 30% of patients with disseminated malignancy (particularly in association with breast, prostate and lung cancers) and should be treated as an emergency, as early diagnosis and treatment reduces permanent disability.[50] Back pain precedes neurological impairment in over 90% of cases and should, therefore, always be thoroughly investigated in any patient with a history of cancer.[51] The pain is typically exacerbated by movement or coughing and is usually associated with focal tenderness on examination. Once cord compression is present, there is a relentless progression towards increasing neurological impairment with development of motor weakness, hyperreflexia, dermatomal sensory loss and sphincter disturbance. 70% of patients experience such deterioration in function between the first onset of symptoms and treatment. Those patients who become paralysed prior to treatment have little chance of regaining mobility. Dexamethasone should be started once cord compression is suspected clinically and the patient confined to bed. A hard collar should be used if the cervical spine is involved. DVT prophylaxis should also be considered, as immobilized patients with active malignancy are at very high risk of thromboembolic events.

The investigation of choice is MRI but if this is contraindicated, CT myelography may be helpful. Once the level of compression has been identified, the patient should usually be discussed with the spinal or neurosurgeons. There is increasing evidence to show that full surgical decompression with reconstruction and spinal stabilization followed by adjuvant radiotherapy is more effective than radiotherapy alone in relieving pain and preserving or regaining neurological function.[52] If surgery is thought to be inappropriate because of overall life expectancy (< 3 months), widespread disease throughout the spinal column, poor performance status or other comorbidities, then the patient should be offered palliative radiotherapy. Patient morbidity is significantly increased if surgery is performed after radiotherapy, predominantly due to the effect of radiotherapy on wound healing. Maintenance dexamethasone should be continued during radiotherapy and then tailed off slowly over several weeks.

....

50 Abeloff *et al. Clinical Oncology.* 3rd Ed, Churchill Livingstone, 2004.

51 Loblaw *et al.* Clin Oncol (2005) 23: 2029–2037.

52 Patchell *et al.* Lancet (2005) 366: 643–648.

Chapter 14

Katherine Lowndes and David Perry

HAEMATOLOGY

While most physicians are familiar with red cell indices, and have the ability to confidently palpate a spleen, it is the haematologist that is in a unique position to combine use of the laboratory and clinical findings to guide the diagnosis and management of blood disorders. Knowledge of the laboratory's scope is as important as an understanding of its limitations; we hope to draw a little attention to both in this chapter.

THE PANCYTOPENIC PATIENT

Pancytopenia, the combination of anaemia, leucopenia (most commonly neutropenia) and thrombocytopenia, often makes clinicians think immediately of bone marrow failure or infiltration. This may be the case, however, it is useful to remember that pancytopenia may also be due to the production of abnormal cells that have a shortened survival (e.g. myelodysplasia) or the production of normal cells that are exposed to an abnormal environment (e.g. hypersplenism). Bone marrow failure can present as either pancytopenia due to a defect in the pluripotent stem cell, namely aplastic anaemia, or a defect with one of the committed cell lines producing a single cell cytopenia. There is also considerable overlap, as a single cell cytopenia can progress to total marrow failure and aplastic anaemia can partially recover to a single cell cytopenia.

When presented with a patient who is pancytopenic, the cause may be readily apparent from the clinical history (most notably the drug history) and the physical examination. However, it is often helpful to initially clarify whether this is a problem of increased destruction or decreased production. Increased destruction is indicated in the full blood count (FBC) if there is a raised mean cell volume (MCV), red cell distribution width (RDW), and a raised reticulo-cyte count. This reflects the fact that the bone marrow is pushing out more immature red cell precursors, which are larger than mature cells, to keep up with demand. There will also be an increase in the number of large immature platelets which will be reflected by a raised mean platelet volume (MPV). Conversely, decreased production leads to a decreased reticulocyte count and decreased MPV.

The next step is to ascertain the appearance of the blood film. The presence of abnormal cells such as blasts, lymphomatous or myelomatous cells is infrequent but obviously significant. The combination of immature granulocytes and nucleated red cells (a leucoerythroblastic film) is most commonly associated with either bone marrow infiltration or idiopathic myelofibrosis. Other helpful features are dysplasia in any cell lineage, seen in myelodysplasia (MDS), megaloblastic anaemia and some acute infections. The presence of macrocytosis is also useful, but can be seen in a number of conditions including liver disease, alcohol abuse, megaloblastic anaemia, aplastic anaemia and MDS.

Inevitably, most cases require a bone marrow examination, both an aspirate and trephine. This allows the identification of any infiltration of haematological or non-haematological cells, dysplasia (as in MDS), hyperplasia (indicative of increased peripheral destruction) or aplasia/hypoplasia.

Liver function tests and hepatitis serology should be performed routinely to detect antecedent hepatitis. Aplasia may also occur 2–3 months after an episode of acute hepatitis. Although more common in young males, the serology is most often negative for all known hepatitis viruses. Cytomegalovirus (CMV), Epstein–Barr virus (EBV) and parvovirus should also be screened for, although the latter tends to cause an isolated red cell aplasia. Vitamin B12 and folate deficiency, when severe, can also cause pancytopenia. As the commonest autoimmune condition associated with aplasia is systemic lupus erythematosus, the autoantibody screen should include anti-nuclear antibody and anti-dsDNA antibody.

The term aplastic anaemia is rather a misnomer because the disorder is defined as pancytopenia with a hypocellular bone marrow. The anaemia is much less of a clinical problem than the neutropenia (which defines its severity) and thrombocytopenia. More than 80% of cases will be acquired and there is increasing clinical and biochemical evidence that this has an autoimmune mechanism. Treatment is initially supportive and includes transfusions and prompt treatment of infections. It is suggested that 20% of patients will spontaneously recover, however, there is a 70% mortality if left with supportive therapy alone so this is rarely done. If the patient has a matched sibling donor, then a bone marrow transplant (BMT) is the treatment of choice with a 90% 5-year survival. In the absence of a sibling donor, treatment involves immunosuppression with anti-lymphocyte globulin and ciclosporin which has a 75% 5-year survival. Only in the setting of failed immunosuppression would an unrelated donor BMT be considered, and in this case only if the donor was fully HLA-matched.

FALLING PLATELETS

A very common problem in the hospital setting is that of thrombocytopenia. This is not surprising considering that many systemic illnesses, drugs and infections can be associated with low platelets, leaving aside the primary haematological disorders.

The normal range for platelets is $150–400 \times 10^9/l$, but of course 2.5% of the population will have a level beneath this range. However, a recent fall in platelet count is significant and should be investigated. If confirmed on a second sample then a blood film should be examined. Two situations falsely lower the count. Inadequate anticoagulant in the sample may cause the platelets to clump and therefore not register on the analyser. Second, 0.1% of the normal population have EDTA-dependant agglutinins which will also cause the platelets to clump. These platelet autoantibodies are directed against an epitope on the platelet membrane glycoprotein IIb/IIIa (and can also develop after administration of abciximab, the GpIIb/IIIa monoclonal antibody). In both situations the FBC should be repeated in lithium heparin or sodium citrate. Platelet clumps will be seen on the blood film.

Once platelet clumping has been excluded, the next step is to decide whether there is decreased platelet production or increased destruction. Drugs and infections can have their effect through either mechanism. Reduced production is suggested by the presence of small platelets, associated anaemia or neutropenia, immature granulocytes (e.g. blast cells) or a leucoerythroblastic blood film. A macrocytosis is indicative of B12/folate deficiency which can also lead to decreased platelet production. Large platelets, on the other hand, imply increased destruction. If associated with fragmented red cells and haemolysis, it is suggestive of thrombotic thrombocytopenic purpura–haemolytic uraemic syndrome (TTP–HUS). At this point, if the diagnosis is not clear, a bone marrow aspirate is indicated.

There are a few conditions that warrant specific mention. These include heparin-induced thrombocytopenia and thrombosis (HITT), idiopathic thrombocytopenic purpura (ITP) and disseminated intravascular coagulation (DIC).

Heparin-induced thrombocytopenia and thrombosis (HITT)

Two types of thrombocytopenia are associated with the use of heparin. Type I is mild, occurs in the first few days after heparin is started and will resolve despite the continuation of heparin. The platelet count does not tend to drop below $100 \times 10^9/l$ and the condition is clinically insignificant. Type 2, however, is much more serious because of the high risk of death from associated venous or arterial thrombosis. It is immune-mediated due to the formation of antibodies against the heparin–platelet factor 4 (PF4) complex. PF4 is a platelet-specific chemokine that is released in high concentrations at sites of platelet activation. Binding of heparin to PF4 exposes new antigenic epitopes that lead to antibody formation. All classes of antibodies have been detected, but it appears that those patients that develop high-titre IgG antibodies are at greatest risk of developing clinical disease. The formation of this complex causes further platelet activation and amplification of the process. The resulting thrombin activation promotes a systemic hypercoagulable state.

The platelets usually fall 4–10 days after starting heparin, but can fall earlier if the patient has been exposed to heparin in the previous 3–4 months due to the persistence of antibodies. The average fall is to levels of $30–50 \times 10^9/l$. It is estimated that up to 3% of patients exposed to unfractionated heparin for more than 3 days will develop type 2 HITT. It can occur with any dose of heparin and has even been described after using heparin to flush an intravenous cannula. HITT is about 10 times less common with low molecular weight heparin than unfractionated heparin. Affected patients very rarely bleed, the main risk is actually that of thrombosis that can occur before the platelets fall significantly due to the hypercoagulable state. HITT remains a clinical diagnosis which can be challenging as those affected are often critically ill or post-surgery, and may have alternative reasons for thrombocytopenia.

A clinical scoring system has been developed to aid patient assessment, the results of which are supported by confirmatory laboratory testing. [1] The scoring system uses the degree of thrombocytopenia, the timing of the fall in platelet count, the presence of thrombosis or other sequelae (e.g. skin necrosis) and the presence or absence of other causes for thrombocytopenia. The most commonly used confirmatory test is an immunoassay that measures the presence of heparin–PF4 complex antibodies, but there is a problem with false positives. Many patients who have been exposed to heparin will develop non-neutralizing antibodies but will not become thrombocytopenic or develop further thromboses. This is seen in 1–3% of dialysis patients, 10–15% of medical patients and > 20% of patients receiving heparin for peripheral vascular surgery. In contrast, bioassays detect the degree of platelet activation by the patient's plasma when exposed to low levels of heparin: these are specific,

---

[1] Warkentin, BJH (2003) 121: 535–555.

but not very sensitive and require particular skill in performing and interpreting so should only be undertaken in experienced laboratories. In certain populations (such as intensive care units) where there is widespread heparin exposure and multiple possible aetiologies for thrombocytopenia, there is an argument for performing both an immunoassay (ELISA) and platelet activation assay. If both are positive the likelihood of HITT is high. However, it remains that if the pretest probability of HITT is low, then the positive predictive value of the immunoassay is low and probably represents a false positive. If the pretest probability is high or both tests are positive, then it should be treated as HITT, as the consequences of missing a true positive case could be catastrophic.

Obviously, management includes stopping the heparin (including low molecular weight heparin) and starting an alternative anticoagulant, such as danaparoid or lepirudin.[2] Warfarin alone is contraindicated initially because it has been associated with massive thrombosis and skin necrosis, probably secondary to initial low levels of protein C. Danaparoid has a theoretical risk of cross-reactivity as it consists of a mix of heparan sulphate, chondroitin sulphate and dextran sulphate, however, in practice this is rare. It should be given in treatment, not prophylactic doses, and is renally cleared so care must be taken not to overanticoagulate those patients with renal impairment. This can be monitored with the anti-Xa level, usually on day 3 and every other day thereafter. Lepirudin is a direct thrombin inhibitor and is the recombinant form of the anticoagulant protein hirudin found in leeches. It is also renally cleared. The effects are monitored using the activated partial thromboplastin time (APTT) ratio, aiming for 1.5–2.5. The risk of haemorrhage is directly related to the APTT ratio. Warfarin can then be introduced when adequate anticoagulation has been achieved and the platelet count has normalized. The risk of new thromboembolic events due to HITT lasts for about 1 month. Patients usually become antibody negative 50–80 days after diagnosis. These antibodies do not show an anamnestic response (in other words, they do not retain memory), so heparin can be used again. The current recommendations are after 100 days.

Immune thrombocytopenic purpura (ITP)

The two main issues in ITP for the general physician concern indications for bone marrow biopsy and the management of such patients who require a surgical procedure. In ITP, anti-platelet antibodies are directed against platelets, or T-cells are directed against the platelets or megakaryocytes. In children,

---

[2] BCSH Guidelines on the management of heparin induced thrombocytopenia, 2005 (www.bcshguidelines.com)

this is most commonly associated with a previous viral infection and the vast majority will resolve spontaneously, but in adults there is often no precipitant and it rarely resolves without treatment. Until recently, a bone marrow biopsy was performed routinely to exclude aplasia, leukaemia or other clonal or infiltrative processes, but this has become a contentious issue as other conditions very rarely present with an isolated thrombocytopenia (i.e. with a normal Hb, white cell count, blood film and physical examination). A retrospective Chinese study evaluated 83 patients with suspected ITP, all of whom underwent a bone marrow examination. It did show 11 patients in whom there was reduced or absent marrow iron, but the bone marrows were otherwise normal.[3] In their guidelines for ITP, the British Committee for Standards in Haematology (BCSH) states that bone marrow examination can be reserved for those patients who are older than 60 years of age, have atypical features, respond poorly to first-line treatment, or are being considered for splenectomy.[4] In elderly patients, MDS is an important differential as 1% of these patients will present with an isolated thrombocytopenia.

Platelet antibodies can be present in a variety of conditions in the absence of thrombocytopenia. They are, therefore, unhelpful in the diagnosis of ITP. It is worth determining the presence of *H. pylori* in patients refractory to therapy since some patients have shown improvement in platelet counts following eradication therapy.[5,6]

Bleeding in ITP is rare unless the platelets are consistently < 10 × 10⁹/l, and patients do not require treatment if their platelet count is consistently greater than 30 × 10⁹/l. Until recently, many patients have been over-treated and the major cause of morbidity has been infection rather than bleeding. Of course surgery, dentistry and delivery are situations where platelet counts may need to be higher; recommended platelet levels for certain procedures are below.

Platelet counts and interventions in ITP

General dentistry	≥ 10 × 10⁹/l
Dental extractions or regional dental block	≥30 × 10⁹/l
Minor surgery, vaginal delivery, Caesarean section, lumbar puncture or spinal anaesthesia	≥ 50 × 10⁹/l
Major surgery or epidural anaesthesia	≥ 80 × 10⁹/l

[3] Mak *et al*. Clin Lab Haematol (2000) 22: 355–358.

[4] BCSH Guidelines, BJH (2003) 120: 574.

[5] Emilia *et al*. Blood (2001) 97: 812–814.

[6] Kohda *et al*. BJH (2002) 118: 584–588.

First-line therapy comprises oral corticosteroids and intravenous immunoglobulin (IVIG), but there are no randomized studies comparing these two agents against placebo. A third of patients will have a long-term response to oral prednisolone (1 mg/kg per day for 2 4 weeks followed by a gradual tapering off over several weeks). Pooled IVIG will transiently elevate the platelet count in 75% of patients, 50% of whom will achieve normal counts, but 3–4 weeks later, counts will drift back to pre-treatment levels. It is useful in situations when the platelet count has to be raised because of bleeding or when there is likely to be predictable bleeding (e.g. dentistry, surgery or labour). IVIG is a pooled blood product so there is always the theoretical risk of transmission of infectious agents.

Intravenous anti-D given to Rh positive patients has also been shown to transiently increase platelet levels in a similar proportion of patients. This is thought to occur by the preferential removal of opsonized Rh (D) positive cells by the spleen, blocking Fc receptors on macrophages and sparing the autoantibody-coated platelets. This is obviously not an option for patients without a spleen.

Second-line therapy usually involves splenectomy, although high-dose corticosteroids with or without cyclophosphamide, high-dose IVIG, vinca alkaloids, danazol, azathioprine and ciclosporin have also been used. Campath-1H and rituximab may be useful in patients where other therapies have failed and there is a definite need to elevate the platelet count. In an emergency situation a transfusion of random donor platelets is appropriate, but the response will be extremely short lived.

Disseminated intravascular coagulation (DIC)

Conditions that promote the expression of tissue factor such as gram negative septicaemia (endotoxin-mediated endothelial damage), trauma, malignancy, hypoxia and obstetric complications such as placental abruption and retention of a dead foetus may cause DIC. The tissue factor combines with factor VII to initiate coagulation. Excess thrombin is then generated with subsequent conversion of fibrinogen to fibrin (causing the consumption of fibrinogen). Fibrin polymerizes and forms microcirculation deposits and thrombin promotes platelet aggregation, consumption and subsequent thrombocytopenia. The result is bleeding, as well as end organ damage due to the deposition of microthrombi.

Decreased fibrinogen and platelets with a prolonged prothrombin time (PT), APTT and thrombin time (TT) are seen, whereas fibrin degradation products (FDP) are increased. The earliest laboratory sign comes from the waveform produced by the APTT assay. The automated APTT analysers measure the optical density of the patient sample as it clots. This produces a waveform. In some patients with impending DIC there is a rise in calcium-dependent C-reactive protein, which complexes with very light density lipoprotein (VLDL) in the serum causing the waveform to become biphasic. This is particularly sensitive and specific for DIC associated with sepsis, such that a normal waveform has a high negative predictive value in excluding DIC.

Treatment of DIC is obviously aimed primarily at treatment of the underlying disorder, and correction of the coagulopathy is only required if the patient is bleeding. In this case, platelets can be transfused to keep the level above $20 \times 10^9/l$, fresh frozen plasma is used to replace the clotting factors and cryoprecipitate should be given to replace fibrinogen if it is less than 1.0 g/l. In patients with ongoing consumption despite rigorous replacement, the coagulation system can be blocked by the use of heparin, but this is controversial. Some patients will be resistant due to low levels of antithrombin (which has been consumed), in which case activated protein C may be of use. Heparin may be of use in those patients with chronic DIC (perhaps due to malignancy) as it is better at suppressing the associated chronic activation of coagulation than warfarin.

THE BLEEDING PATIENT

The most common forms of presentation are those of a patient with acute unexpected peri/post-operative bleeding, or a patient with increased bruising, epistaxis or mucosal bleeding progressing over several months. One approach is to assess whether the bleeding has a haematological cause or not.[7] The PT and APTT are relatively insensitive to mild, but clinically significant conditions such as von Willebrand's disease (vWD) and platelet disorders. These are most likely to be picked up in the history, in particular the patients' response to previous haemostatic challenges such as dental extraction, surgery and menstruation, and the family history of any bleeding problems. A history of easy bruising and childhood epistaxis is notoriously difficult to quantify and has a low predictive value for an underlying bleeding disorder. If the clotting screen (PT and APTT) is normal then more complex laboratory assessment of haemostasis is required, as long as a non-haematological cause for bleeding has been excluded. The commonest inherited bleeding tendency is that of a low von Willebrand protein, as it acts as a carrier protein for factor VIII and mediates platelet adhesion to the vascular endothelium. This can be caused by genetic mutations (vWD) or be present in those people with blood group O.

---

[7] Baglin, Clin Med (2005) 5: 326–328.

The von Willebrand protein is increased as part of the acute stress response, so normal levels immediately post-operatively may need to be re-checked at a later stage.

Anticoagulant therapy is the most common cause of an acquired bleeding disorder and over-anticoagulation is responsible for the majority of life-threatening bleeds. Drug-induced bleeding is also precipitated by anti-platelet drugs and drugs causing thrombocytopenia. The response to anti-platelet therapy can be highly variable between individuals, in some producing a significant bleeding tendency. Many drugs cause a mostly mild, reversible and idiosyncratic thrombocytopenia, however sometimes it can be profound (as with quinine and gold). Others cause generalized bone marrow suppression (azathioprine and methotrexate). A few days without nutrition in critically ill patients is all that is needed to develop vitamin K deficiency resulting in a coagulopathy. Massive transfusion causes a dilutional coagulopathy and DIC always needs to be considered. Rarely patients can develop acquired inhibitors (autoantibodies) to specific factors such as factor VIII resulting in a severe bleeding disorder. Management requires the offending drugs to be stopped, non-haematological causes of bleeding to be corrected and vitamin K to be supplemented in those likely to be deficient. Haematological support is available in the form of FFP, cryoprecipitate and platelet transfusions. Drugs such as desmopressin (DDAVP) for vWD and antifibrinolytics such as aprotinin and tranexamic acid should be used following consultation with a haematologist.

Recombinant factor VIIa is being used with increased frequency, especially within the intensive care setting. It is only licensed for those patients with haemophilia who have developed an inhibitor, acquired haemophilia, patients with factor VII deficiency and patients with Glanzmann's thrombasthenia (a defect in the platelet GPIIb/IIIa receptor), but its uses off-license are more extensive.[8] It acts by binding to the surface of locally activated platelets causing direct activation of factor X. This in turn provides a burst of thrombin which leads to the formation of a stable fibrin clot, an action which is independent of factors VIII, IX and tissue factor.

THE 'CLOTTING' PATIENT

Thrombophilia

After completing a course of anticoagulant therapy for venous thromboembolism (VTE), 10–25% of patients will suffer a recurrence in the first 1–2 years

---

[8] Ghorashian et al. Blood Rev (2004) 18: 245–259.

off therapy. The initial rationale for thrombophilia screening is to detect those at greatest risk of recurrence, therefore requiring prolonged or lifelong anticoagulation, and those patients with a strong family history of VTE who may need to take precautions at times of unavoidable high risk.

In consecutive patients presenting with a first VTE, approximately 5% will have a protein C, S or antithrombin deficiency, 15% will have the factor V Leiden mutation and 3–5% will have the prothrombin gene mutation (F2G20210A). Despite this, a prospective study in Cambridge showed that the risk of recurrence related to the clinical circumstances at the time of the first event, rather than thrombophilia testing which had no predictive value.[9] The Leiden thrombophilia study group reported similar findings with long-term follow-up.

In practice, if there is a clear precipitant to the VTE (such as surgery or immobilization), then there is no benefit in testing the patient and anticoagulation is only required for 3 months (although most centres will suggest 6 months treatment). If, however, the VTE is unprovoked and one of the following factors is present; age < 45 years, an unusual site (e.g. mesenteric veins, dural sinus), history of recurrent foetal loss, strong family history of VTE, 2 or more events with no clear precipitant or neonatal thrombosis/stroke, then thrombophilia testing is reasonable.

This testing should take place once the initial period of anticoagulant therapy is completed as warfarin and heparin interfere with natural anticoagulant levels (protein C, S and antithrombin). The current screen includes lupus anticoagulant, anticardiolipin antibodies, functional measurements of protein C, S and antithrombin levels and genetic analysis for both the factor V Leiden and the prothrombin gene mutations. Thrombophilia testing has no role in influencing the intensity of heparin or warfarin therapy, or the duration of anticoagulation in symptomatic patients.

The results of the screen have to be interpreted in conjunction with the clinical situation. Patients with persistent antiphospholipid antibodies (lupus anticoagulant, anticardiolipin antibodies) are at increased risk of both arterial and venous thrombosis during and after anticoagulant therapy, so should remain therapeutically anticoagulated lifelong. Similarly patients with antithrombin deficiency who have had a DVT appear to be at increased risk of recurrence, but they may not merit indefinite anticoagulation. Protein C and S deficiencies are even less clear-cut: the levels are affected by different situations (including pregnancy and warfarin treatment), so they really have to be low on repeated

[9] Baglin *et al.* Lancet (2003) 362: 523–526.

testing before they can be considered as significant. Whether the associated risk is great enough to keep patients on lifelong anticoagulation is also unclear. Heterozygous states for the factor V Leiden or prothrombin gene mutation do not appear to be clinically important unless there is a strong family history of VTE, or the patient is taking the combined oral contraceptive pill. Compound heterozygotes for both mutations and homozygotes for the factor V Leiden mutation do have a higher relative risk for recurrent DVT, but there are only a small number of these patients in clinical trials so the absolute risk is not certain. Elevated factor VIII levels appear to be a risk factor, although as it is an acute phase protein it may be that the initial insult causing the elevated levels is more significant. Finally, hyperhomocysteinemia (hereditary or acquired) does appear to be associated with increased recurrent VTE, but lowering it with vitamin therapy does not reduce the frequency of recurrence.

MALIGNANCY

The majority of acute haematological malignancies are treated solely by haematologists, although the initial diagnosis is not infrequently made by general physicians. The more common of these malignancies include multiple myeloma, chronic lymphocytic leukaemia, MDS and the myeloproliferative disorders.

Multiple myeloma and paraproteinaemia

One of the commonest routes of referral for patients with a new diagnosis of multiple myeloma is via the general physician, be it through the investigation of back pain, hypercalcaemia or renal failure. It remains a disease of older age with only 15% of cases diagnosed in those under the age of 60 and less than 2% under 40 years of age. This has implications for the population eligible for specific types of treatment such as high-dose chemotherapy and stem cell transplantation. The diagnosis of myeloma is confirmed by the presence of a monoclonal paraprotein (M-protein) in the serum or urine and/or lytic bone lesions with increased plasma cells in the bone marrow. M-proteins can also be present in monoclonal gammopathy of undetermined significance (MGUS), chronic lymphocytic leukaemia, B-cell non-Hodgkins lymphoma (including Waldenstrom's macroglobulinaemia), amyloidosis and solitary plasmacytoma. The majority of patients with an M-protein will have MGUS detected through the increasingly common use of protein electrophoresis.

A new classification has recently been proposed, based on the level of M-protein, the percentage of plasma cells in the bone marrow and the presence or absence of myeloma-related organ or tissue impairment (ROTI).[10] The categories include MGUS, symptomatic myeloma and asymptomatic myeloma. The latter term incorporates most patients that might previously have been termed as indolent, equivocal or 'smoldering' myeloma. In addition, some patients who have no symptoms would still be classified as symptomatic because they have evidence of end organ damage (such as anaemia, lytic bone lesions or renal impairment). This new classification really isolates those patients that require immediate treatment (those with symptomatic myeloma) which is useful, as early intervention in patients with asymptomatic myeloma has shown no benefit.

When the M-protein is less than 30 g/l, the bone marrow plasma cell percentage is less than 10%, there is no evidence of end organ damage and no other reason for an M-protein, the patient has MGUS. Asymptomatic myeloma patients have an M-protein level of more than 30 g/l, bone marrow plasma cell percentage of more than 10% but no evidence of myeloma-related end organ damage. There must be evidence of myeloma-related end organ damage for the diagnosis of symptomatic myeloma and an excess of plasma cells in the bone marrow, but the precise percentage is not important. An M-protein may be detected in the serum or urine, but this is not obligatory for the diagnosis as there is a small population of patients with symptomatic myeloma that do not produce a paraprotein. These cases are termed non-secretory.

One caution, however, is the over-investigation of healthy patients with a low level paraprotein. It is not reasonable or practical to perform a bone marrow examination in asymptomatic, elderly patients with a low level of M-protein and no evidence of end organ damage, as the results are very unlikely to change management. The extent of diagnostic procedures should take into account the age of the patient, the level of M-protein and the presence of other diseases. A number of patients with MGUS will also have a low level Bence-Jones proteinuria and a reduced polyclonal IgG, and so these are not necessarily a marker of malignancy. Current recommendations are that bone marrow biopsy and skeletal surveys should be reserved for younger patients and older patients with a paraprotein of > 20 g/l.

On average, 1% of patients with MGUS will progress to symptomatic myeloma per year, with the only proven prognostic factor being the level of the M-protein. A useful rule of thumb is that the percentage risk of progression in 10 years equates roughly to the level of M-protein (so 20 g/l is associated with a 20% risk). The M-protein level of 20 g/l is also the level that should prompt

---

[10] BSCH UK-Nordic Myeloma Guidelines, 2005 (www.bcshguidelines.com)

a bone marrow biopsy. The median time to progression from asymptomatic to symptomatic myeloma is 12–32 months.

Survival in symptomatic myeloma can range from weeks to more than 20 years. A number of attempts have been made to stage patients using various prognostic markers. The Durie/Salmon staging system is the one in common usage, but this does not include the β2-microglobulin or albumin levels that have the best correlation with survival. These have now been incorporated in the new International Staging System (below). [11]

Mortality in myeloma

Stage	Criteria	Median survival
I	Serum β2-microglobulin < 3.5mg/l Serum albumin > 3.5g/dl	62 months
II	Neither I nor III	45 months
III	Serum β2-microglobulin > 5.5mg/l	29 months

These survival figures are in treated patients, but importantly are irrespective of the type of treatment. Renal function is only indirectly represented in this scoring system via the serum β2-microglobulin which is increased in renal failure. So, if a patient requires renal replacement therapy at diagnosis they can still be expected to survive at least 2–3 years with treatment and maintain a reasonable quality of life.

The management of myeloma patients has been significantly improved with the introduction of evidence-based guidelines.[10] These include the use of long-term bisphosphonate therapy to improve bone disease and autologous stem cell transplantation to improve survival. Over the last few years a number of novel agents have shown considerable promise in treating relapsed myeloma. These include thalidomide and its derivatives, bortezomib (a proteosome inhibitor) and arsenic trioxide. These drugs act both alone and synergistically in combination with other active drugs, so current trials are investigating the best time to introduce them and in which combination. The hope is that they will lead to an improvement in prognosis.

Chronic lymphocytic leukaemia (CLL)[12]

CLL is the commonest of all leukaemias in patients over 65 years of age. It is most often diagnosed on a routine FBC which shows a lymphocytosis with the

---

[11] Griepp et al. J Clin Onc (2005) 23: 3412–3420.

[12] BCSH Guidelines on the diagnosis and management of CLL, BJH (2004) 125: 294–317.

typical lymphocyte morphology on the blood film. In the first instance, if there is no lymphadenopathy, the lymphocytosis should be greater than $5 \times 10^9/l$ to attract the label of CLL. Patients that require treatment are those with progressive marrow failure (anaemia, thrombocytopenia), massive (> 10 cm) or progressive lymphadenopathy, massive (> 6 cm below costal margin) or progressive splenomegaly, a lymphocyte doubling time of < 6 months or systemic symptoms. The development of an autoimmune cytopenia is also an indication for treatment, but this need not be cytotoxic therapy. Some patients can have exceedingly high, but slowly progressive lymphocyte counts and are otherwise asymptomatic. Unlike patients with myeloproliferative conditions these patients are not at an increased risk of thrombosis or leucostasis. Their main complication, if any, is likely to be an increased risk of infection. Hypogammaglobulinaemia and recurrent infections are indications for regular immunoglobulin replacement. There are no large studies assessing the efficacy of prophylactic antibiotics in CLL whereas the use of prophylactic IVIG in reducing recurrent bacterial infections has been well documented.[13] Annual influenza vaccinations are also recommended, although they may not be wholly efficacious. Vaccination against influenza has been shown to increase the baseline immunity in patients with CLL, however the same effect has not been shown with pneumococcal vaccination.

Myeloproliferative disorders

Increased arterial and venous thrombosis together with bleeding constitutes the major morbidity and mortality in these primary bone marrow disorders. They may also progress with increasing splenomegaly, bone marrow fibrosis and failure, or occasionally acute leukaemia. In the majority of patients however, polycythaemia and thrombocytosis will simply be due to reactive causes and here the thrombotic risk is not as exaggerated. Similarly, there is no risk of disease progression so the treatment is obviously different.

Polycythaemia[14]

A raised haemoglobin (Hb) and haematocrit (Hct) is often present in patients admitted acutely. In the majority of these cases, increases are transient and do not require further investigation. However, patients who have a persistently

---

[13] Chapel *et al.* Semin Hematol (1987) 24: 291–296

[14] BCSH Guidelines on the diagnosis, investigation and management of polycythaemia/ erythrocytosis, 2004 (www.bcshguidelines.com)

raised venous Hct (> 0.52 in males, > 0.48 in females) for more than 2 months should cause concern. Investigation starts with a measurement of the red cell mass, which will sort out those patients who have a true polycythaemia from those with an apparent one due to reduced plasma volume (also known as spurious or stress polycythaemia or Gaisbock's syndrome). Males and females with Hct values above 0.60 and 0.56 respectively can be assumed to have a true polycythaemia and do not require a red cell mass for further confirmation. The WHO criteria accept a Hb of greater than 18.5 g/dl in males and 16.5 g/dl in females, but this has not been verified.

Once an erythrocytosis has been confirmed, causes of secondary polycythaemia should be considered. Most acquired forms are mediated by increased erythro-poietin (EPO) levels, often driven by hypoxia, either central (chronic lung disease, sleep apnoea, right to left shunt or smoking) or within the renal vasculature. Pathological EPO production (tumours such as hepatocellular carcinoma) or exogenous EPO administration (following a renal transplant or in the miscreant sportsman) also occurs. Congenital causes are much less common but include the high oxygen-affinity Hbs and EPO receptor abnormalities. The majority of cases will be diagnosed on the basis of initial investigations that include, FBC and film, arterial oxygen saturation, renal and liver function tests, ferritin and serum erythropoietin levels, abdominal ultra-sound and chest X-ray. More specialized tests are sometimes required, such as a bone marrow aspirate and trephine, EPO receptor gene analysis and p50 (oxygen dissociation curve to detect high oxygen-affinity Hbs).

Untreated Polycythaemia Vera (PV) has historically had a dismal prognosis with a median survival of 18 months, thrombosis being the commonest cause of death. Treatment with aspirin and either venesection or cytoreduction with chemotherapy (usually hydroxyurea) can return the life expectancy of the average patient to normal, or near normal. If diagnosed before 40 years of age the median survival of patients is greater than 15 years.

Treatment of patients with secondary polycythaemia is a little more controversial. If the polycythaemia is hypoxia-driven then the erythrocytosis is a physiological response. Aggressive venesection will then have the deleterious effect of driving the process even harder. This has to be balanced against the thrombotic risk of allowing the Hct to get too high. In practice, venesection is performed at a higher Hct (> 0.54) compared with PV (HCT > 0.45), or if the patient has symptoms of hyperviscosity.

Thrombocytosis

The diagnosis of essential thrombocythaemia (ET) as the cause of a persistently raised platelet count is one of exclusion. Most commonly this is a reactive condition associated with iron deficiency, blood loss, inflammation, surgery, trauma, infection, malignancy or splenectomy. It can also be seen with other myeloproliferative disorders and MDS, but even then, only 10% of platelet counts > $1000 \times 10^9/l$ will be due to this.[15] A reactive cause is usually apparent from the history and is often accompanied by raised inflammatory markers. Typically the blood film in this situation just reveals an excess of normal platelets in contrast to the blood film in myeloproliferative conditions when platelet size and granularity are usually variable.

The diagnosis of ET confers a relative risk of death 4 times greater than that in age-matched controls, but if major thrombotic and bleeding complications are avoided, the patient can expect a normal lifespan. Therapy involves regular low-dose asprin and cytoreductive chemotherapy to keep the platelet count within the normal range. In patients with a reactive thrombocytosis regular asprin is usually reserved for those with platelet counts greater than $1000 \times 10^9/l$. Here the risk of thrombosis is proportional to the platelet count, whereas this is not necessarily the case in a patient with ET.

Myelodysplasia (MDS)

Patients with MDS have myeloid progenitors within the bone marrow but they are unable to mature and differentiate properly leading to peripheral blood cytopenias in the presence of a hypercellular bone marrow. In some patients the cells mature and the peripheral counts are normal but they acquire a functional defect causing increased infection and bleeding. The myelodysplastic syndromes (MDSs) are a heterogeneous group of disorders. They are considered to be preleukaemic, but the natural history of progression can range from months (rarely) to many years. As a result, the majority of patients will die of complications of the cytopenias or other comorbidities unrelated to the MDS. The most important aetiological factor is age and as only 20% of patients will present with an isolated anaemia, the majority of patients will be elderly, anaemic and neutropenic or thrombocytopenic. The presence of MDS can be alluded to on the blood film with the presence of hypogranular neutrophils and giant platelets, with oval macrocytic red cells, but these features are not specific. There are some conditions that produce very similar dysplastic features in the bone marrow and peripheral blood and should therefore be excluded first. These include vitamin B12 and folate deficiency, some viral infections, HIV-related infections and drugs including antibiotics, alcohol and chemotherapy.

---

[15] Bain, *Blood Cells, A Practical Guide*. 3rd Ed, Blackwell, Oxford (2002).

For younger patients, allogeneic stem cell transplantation will be offered if there is a matched sibling donor. The upper age limit for this is gradually increasing with the use of pre-transplant chemotherapy regimens that are less myeloablative. However, the mainstay of treatment in the elderly population is supportive care. This includes regular blood and platelet transfusions and prophylactic antibiotics and antifungals. Erythropoeitin therapy will increase the Hb in about 25% of patients. When combined with growth factors (such as G-CSF) about 45% of patients will respond. This can often maintain counts for an extended period of time minimizing the patient's transfusion requirement and importantly, maintaining their quality of life.

Chapter 15

Chi Chi Cheung and Bee Wee

PALLIATIVE CARE MEDICINE

'It hath been often said, that it is not death, but dying, which is terrible'
Henry Fielding (1707–1754)[1]

At times, the work of the palliative physician and the acute medical take seem poles apart. Often, though, these two worlds meet, and general physicians find themselves needing to make sure that a terminally ill patient is comfortable. Access to specialist palliative care services is patchy. The historical funding of the hospice movement and the fact that policy makers have not always regarded palliative care as a core NHS function mean that this is likely to continue to be the case. All physicians, therefore, have a duty to the terminally ill – it is not 'someone else's problem'. Palliative care can be challenging but also deeply satisfying. So what is it all about?

Broadly speaking, palliative care is about improving the quality of life of patients with life threatening illnesses and that of their families. It attempts to relieve suffering by prevention, identification, assessment and treatment of pain and other problems, whether physical, psychosocial or spiritual.[2] It is not just about cancer, nor is it merely the treatment of a single symptom; it involves placing that symptom in the overall context of someone who is recognized to be seriously ill, perhaps even dying. As with any other patient, a shrewd clinical assessment, carefully targeted investigation and a pragmatic approach to management are all important. One must not forget the family who may be even more distressed and anxious than the patient. All this can be done quickly. That palliative care requires aeons of time is just a myth,

[1] MacDonald, *Oxford Dictionary of Medical Quotations*. OUP, Oxford, 2004.

[2] WHO Expert Committee, Cancer pain relief and palliative care (1990) (www.who.int/cancer/publications)

though more time is certainly needed at critical points in the progress of the illness: at diagnosis, the point of first recurrence and when other major setbacks occur. [3] The other occasion when lengthy discussions may need to take place is when previous communication has, in the view of the patient or family, been inadequate or confusing.

Palliative care requires teamwork. This does not mean having too many cooks, which can overwhelm the patient, nor does it mean 'passing the buck' to yet another team. It means thinking through who should be involved now, what one is asking of them and how all this feeds into the clearly identified goals that have been negotiated with the patient.

SYMPTOM MANAGEMENT

Getting comfortable

The basic tenets of symptom management include identifying each problem as the patient sees it, seeking the cause or contributing factors and deciding whether these are reversible. One then decides what could and should be done now. Symptoms may be related to the disease, its treatment or an unrelated condition.

Common symptoms in patients with advanced cancer and nonmalignant disease include anorexia, fatigue, pain, breathlessness, dry mouth, nausea and vomiting.[4] Start by allowing patients to volunteer what is troubling them, and then check routinely about symptoms that may seem trivial or embarrassing (such as sleeplessness or constipation). See if the cause of the problem can be reversed or diminished, but otherwise focus on improving the symptom itself. In all situations, regular review gives the opportunity to modify plans, inspires confidence and avoids patients continuing with unnecessary, unhelpful interventions. As always, compliance improves when patients share ownership of their treatment plan. Sensible warnings should be given about the likely side effects of certain drugs.

Most patients prefer oral medication. Where this is not possible (perhaps on account of vomiting or decreased consciousness), subcutaneous administration of drugs is more comfortable than intramuscular, either as 'stat' injections or an infusion. Syringe drivers (for instance, the Graseby) are particularly useful for subcutaneous infusion in these patients. They are battery operated, relatively small and can be carried in a 'money belt' round the waist or discretely

[3] Cancer Service Guidance (March 2004) (www.nice.org.uk)

[4] Tranmer *et al.* J Pain Symptom Manage (2003) 25: 420–429.

placed under the covers or pillow. However, these useful devices are often misunderstood: a patient who has a syringe driver is not necessarily dying, and a patient who is dying does not necessarily require a syringe driver. They simply offer an alternative route of drug administration. Up to four drugs may be combined in a syringe driver but it is worth checking compatibility if less common drugs are used.[5]

Drugs for symptom relief are often used in ways or by routes that are beyond their licence. This is acceptable provided that use and dose range are consistent with clinical practice. If in doubt, check with the local specialist palliative care team.

Easing pain

Pain assessment should be thorough, taking into account all the usual features of pain: timing, quality, severity and exacerbating and relieving factors. Ask about analgesics tried and their beneficial and unwanted effects. Following an appropriate physical examination, a clinical diagnosis can usually be made. Radiological investigations may be helpful, usually to confirm or refute a diagnosis that might lead to further intervention, such as radiotherapy for bone pain or surgery for pathological fracture. Pain management tends to be limited in its effectiveness if the whole situation is not taken into account. For example, one must always consider the patient's fears and concerns, such as what the pain represents and what it will mean for their future and that of those caring for them, especially in a busy hospital environment.

Using the ladder

The World Health Organization's analgesic ladder is a good starting point in pain management.[2] This requires a working knowledge of at least one drug at each step and a willingness to move up and down the ladder when needed and to add adjuvant medications as required. The usual starting dose for strong opioids is 5–10 mg of immediate-release morphine every 4 h, but a slightly higher dose may be needed if the pain has not been controlled on step-two analgesia, and a slightly lower dose may be needed in elderly opioid-naïve patients or in those with renal compromise. In addition, a short-acting analgesic should be prescribed, as required (prn), for breakthrough pain. If the patient is on regular morphine (modified or immediate release), the prn dose of immediate-release morphine should be one-sixth of the total daily dose,

[5] Twycross et al. Palliative Care Formulary. 2nd Ed, Radcliffe Medical Press, 2003.

and this can be given hourly if needed. Thereafter, the regular daily dose requires upward titration to ensure optimum pain control. The prn dose should also be adjusted accordingly.

There is an increasing range of opioids hitting the market, bewildering clinicians who do not prescribe these drugs on a regular basis. Morphine remains the gold standard. It is cheap, and there is no hard evidence that any other opioid is more effective, despite claims by enthusiasts. The indication for switching to an alternative opioid is intolerable side effects, not superior efficacy. Usually, careful titration of the dose of morphine and treatment of side effects are sufficient to enable patients to continue with morphine.

Fentanyl is one of the alternative opioids that the general physician will encounter, because it is available as a transdermal patch. The patch lasts 72 h and should only be used once pain control has been achieved: a shorter-acting prn analgesic (such as immediate-release oral morphine) should be employed for breakthrough pain. The lowest patch dose is 25 mcg/h, equivalent to up to 120 mg morphine over 24 h, making fentanyl inappropriate for patients who only require low-opioid doses. Other opioids on the market include oral and subcutaneous oxycodone, hydromorphone, tramadol, methadone, transmucosal fentanyl and transdermal buprenorphine. Although marketed with great enthusiasm, evidence of superiority over traditional opioids is lacking.

When an injectable opioid is required, diamorphine is the drug of choice because of its greater solubility. To convert oral morphine to diamorphine, the total daily morphine dose should be divided by three. If there is a shortage in diamorphine stocks, parenteral morphine can be used instead, in which case, the total daily oral morphine dose should be divided by two to work out the dose of parenteral morphine required per 24 h.

Bone pain

Strong opioids, nonsteroidal anti-inflammatories (which are available parenterally) and radiotherapy are the mainstays of pain management for bone metastases. Bisphosphonates have a place in managing widespread bone pain from myeloma, breast and prostate cancer — so far, there is no evidence of their efficacy in other cancers.

Hitting a raw nerve

Classically, neuropathic pain is pain in a numb area. It may also be shooting, lancinating or burning in character. Treatment should start on the WHO analgesic ladder but this is likely to be inadequate, and adjuvant treatments can be added in. There is good evidence that tricyclic antidepressants (including amitryptiline) and anticonvulsants (such as gabapentin) are effective. Steroids, nerve blocks and radiotherapy may help.

Spinal cord compression

Any patient who complains of back pain accompanied by limb weakness, sensory changes or simply nonspecific feelings in the arms or legs may have cord compression. It is easy to miss in ill or bed-bound patients. High-dose dexamethasone (16 mg at once, then 8 mg twice daily) should be commenced immediately and an MRI scan arranged without delay. Radiotherapy is usually the treatment of choice but fit patients with a solitary metastasis may be eligible for surgery. Cord compression is always a medical emergency as early treatment can prevent or reduce paralysis. About 70% of patients who are ambulatory prior to treatment remain so, whereas only 5% of those who are paraplegic at that point regain some mobility. Rehabilitation is essential – it maximizes function and quality of life. In those who remain bed- or wheelchair-bound, basic measures, such as good bowel and pressure-area care, can also have a significant impact on comfort and well-being.

Nausea and vomiting

The patient who vomits provokes a quick journey to the sluice or drug cupboard. Conversely, the patient who is nauseated often has difficulty drawing attention to their plight. Faced with a patient who has one or both symptoms, where does the general physician begin?

As always, one should identify the probable cause. This enables appropriate intervention and saves the patient and physician from wading through a series of potentially demoralizing, ineffective manoeuvres.

Having considered reversible causes of nausea and vomiting, attention should move to the symptom itself. As a rule, first-line antiemetics such as cyclizine, low-dose haloperidol or metoclopramide should be targeted at the probable cause. [6] If unsuccessful, addition of another antiemetic that works on different receptors may be helpful (a combination might be cyclizine plus haloperidol). The prokinetic action of metoclopramide is antagonized by cyclizine, so these drugs should not be used together. Alternatively, a broadspectrum antiemetic, such as levomepromazine, can be useful. Although 5-HT$_3$ antagonists (such as ondansetron and granisetron) are useful in

---

[6] Twycross et al. Symptom Management in Advanced Cancer, 3rd Ed, Radcliffe Medical Press, 2001.

chemotherapy- and radiotherapy-induced vomiting, they are usually ineffective for nausea and vomiting from other causes.

Those who vomit may not be able to retain oral medication. This is where syringe drivers come into their own by offering an alternative route, allowing the upper gastrointestinal tract 'a rest' and ensuring that essential analgesics and antiemetics have the opportunity to be absorbed. Once the symptom is under control, a switch to oral drugs can easily be made.

Hypercalcaemia in malignancy

A cause of vomiting that is often missed is hypercalcaemia related to cancer, especially in those with multiple myeloma or cancer of the lung (squamous cell), breast or prostate. Patients may complain of nausea, vomiting, increased pain, constipation and confusion, all of which are common in advanced cancer. Treatment consists of rehydration and intravenous bisphosphonates. Patients with mild hypercalcaemia may respond to rehydration alone. In others, bisphosphonates will take at least 2–3 days to take effect, so it may not be necessary to check serum calcium levels until a few days have passed. The patient's symptoms may respond dramatically, and this can be very rewarding, given the simplicity of the intervention. However, active treatment may be inappropriate if the patient is imminently dying, and other methods of symptom control may be preferable. Hypercalcaemia is a poor prognostic indicator in the context of malignancy, and 80% of such patients will die within a year.

Malignant bowel obstruction

Malignant bowel obstruction is most common in carcinoma of the colon or ovary. If a single site of obstruction is likely and the patient is fit enough, a surgical opinion is required. If surgery is not planned, there is no need for a 'drip and suck' approach, as this is both uncomfortable and usually unhelpful. Instead, the focus should be on symptom control, usually of abdominal pain, colic, vomiting and constipation. Drug absorption will be compromised, so a syringe driver is often required. Diamorphine is useful for background abdominal pain, and hyoscine butylbromide relieves colic. Cyclizine and haloperidol are suitable first-line antiemetics. Softening laxatives (sodium docusate) and suppositories (glycerine) are helpful. If patients wish to eat or drink, they should be allowed to do so.

Breathlessness

Dyspnoea is a common and frightening symptom in patients with lung disease. As always, the golden rule is to look for the cause and, where appropriate, treat anything that is reversible, such as infection, cardiac failure, pulmonary embolism, pleural effusion or anaemia. Lymphangitis carcinomatosis is sometimes associated with metastatic breast cancer, and symptoms may be alleviated with high-dose dexamethasone.

Once reversible causes have been considered, symptom management is required. This consists of reducing the respiratory drive with morphine and treating anxiety with benzodiazepines. A suitable starting dose of morphine for breathlessness would be 2.5 mg immediate-release oral morphine every 4 h. Nebulized morphine is not effective. Short-acting benzodiazepines such as lorazepam are helpful in an acute attack, especially where panic is a component. The longer-acting diazepam is more useful for chronic anxiety. Contrary to popular opinion, patients with lung cancer or COPD do not choke or suffocate to death; effective reassurance can be life changing for many patients.

Relaxation techniques and breathing exercises can also be effective. Even simple counting exercises such as breathing in on 'one', and breathing out on 'two' and 'three', can help increase breathing efficiency and distract the patient. Oxygen is probably overused. It restricts mobility and, in those who are not hypoxic (oxygen saturation > 90%), a fan can be just as effective. Advice from physiotherapists (breathing techniques) and occupational therapists may be invaluable.

Superior vena caval obstruction

Superior vena caval obstruction may come on acutely in patients with cancer of the lung or breast, or lymphoma. It classically presents with breathlessness and headache, being accompanied by swelling of the head, upper trunk and arms with periorbital oedema and injected conjunctivae. Dilated collateral veins in the neck and chest are common. High-dose dexamethasone should be commenced immediately and an urgent oncology opinion obtained. It is unsurprisingly a poor prognostic sign in patients with cancer.

The terminal phase

Amidst the frantic activity of an acute hospital ward, with pagers and pumps beeping, it is sometimes difficult to recognize that a patient's failure to respond to treatment is because he is now dying. It is time to take a step back and reevaluate the whole situation. Once dying has been recognized, everything else falls into place much more easily. The Liverpool Care Pathway for the Dying was developed to guide those who are not familiar with looking after dying patients.[7] It is a useful tool but focuses only on the last 48 h of life. Recognizing when somebody is dying (in order to start them on this pathway) and ensuring that each patient continues to receive individualized care remain the more difficult challenges that have to be tackled.

In reality, diagnosing imminent death is about piecing together a clinical impression based on disease progression, one's knowledge of the patient, a rapid increase in weakness and drowsiness and diminishing interest in surroundings, food and fluids. Attempts to identify reliable prognostic indicators continue but, for now, clinical judgement remains paramount.

Should dying patients remain in hospital? Approximately 70% of terminally ill cancer patients state that they wish to die at home, yet only 25% realize this goal.[8,9,10] Timely exploration of the patient's wishes and discussion with the family may help achieve this. Early discussions with the general practitioner, district nurses and social services are essential. Even if the patient is deteriorating and the window of opportunity is narrow, hands-on care, equipment, drugs (subcutaneous as well as oral) and transport can generally all be accessed within 24–48 h if the discharge is prioritized and well coordinated. However, unfortunately, many patients do die in hospital, either by choice, necessity or chance, so acute teams need to be skilled in handling this final phase of care.

Although our primary duty is to the patient, it is obviously sensible to communicate effectively with the family (with the patient's permission) at each stage. If the family is part of the team, this may help with the patient's care and assist relatives in their bereavement.

Prescribing

In terms of managing the dying patient, what needs to be considered? First, there needs to be a 'gear change'. Stop and reprioritize. At this point, the focus is comfort. Futile treatments (any treatment not connected with symptom control, such as antihypertensives and, often, antibiotics) should be discontinued. Patients who have difficulty swallowing medication may need to have essential drugs (such as analgesics) administered via a syringe driver or rectally. Titration of symptom relief medication against effect remains as important as ever.

[7] Ellershaw et al. Care of the Dying. A Pathway to Excellence. Oxford University Press, Oxford, 2003.

[8] Higginson et al. J Palliat Med (2000) 3: 287–300.

[9] Thomas et al. Soc Sci Med (2004) 58: 2431–2444.

[10] Higginson et al. Palliat Med (1998) 12: 353–363.

Restlessness or agitation is common in those who are dying. If no reversible cause can be found (urinary retention and constipation are prime candidates), symptom management is required. Subcutaneous midazolam is the treatment of choice. Haloperidol may be useful if delirium or paranoia is present. Occasionally, sedation is needed in dying patients who remain in distress when all other symptom relief measures have been exhausted. Euthanasia is illegal: sedation, if needed, should always be targeted at the anxiety and not simply escalated. These decisions should never be taken without senior medical involvement. It is advisable to contact the specialist palliative care team in these situations.

Another problem unique to the dying phase is the onset of 'death rattle' or noisy, rattling breathing. It is assumed to be due to an accumulation of secretions in the oropharynx, which oscillate with respiration but there is no firm evidence that this is the case. Intervention includes repositioning, gentle suction and antimuscarinic agents (hyoscine hydrobromide, hyoscine butylbromide or glycopyrronium) to inhibit secretions. Generally, patients do not seem troubled by death rattle. In the absence of patient distress, the rationale for intervention is often said to be the comfort of attending relatives. However, evidence is emerging that relatives are not always disturbed by the death rattle: sometimes their visible distress is simply related to their imminent loss or misperceptions that the sound of death rattle is that of the patient 'drowning'.[11] Careful explanation, clarifying the relatives' perceptions and ensuring that they realize this is a sign of impending death, should be carried out before resorting to drugs that cause adverse effects (such as excessively dry mouth).

If the patient is being discharged to die at home, medications should be prescribed and dispensed preemptively, so that they are available without delay. This may mean providing analgesia and some parenteral preparations while liaising with the primary care team. Relatives should be informed of whom to contact if a problem arises, so as to avoid undue distress: a panicked call for an ambulance is likely to result in readmission, when it may be possible to manage the problem at home. It is worth checking the availability of out-of-hours district nursing and specialist palliative care services locally.

Being fed and watered

Patients and their families sometimes worry about dying of dehydration or starving to death. There is no evidence that parenteral fluids improve the symptoms of thirst and dry mouth, nor do they affect prognosis during the

---

[11] Wee, *Death Rattle: an exploration* (PhD thesis, University of Southampton) (2003).

last days of life.[12] Thirst 'ends at the mouth'; so dry mouth should be obviated by good mouth care, including sips and artificial saliva. Relatives often benefit by participating in this care. However, someone who is losing fluid excessively (perhaps through profuse diarrhoea or vomiting) may gain from intravenous or subcutaneous fluids, if death is unlikely to be imminent.

Artificial nutrition involves nasogastric tubes, gastrostomies or central or peripheral venous lines. These are invasive in the final phase of life and achieve little by way of comfort or physiological benefit. The catabolic nature of advanced cancer and other diseases such as heart failure means that artificial supplementation of calories makes little difference to the resulting cachexia.[13] Artificial feeding of dying patients who are not hungry is unnecessary and may be inhumane. However, patients who have a prognosis of several months and cannot swallow, due to cancer or another disorder, may benefit from percutaneous gastrostomy feeding.

Acute terminal haemorrhage

Most patients with chronic progressive diseases deteriorate gradually and have a peaceful death. Sometimes, something catastrophic occurs, such as major haemorrhage. This can be frightening for patients and cause panic in relatives and inexperienced staff. Rapid sedation with midazolam (10 mg slow iv, or intramuscular if no intravenous access) calms the patient and, hence, the situation. Opioids may be used (at twice the usual breakthrough dose). Calmness in staff handling the event goes a long way towards reassuring patients and families. Relatives should be kept briefed and reassured, with no attempt to either exaggerate or minimize the seriousness of the event. Afterwards, relatives, staff and other patients who have witnessed this may require time to talk things over.

UNFINISHED BUSINESS

Decision-making in palliative medicine is imprecise, emphasizing the constant need to weigh up benefits against burden and risks in clinical decisions. For example, depression is underdiagnosed (and therefore undertreated) in patients with advanced cancer. It can be difficult to distinguish between understandable sadness and clinically treatable depression. Another difficult

---

[12] National Council for Hospice and Specialist Palliative Care Services, Eur J Pall Care (1997) 4: 124.

[13] Inui, CA Cancer J Clin (2002) 52: 72–91.

decision facing the general physician is whether or not to pursue plans for discharging a patient home. If the physician hesitates too long, the window of opportunity might be shut. If one moves too hastily, the patient might have to be subsequently readmitted for physical, psychological or social reasons, to the distress and dissatisfaction of all concerned.

When faced with a life-threatening condition, some patients adopt a proactive stance, getting 'their house in order' and ensuring that wills and other legal affairs are sorted out. However, some also feel that by writing a will, they are 'giving up', or, worse still, 'tempting fate'. Relatives may find the subject too distressing to discuss (although the consequences of dying intestate are usually even more distressing for the family later on). Health care professionals can sometimes help by gently prompting this. Wills are best written when the patient is feeling well, can bring peace of mind, and of course, can be changed at any time. Some patients draw up advance directives, in which they specify interventions that they would refuse if they were in a particular situation. To be considered legally binding, such documents should be signed, witnessed and dated. Communication is imperative, and it is, therefore, useful to have a copy of the advance directive in the hospital notes, with the GP and with a relative (as well as with the patient). The current legal position of advance directives is that if a situation defined by that individual were to occur (for instance, advanced cancer or a cerebrovascular accident), it would be unlawful to consciously carry out interventions that they had ruled out in the advanced directive. At the same time, health professionals have no obligation to carry out requested interventions that are against the patient's best interests. The Mental Capacity Act comes into force on April 1, 2007, and enables patients to name a proxy to make health, welfare and other decisions ('Lasting Power of Attorney'). A code of practice is currently being developed and will be very relevant for all clinicians when a patient does not have full capacity, including those who are confused or have a decreased level of consciousness.

The journey of a terminally ill patient is not all doom and gloom, although there are certainly low points that may be predicted. Facing death may trigger patients to reprioritize and focus on more important aspects of life, and, as such, gain a greater sense of meaning. Palliative care is provided both by specialist palliative care teams and by all health professionals involved in the patient's care. Good communication, empathy and a pragmatic approach to the clinical situation may not be hi-tech, but they go a long way to improve the quality of dying – something we may all one day come to appreciate.

Chapter 16

Matthew Giles and Andrew Coull

GERIATRIC MEDICINE

Setting the scene – the time bomb has arrived

The problem of the demographic time bomb – our ageing population – is here and will only get worse. The statistics are both impressive and deeply worrying. More than 20% of the population are now aged over 60 years, and the number over 90 years of age is set to double in the next two decades. The elderly are not a homogeneous entity. It is patronizing, ageist and incorrect to treat them as a uniform group. The large majority of community-living people over 65 years are mobile (90%), in full control of their mental faculties (90%), independent in self-care (97%), independent in domestic care (82%) and, in fact, caring for others (60%). This has major implications for both the general practitioner at the frontline and the general physician on the acute medical take. Rates of admission in the elderly have risen faster than the demographic change, suggesting the inclusion of multiple admissions of individual patients. Geriatrician involvement on the acute take remains variable, and a minority of older patients are cared for solely by geriatricians in the acute phase. Therefore, it is all the more important to identify the subgroup, particularly of the very elderly, who require extra consideration and time to identify a problem that they may find hard to describe and the doctor may find hard to define. Current pressures on acute beds do not favour the optimal care of older people with the ever-present tension between bed management, discharge and quality care. Never has there been a greater need for geriatricians at the front door.

What do geriatricians do, and why do we have them?

Those looking for an evidence base for geriatrics should start by reading on the classic 1984 randomized controlled trial of comprehensive geriatric care which showed elegantly that multidisciplinary assessment in a dedicated geriatric evaluation unit reduced mortality and admission to nursing homes.[1] Geriatricians are often best placed to assess those with nonspecific presentations, multiple comorbidities and pre-existing disability. These skills are utilized throughout the patient journey from acute assessment at the hospital front door to post-acute care and rehabilitation. Equally important are those skills in caring for the frailest of the frail awaiting placement. This is an ever-increasing number, with some estimates suggesting that such patients occupy up to 10% of acute sector beds.

A geriatrician is similarly adept in making an early decision to admit and directing to an appropriate bed, or indeed to early supported discharge. It is often said that it is easier to admit than discharge, and this is especially so in the elderly and frail. However, hospitals are not necessarily the safest of places for older people prone to succumb to potentially misplaced investigations, invasive interventions, hospital-acquired infections or falls. Older people (like younger ones) do not want to be in hospital. Every attempt should be made to consider whether patients can be managed in the community and the skills of a geriatrician are particularly relevant in this area. Assessments are not made in isolation and involve multidisciplinary teams working in close collaboration with the primary and secondary care interface. Having a working knowledge of the local resources is half the battle won. Consideration should be given to using heart failure specialist or respiratory liaison nurses. Ambulatory care and hospital-in-the-home services have been set up with varying success across the country. Complementing these services, there should be rapid response and community rehabilitation teams. Access to urgent outpatient slots, day hospital, speciality clinics for falls, funny turns, memory and continence problems should all be readily available. In collaboration with these services, access should be provided to beds in community hospitals or care homes for time-limited assessment. Medical input to such services is a must.

Another group of regular attendees are those usually residing in care homes, often producing a sinking feeling in the admitting doctor. It is terribly important, however, to get the facts right. Many care homes may look after patients with varying needs, from those requiring simple supervision with personal care to those who are bed bound. At times, a request for admission may represent a call for help from a home that has insufficient resources to provide safe, quality care. The importance of obtaining correct premorbid

---

[1] Rubenstein et al. N Eng J Med (1984) 311: 1664–1670.

information by talking to a carer cannot be overemphasized. Early contact with the care home manager is critical in setting achievable goals and an early discharge date. As with most geriatric practice, the devil is often in the detail.

The skill to recognize a dying patient is as important as the ability to make a comprehensive assessment. This is sometimes extraordinarily difficult, particularly at an initial encounter on a busy post-take ward round. However the clues to making the diagnosis of 'dying' are often present if the opportunity is taken to talk with carers or relatives about pre-existing disability. Geriatricians may be most familiar and experienced with such sensitive and difficult discussions. An early senior assessment might prevent further inappropriate and potentially distressing investigations or futile treatments. A good death is definitely worth striving for, and carers will often thank one for it.

THE GERIATRIC SYNDROMES

Old people may not behave like young ones. They may not give good case histories. Examination findings may be complex and contradictory, with the signs of pre-existing disability often clouding the picture. A unifying diagnosis is commonly elusive. A threshold is often seen in age-related degenerative diseases in which the amount of additional pathology needed for clinical presentation declines due to the accumulation of subclinical pathology. Multiple pathologies may converge on one area of function, along with extrinsic factors, to produce a geriatric syndrome such as falls, cognitive impairment, 'inability to cope', incontinence or, indeed, any combination of these. The skill of geriatric practice is to unpick that tangled web focusing on the relevant precipitants while carefully assessing and accounting for the potential comorbidity in order to develop a multidisciplinary management plan to achieve patient and carer goals. Terms such as 'off legs', 'acopia' and 'social admission' irritate the practising geriatrician. Unfortunately, all are recognizable even to the medical student on their first take. Importantly, these labels can hide potentially reversible illness that has led to significant functional decline.

All fall down

The 'fall' statistics are frightening. Every 5 h, an older person dies as a result of a fall. Many first fallers will become recurrent fallers with one-third subsequently suffering from an incapacitating fear of falling that interferes with daily activities. Alongside falls must be considered osteoporosis, as fracture is often associated with loss of independence and chronic pain. There are now clear guidelines on who should be referred on to a specialist falls service.[2]

Falls have multiple causes but the most common is accidental or the 'simple trip', typically on an uneven pavement or a loose rug. However, beware of the recurrent 'accidents' that require further examination. A careful history, corroborated if possible, is critical in all assessments. Those with 'recurrent accidents' often have undiagnosed pathology. Gait and balance problems occur in more than 25% of over-75-year-old community dwellers in the apparent absence of neurological or musculoskeletal cause. These patients present in a variety of ways including with 'dizziness', falls and fractures, loss of independence or a need for increasing social support. Such presentations should alert the physician to a potentially reversible diagnosis. It may be very revealing and worthwhile to ask the patient to get up and walk on a post-take ward round. Characteristic gait disorders are immediately recognizable, including: the slow shuffling extrapyramidal gait of Parkinson's disease; an ataxic cerebellar gait with unsteadiness on turning and poor heel-to-toe that may be related to alcohol; the stiff and spastic gait of those with multiple strokes or cervical myelopathy; the small-stepped, feet-stuck-to-the-ground 'marche à petit pas' of multiple lacunar strokes; the difficulty in rising from a chair of proximal myopathy; or the foot-slapping gait of a peripheral neuropathy. Risk factors for falls should be identified. These include previous falls, gait or balance deficits associated with joint disease, stroke or neurodegenerative conditions, visual impairment and cognitive impairment.[3] Intercurrent illness may temporarily worsen gait disorder. Drugs may commonly be implicated, and those taking four or more culprit medications are particularly at risk. Almost any drug may be responsible but particularly those acting on the central nervous or cardiovascular system.

Cognitive impairment leading to lack of insight and safety awareness is an important factor in many falls particularly in institutional settings and should be screened for routinely with an abbreviated mental test score. Multidisciplinary specialist services identify intrinsic and extrinsic risk factors in order to provide interventions to prevent further falls or strategies to manage further falls, to identify and manage any psychological consequences of falls and manage the risk of osteoporotic fracture. A Cochrane systematic review has recently examined the accumulating evidence in falls prevention.[4] Effective interventions include

[2] Department of Health, National Service Framework for Older People (2001).

[3] American Geriatrics Society, JAGS (2001) 49: 664–672.

[4] Gillespie et al. Cochrane Database Syst Rev (2005) Issue 3.

multidisciplinary assessment with modification of environmental hazards, exercise programs including gait and balance retraining with muscle strengthening and education on appropriate use of walking aids. One recent paper hypothesizes that some types of exercise in particular (such as sculling) may be important in reducing the risk of hip fracture, by strengthening specific (superolateral) areas of the bony cortex: an idea supported by the low rates of hip fracture reported in countries where squatting (for toileting, dining or to work the fields) is commonplace.[5] Critically, there should be review, modification and removal of medication. Identification and management of postural hypotension and cardiovascular disorders such as arrhythmias or carotid sinus hypersensitivity may be important.

Out for the count

Syncope and 'collapse' are a common reason for those over 65 years of age to be admitted. There is a considerable overlap between those presenting with recurrent falls and syncope. The incidence of syncope in those over 70 years of age is approximately 6% with a 2-year recurrence rate of 30%. Amnesia for loss of consciousness is a common reason why patients present giving an account of falls rather than syncope. The commonest causes of syncope in older people are orthostatic hypotension, carotid sinus syndrome, vasovagal syncope and cardiac arrhythmias. Approximately half of all cases will be diagnosed on history and examination, orthostatic blood pressure measurement and upright and supine carotid sinus massage. Echocardiography is of limited help in the absence of clinical and ECG evidence of cardiac disease. Although up to 20% of syncope in older patients is due to cardiac arrhythmia, the yield with Holter monitoring is only 1%. The presence of structural heart disease is the most important predictor of further problems. In those older than 45 years, history of congestive cardiac failure, history of ventricular arrhythmias and an abnormal ECG have been identified as risk factors for further syncopal attacks. With no risk factors, subsequent arrhythmia or death occurs in 4–7% over 1 year, whereas in those with three or more risk factors, this figure progressively increases to 58–80%. Importantly, over 30% will have more than one possible attributable cause.[6]

Stand up, fall down

Orthostatic hypotension refers to syncope in which the upright position causes arterial hypotension. Prevalence varies between 6% in community dwellers

---

[5] Mayhew *et al.* Lancet (2005) 366: 129–135.

[6] ESC Task Force on Syncope, Europace (2004) 6: 467–537.

and 30% in inpatients. Orthostatic hypotension usually occurs in the mornings, either post-prandially or after medication. Supine systolic hypertension is often present. Primary autonomic failure may be isolated or associated with multisystem atrophy or Parkinson's disease. Secondary autonomic failure may occur with diabetes, kidney or liver failure and alcohol abuse. Drugs are a major cause of orthostatic hypotension. Volume depletion and Addison's disease should also be considered in the acute setting. No cause is found in a quarter of patients. It is not always reproducible and may require repeated morning measurements or 24-h ambulatory blood pressure monitoring. Upright tilt testing for 5 min may pick up previously undiagnosed postural hypotension. Patients should be advised and educated on factors that influence blood pressure. Encouraging fluid and salt intake, support hosiery if tolerated, frequent meals with reduced carbohydrate content, physical countermeasures such as leg crossing, squatting and hand grip exercises should all be considered. Fludrocortisone may be required but its use is limited by the presence of supine or nocturnal hypertension, where it should be avoided. Prognosis is largely related to comorbidity.

Necks on the line

Patients with carotid sinus hypersensitivity have an exaggerated baroreceptor-mediated reflex that may lead to dizziness, syncope or falls.[7] It predominantly affects older people and males and is associated with hypertension and athero-sclerotic disease. Precipitating factors include head movements, prolonged standing and heavy meals. Diagnosis is confirmed by performing carotid sinus massage (CSM) in supine and upright positions in controlled conditions. Cardioinhibitory carotid sinus hypersensitivity is an attributable cause of symptoms in up to 20% of elderly patients with syncope and is diagnosed if CSM produces asystole for 3 s or more. The treatment of choice is a dual-chamber pacemaker. Vasodepressor carotid sinus hypersensitivity is diagnosed on CSM with a fall in systolic blood pressure of over 50 mmHg, or 30 mmHg with symptoms. Treatment is medical, complex and mostly unrewarding. Mixed forms do occur, and pacemaker therapy is less effective in this group. The syndrome is missed in half of all cases if massage is not performed in the upright position.

Vasovagal syncope

Up to 15% of syncope in the elderly is vasovagal with half related to cardio-vascular drugs. There is usually a prodromal warning, and precipitating factors

[7] Kenny, J Cardiovasc Electrophysiol (2003) 14: S74–S77.

include standing, stress, pain, heavy meals and warm weather. Post-syncope, there may be nausea and headache. Prolonged head-up tilt testing, monitoring heart rate, blood pressure and symptoms are the widely accepted methods of diagnosis. Avoidance of precipitating factors and taking abortive action in the context of warning symptoms should be advised. Discontinuation of vasodilator drugs, increased fluid intake, exercise training, tilt training and leg crossing manoeuvres should be considered. Pharmacological interventions are often unhelpful. Pacemaker therapy may be appropriate for a very small, select, severely affected group. Prognosis is good.

Acute confusional state

It is easy to gain the impression on a busy medical take that confusion might be a normal accompaniment to old age. It is worthwhile reinforcing that if 20% of those over 80 years have cognitive impairment, 80% do not. Confusion, therefore, is often a danger sign and requires a rapid diagnosis and early treatment. Indeed, if there was awareness that delirium has a worse outcome (up to 15% in-hospital mortality) than the troponin-positive acute coronary syndromes, then the management of the confused older person would perhaps be regarded as rather more pressing.

Delirium is extremely common, affecting up to 30% of all elderly medical patients.[8] It classically manifests itself as inattention leading to distractibility. There is often memory impairment, disorientation, language disturbance and perceptual impairment. It has an onset over hours or days and varies during the day. There may be disturbances of the sleep–wake cycle with complete reversal. Delirium is usually a direct consequence of a general medical condition, drug withdrawal or intoxication.[9] It is often missed, and nondetection rates as high as 60% have been reported. A corroborative history is critical. Two subtypes may be recognized: those who are hyperactive and characterized by psychomotor overactivity (displaying aggression or plucking at bedclothes) who are often at risk of falls and fracture; and those who are hypoactive, apathetic and at risk from the complications of immobility. A nonspecific but simple bedside test of impaired attentiveness is asking the patient to count backwards from 20. It is often said that patients are never the same after an episode of delirium, and this has been put down to the 'unmasking' of a dementing illness. Increasingly it is being hypothesized that delirium causes

---

[8] Brown *et al.* BMJ (2002) 325: 644–647.

[9] Burns *et al.* J Neurol Neurosurg Psychiatry (2004) 75: 362–367.

brain damage. Overall, the outcome for survivors is poor with a third staying the same, a third partially improving and a third returning to their previous state. There is a high risk of institutionalization.

Patients at risk can be identified as they are often older, severely ill, have a history of prior cognitive impairment, may be physically frail, visually or hearing impaired, on excessive drugs or have a background of alcohol excess. Pain can also precipitate delirium. Patients should be thoroughly examined. Core temperature should be measured, as sepsis, occasionally occult, is a common cause. However, asymptomatic bacteriuria is common in older people and may not signify frank urinary sepsis. Dehydration can also cause delirium, often in the setting of vomiting or diarrhoea in the face of continued diuretic use. A careful cardiorespiratory examination is required as delirium may be a presenting feature of myocardial infarction, heart failure, pneumonia or pulmonary embolus. Urinary retention may both cause and be a complication of delirium. Constipation may need to be excluded with a rectal examination. If patients are drowsy, have focal neurological signs or a history of falls, brain imaging is mandatory. Medication is a very common precipitant, typically those with anticholinergic activity.

The aetiology of delirium in up to a third of patients may remain elusive. In difficult cases, further investigation should be guided by thorough and repeated clinical examination. Atypical infection may be relevant including endocarditis, tuberculosis and syphilis. HIV-related delirium may be seen more often in the future in certain groups. Neurological abnormalities should stimulate brain imaging to exclude nondominant parietal stroke or subdural haematoma. Head injury in patients with pre-existent brain disease may precipitate delirium. Nonconvulsive seizures should be considered, and EEG may be helpful in selected cases. Occasionally a lumbar puncture is necessary. Endocrinopathies such as hypo- or hyperthyroidism, hyperparathyroidism and hypopituitarism should be considered in difficult cases. A careful search for neoplastic disease may also be fruitful. Prescribed drugs are implicated in 40% of delirium, such as opioids, sedatives and tricyclics.

The early diagnosis and treatment of precipitating factors with the provision of a supportive environment that is quiet, warm, well lit and has reassuring trained staff is important.[10] Early mobilization, maintenance of nutrition, hydration and attention to bladder and bowel care are critical. Spectacles and hearing aids should be used to minimize sensory deprivation. Families should

---

[10] British Geriatrics Society, Guidelines for diagnosis and management of delirium in the elderly (2005).

be encouraged to provide clocks and calendars and familiar clothes or pictures to assist in reorientation. Inter- and intra-ward transfers should be avoided. Such a strategy has been shown to prevent delirium in high-risk patients.[11] Rambling and confused speech should be tactfully disagreed with and the subject changed while acknowledging the expressed feelings but ignoring the content. Interventions such as bladder catheterization should be avoided if possible. Restraints including bed rails are potentially dangerous. Psychotropic drugs are best avoided. Neuroleptics such as haloperidol are occasionally needed. They should be used in low dose and titrated to effect rather than using a high dose 'chemical cosh'. They should be withdrawn as soon as possible. Benzodiazepines are appropriate in alcohol withdrawal. There are ongoing trials looking at cholinesterase inhibitors such as donepezil in delirium. In difficult cases, a trial of empirical broad-spectrum antibiotics may be warranted. Many patients with a delirium have underlying cognitive impairment, and consideration should be given to a referral to the Old Age Psychiatrists on discharge.

WHEN TO INVESTIGATE, AND WHEN TO STOP?

Patient wishes are paramount. Many place symptom control and quality of life ahead of life expectancy. Of course, quality of life is intensely subjective. Discussions with the patient about their goals will guide appropriate management. Many patients in fact rate the outcomes of severe physical disability and dementia as worse than death. If patients are unable to communicate their wishes, it is good medical practice to discuss the situation with the next of kin. Guidelines and a 'cookbook approach' rarely help in the management of frail older people with multiple comorbidities.[12] An advance directive made by a competent adult on the basis of adequate information is legally binding if it is applicable to the particular circumstances, and there is no evidence that the patient has changed their mind.

If there are multiple comorbidities, it is helpful to use a process of identifying problems rather than seeking a unifying diagnosis. Problems having greatest effect on quality of life or, if relevant, problems that will be most limiting of life expectancy should be prioritized. However, one needs to be careful in predicting life expectancy. Clearly, if the prognosis for a specific disease indicates a short life span, planning investigation or treatment in terms of life

---

[11] Inouye *et al.* NEJM (1999) 334: 669–676.

[12] Adler *et al.* Clin Med (2003) 3: 418–422.

expectancy is reasonable. Life expectancy based on epidemiological data is obviously less reliable, given the huge variability among individuals.

Cognitive impairment is associated with significant mortality and impaired quality of life, and investigations should be considered in this context. Physical disability is common in older people and should trigger a shift from the traditional emphasis on cure to improving function, postponing disability using a multidisciplinary assessment and potential environmental modification to improve the quality of life. Such disability makes some investigations inappropriate. There should be thorough and clear documentation of decision-making processes, particularly if further investigation is considered inappropriate. If investigation is refused or felt inappropriate, this should not rule out empirical treatment if available and accepted.

Investigations may be used to guide prognosis even though treatment may not be affected. Such a strategy may allow greater access to home or institutional care or financial support.

SENSIBLE PRESCRIBING IN OLDER PEOPLE

Polypharmacy is one of the most serious problems in caring for older people. Despite this term having a rather negative connotation, there are often legitimate reasons why the elderly may receive numerous medications. Many medications have a greater potential for adverse effects in the elderly as the pharmacokinetic and pharmacodynamic changes with age lead to drugs having more prolonged durations of action and greater risk of toxicity. The greater the number of medications, the greater chance of adverse effects, and these may be severe given a reduced organ reserve. Up to 10% of admissions of older people may be related to adverse drug reactions, commonly presenting as falls or confusion.[13]

Inappropriate drug prescription is that which has greater potential to harm than to benefit the patient. Those treating older people should aim to ensure maximum benefit from as few drugs and with as few adverse effects as possible. Prescription decisions should be individualized. Medications should be prescribed only for appropriate reasons, discontinued when they no longer provide benefit, dosed correctly to reflect alterations with ageing and be monitored closely for adverse effects.

It is well recognized that older people are generally excluded from clinical trials. This is despite the clearly changing demography of the population,

[13] Routledge *et al.* Br J Clin Pharmacol (2003) 57: 121–126.

and the high likelihood of greater absolute benefit or risk that may be evident with different interventions. There is a clear need for trials including older people. However, such lack of data should not be used inflexibly. Absence of data does not mean absence of effectiveness.

Patient choice should be central in prescribing decisions. Many drugs are used based on data (again not including older people) that look primarily at outcomes of mortality. Medications that improve symptoms and relieve suffering may be more important to the individual than simply prolonging life expectancy.

There is often reluctance to manage the vascular risk factors of older people. A strong argument can be made for treating the 80-year old for hypertension or high cholesterol if they are still very active. On the other hand, if an older person is severely disabled then treating vascular risk factors may be less appropriate. In between is a sea of grey that must be left to clinical judgement in consultation with the individual. There is no biological reason why the pertinence of recognized vascular risk factors should change with advancing age but all interventions should be closely monitored for adverse effects. What will change (and the extent of this is not known) is the absolute benefit (and risk) for different interventions in older age groups.

Warfarin is worth a special mention as it is clearly beneficial in thromboembolic prophylaxis for atrial fibrillation. However, the risk of bleeding, including intracranial haemorrhage, rises with age and, therefore, the presence of other major comorbidity, cognitive impairment, risk of falls and worries about concordance should all ring alarm bells.

ASSISTIVE TECHNOLOGY

The cost of caring for swathes of older people in hospital or nursing homes is astronomically higher than caring for them in their own homes. Indeed older people want to stay at home as long as possible, and in those with cognitive impairment the familiarity of home is essential to well being and dignity. If support exists at home, safe discharge might potentially be facilitated. Assistive technology is any product or service designed to enable independence in disabled or older people. It has long been proposed that this technology might prolong older peoples' independence by protecting them from potentially dangerous situations. No longer is this 'pie in the sky', and many projects have been set up across the country. Assistive technology has been highly successful in cases of patients wandering at night, using a bed occupancy sensor that might activate a light if the occupant gets up at night so as to reduce the risk of falls. A timer can be set, and an alarm can be raised if the wanderer has not returned after a preset time. A wandering-client monitor consists of a contact on a doorframe that activates an alert if breached. An infrared detector can activate if someone has walked through the door but not returned around preprogrammed times. 'SMART technology' has been used successfully to avoid catastrophic consequences in the case of people with cognitive impairment who leave gas cookers on. Modern gas sensors can detect this and automatically switch gas off at the mains. Other projects use environmental sensors to monitor the use of the toilet, the state of locks and doors and water taps. In a potentially dangerous situation, the system will first attempt to talk to the client. If this fails, a central 'lifeline' is activated to alert volunteer support. One further exciting development is the 'WISE home', which uses electronic and communication systems to monitor a number of specific parameters. The system 'memorizes' patterns of behaviour so that if there is deviation, an early warning signal can alert carers to a potential problem. There are also technological developments to facilitate patient concordance with medication. In these ways, the homeowner is empowered to maintain independence for as long as possible. Although the limiting factor at present remains the cost, such developments hold great promise for the future.

AT THE END OF THE DAY

There are increasing arrays of life-prolonging treatments but where there is little hope of recovery, their use may cause distress. This paradox raises significant dilemmas. The reader is referred to the General Medical Council, which has issued excellent guidance in this area.[14] Doctors have a duty of care to their patients. The benefits of any intervention should outweigh any risks. If there is no net benefit, then interventions should be avoided. 'Prolonging life' could be considered as always in the patient's best interests but longevity should be seen in context. If there is no net benefit, there is no obligation, ethically or legally, for the doctor to intervene. It is worthy of note that competent patients can also refuse treatments that might be seen to be beneficial if they have the capacity to understand the consequences of their decision. If the patient lacks the capacity, then the physician must make the difficult judgement of what is in the best interests of the patient by weighing up the risks and benefits of an intervention. Such decisions should be taken after discussions with carers or relatives who are best placed to know their loved one's wishes. In difficult cases, where there is no consensus, a second opinion should always

14 www.gmc-uk.org

be sought. In such circumstances, where a treatment is not felt beneficial, there is no legal difference between withholding and withdrawing it.

Decisions involving artificial nutrition or hydration are particularly difficult and emotionally fraught. An assessment of the risks and benefits of these interventions is often difficult as patients may have a reduced conscious level, and there may be concern that distress is caused because nutrition or hydration needs are not met. Negligible oral intake is often part of the dying process. The risk-benefit of different methods of hydration and nutrition should each be considered separately. Communication with families or carers is critical. Before deciding on the withdrawal or withholding of treatment, a formal assessment of the prognosis should be made. If it is clear that death is imminent, a patient's palliative care needs must be identified and met. If death is not approaching, it will usually be appropriate to provide some form of support. However, if it is judged that a patient's condition is so severe and prognosis so poor that interventions would cause distress, such treatment could be withheld or withdrawn, again in consultation with family, if necessary after a second opinion. Such conversations are not for the fainthearted. Detailed documentation is of paramount importance, and regular review of these decisions should be undertaken, as dramatic changes can occasionally occur in the clinical state of a patient when treatments are withdrawn – sometimes for the better!

Chapter 17

Wendy Holden and Joseph Joseph

RHEUMATOLOGY

The days of the general physician with a particular interest in rheumatology seem numbered. As with other areas of medicine, rheumatology has become much more complex and specialized, as both aetiological knowledge and pharmacological possibilities have grown apace. This distancing between rheumatology and general medicine is in some ways a cause for concern, not least for patients. Rheumatological conditions manifest across a multitude of specialties: patients need and deserve holistic care, and all physicians need to remain well briefed.

RHEUMATOID ARTHRITIS

Some doctors may imagine a typical patient with rheumatoid arthritis as an elderly person with gross deformities and pain, obstructing the waiting room with their splints and wheelchair. Such patients are a legacy from the days of the 'pyramid' approach, when non-steroidal anti-inflammatory drugs (NSAIDs) were the mainstay of treatment. Disease-modifying anti-rheumatic drugs (DMARDs) were reserved for those who did not respond to symptomatic relief. Unfortunately for many patients, by the time their treatment was optimized, irreversible joint damage had already occurred and they were destined for a lifetime of progressive disability. Since the routine use of DMARDs and the advent of newer biological therapies, early remission, with the aim of preventing deformity and disability and maintaining a normal lifestyle is now the goal for most patients with early rheumatoid arthritis. Some rheumatologists are even daring to mention the tantalizing possibility of a 'cure'.

Is it rheumatoid?

Rheumatoid arthritis is a clinical diagnosis. There are criteria to be met (as shown in the table on p 374). However, these may lag behind the findings of modern imaging and laboratory tests. Most patients with joint pain, a positive rheumatoid factor (RF) and normal inflammatory markers do not have rheumatoid arthritis. They are much more likely to have either osteoarthritis or a soft tissue problem with an incidentally positive RF. Similarly, most patients with a positive anti-nuclear antibody (ANA) and joint pain do not have lupus (which requires the presence of 4 out of 11 criteria, of which the ANA is just one). Patients with joint pain and either a positive RF or ANA are frequently referred to rheumatologists: most do not need to be. Those who do warrant referral are patients with a raised C-reactive protein (CRP) (rather than a slightly raised ESR which has many benign causes) plus swollen as well as painful joints. Unfortunately there is no agreement on the level of CRP that requires investigation and some patients, particularly with small joint synovitis, have a normal CRP. Pregnancy, the oral contraceptive pill, HRT and obesity (now considered a subclinical pro-inflammatory condition) can also cause a mildly elevated CRP.[1] Assessment and rapid identification of synovitis is necessary, as early diagnosis and aggressive treatment before bony erosions and joint damage occur is likely to improve outcome. As far as investigations are concerned, about 80% of patients with early rheumatoid arthritis have normal radiographic findings but high-resolution musculoskeletal ultrasound can demonstrate synovitis in some such patients. The blood flow within the joint can be assessed with Doppler to help distinguish active from inactive synovitis. MRI can also be helpful in detecting oedematous bone. Anti-cyclic citrullinated peptide (anti-CCP-2) antibodies have been found in the sera of patients with very early RA, sometimes years before clinical symptoms develop. They are much more specific for RA than RF and their presence predicts progression to rheumatoid arthritis in undifferentiated arthritis, the severity of the disease and the development of radiographic joint damage.[2] Anti-CCP-2 antibody testing may replace RF.

American College of Rheumatology diagnostic criteria[3]

- Morning stiffness > 1 h
- Arthritis of ≥ 3 joint areas
- Arthritis of hand joints
- Symmetrical arthritis
- Rheumatoid nodules
- RF positive
- Erosions

4/7 criteria must be met. Arthritis needs to have been present for ≥ 6 weeks.
Reprinted with permission of Wiky-Liss Inc., a subsidiary of John Wiley & Sons, Inc.

[1] Bastard *et al.* Eur Cytokine Netw (2006) 17: 4–12.

[2] Berglin *et al.* Ann Rheum Dis (2005) 65: 453–458.

[3] Arnett *et al.* Arthritis Rheum (1988) 31: 315–324.

Predicting outcome

Most of the damage in RA occurs in the first few years of the disease, so early treatment is critical, especially for those with poor prognostic indicators. Patients who present with bony erosions, are RF positive (or anti-CCP-2 positive), have high levels of inflammatory markers or high levels of disability all have a worse outcome. Genetic advances have also shown that those with the so-called 'shared epitope alleles'(such as HLA-DRB1) will also do worse.

Jumping straight in

The aim of treatment in RA is to control the inflammatory process that drives joint destruction and systemic disease by minimizing synovitis. There is increasing ultrasonographic and MRI evidence that treating synovitis can reduce or even partially heal early bony erosions. DMARDs slow the development of erosions, although they do not prevent damage completely. Although it is important to start DMARD treatment as soon as possible after a diagnosis of RA, it is equally important to avoid unnecessary treatment in patients who have a self-limiting condition such as post-viral polyarthritis. There is a general agreement that polyarthritis persisting for 12 weeks or more probably reflects 'very early' RA and that DMARD therapy should be instituted around this stage.[4] Combinations of DMARDs are more effective than single agents and starting several agents at once, then 'stepping-down' is better than substituting single agents or 'stepping-up'. Various combinations of DMARDs are effective, with methotrexate often the common link: methotrexate can be combined with sulphasalazine and hydroxychloroquine; sulphasalazine and prednisolone; sulphasalazine, hydroxychloroquine and prednisolone; or ciclosporin.[5] Surprisingly, trials of combination therapy have fewer dropouts and no increase in adverse effects, such as myelosuppression or infection, over monotherapy. Frequent monitoring of disease activity (using validated measures), with more aggressive treatment if there is a limited response, can place many more patients effectively into remission (65% versus 15%) than routine care.[6] Whilst monitoring it is very important to always measure the CRP. A slightly raised ESR is often wrongly overlooked especially in elderly patients (since ESR rises with age) but CRP is sensitive and vital for monitoring disease activity.

---

[4] Quinn, Rheum Dis Clin N Am (2005) 31: 763.

[5] O'Dell *et al.* NEJM (1996) 334: 1287–1291.

[6] Grigor *et al.* Lancet (2004) 364: 263–269.

An elevated platelet count is often another indicator of inflammatory activity. Corticosteroids also have a disease-modifying effect and are frequently used for symptomatic relief whilst waiting for conventional DMARDs to take effect. Although DMARDs are widely considered to be immunosuppressive agents, most rheumatologists would regard them as 'immunomodulatory'. The risk of hospitalization for infections (especially of the skin and soft tissues) is increased in RA, particularly if patients are on steroids and have more severe disease. Methotrexate may also increase this risk, although this may reflect disease severity rather than an effect of the drug. DMARDs are also effective in other forms of inflammatory arthritis (such as psoriatic arthritis and the peripheral joint disease of spondyloarthropathy).

The biologics

The immunological basis of inflammatory arthritis is complex and remains only partially understood. Early therapies aimed at single aspects of the immune pathway were not very successful because of this complexity. Much more effective drugs, the 'biologics' have been developed to target the pro-inflammatory cytokines, particularly the ubiquitous tumour necrosis factor alpha (TNF α). These include etanercept (the soluble receptor for TNF α), infliximab (a chimeric mouse–human monoclonal antibody against TNF α) and adalimumab (a fully human monoclonal antibody). For some patients, these drugs have been little short of miraculous, with many anecdotal accounts of severely disabled patients resuming normal life, returning to work and even running marathons. All of these agents seem similar in effect.[7] Biological therapy combined with methotrexate is even more effective.[8] All of these anti-TNF therapies produce a good initial response in about two-third of patients. Switching from one biologic to another (after one has failed) can have a good clinical impact. Other biological agents include anakinra (a recombinant IL-1 receptor antagonist) and novel agents are constantly being developed. Excitingly, if remission of early disease is brought about with aggressive early treatment with biologics, the effect lasts for some time (at least to 2 years) even if the biologic is promptly stopped following the induction of remission.[9]

As well as being of proven efficacy in RA, biologics are also used in other forms of inflammatory arthritis such as psoriatic arthritis and ankylosing

------

[7] Maini *et al.* Lancet (1999) 354: 1932–1939.

[8] Lipsky *et al.* NEJM (2000) 343: 1594–1602.

[9] Quinn *et al.* Arthritis Rheum (2005) 52: 27–35.

spondylitis, juvenile inflammatory arthritis (etanercept), Wegener's granulomatosis (infliximab), as well as other conditions such as Crohn's disease (infliximab, but surprisingly not etanercept).

Widespread use of biologics is limited by cost (about £10,000 per year). As new prognostic biomarkers become available, early therapy can be better targeted. Rationing of expensive treatments is inevitable, and complicated economic arguments need to balance costs to the NHS against savings made by enabling work and reducing dependency. Other issues with biologics include the definite risk of reactivating TB and uncertainty around heightening the chances of future malignancy, particularly lymphoma.

Rheumatoid as a cardiovascular risk

Patients with rheumatoid arthritis have high rates of cardiovascular disease. Many consider that patients with RA who are at particularly high risk of cardiovascular disease should be managed in a similar way to those with diabetes and be treated aggressively, with tight control of hypertension and routine prescription of aspirin and statins. Aggressive control of disease probably reduces this risk because most evidence points to uncontrolled inflammation as the contributing factor towards heart disease.

Patients with rheumatoid arthritis have a standardized mortality ratio of about 2.7.[10] In one series of over a 1000 newly diagnosed patients with RA, 48% had died after a median follow-up of 11 years, a mortality worse than for many forms of cancer.[11] Much of this excess mortality is due to cardiovascular disease. Women who are seropositive have double the risk of cardiovascular disease. Some of the excess cardiovascular mortality is in turn due to the traditional risk factors: patients with rheumatoid arthritis are more likely to smoke, do little exercise and have diabetes. They are often hypertensive, and this can be exacerbated by the use of NSAIDs, leflunomide and ciclosporin. Patients with both early active RA and established disease have normal or low levels of total cholesterol but a disproportionate reduction in the HDL-cholesterol. The atherogenic index can be improved with both combination DMARDS and paradoxically corticosteroids (which can induce hypercholesterolaemia in other populations of patients).

Cardiovascular risks that are more specific for RA include chronic inflammation, hyperhomocysteinaemia, and perhaps the long-term use of

---

10 Symmons *et al.* J Rheumatol (1998) 25: 1072–1077.

11 Goodson *et al.* Ann Rheum Dis (2005) 64: 1595–1601.

corticosteroids and NSAIDs. There are histological similarities between the inflammatory process in synovitic joints and the endothelial processes producing atherogenesis. In RA, endothelial dysfunction is suggested by increased levels of circulating adhesion molecules such as vascular circulating adhesion molecule-1 (VCAM-1), which can predict atherogenesis, and by impaired brachial artery vasodilatation with acetylcholine. Endothelial dysfunction occurs even in young patients with RA and low disease activity.[12] This endothelial dysfunction may be mediated by inflammatory cytokines. A high CRP, even without RA, is a predictor of cardiovascular mortality. It might be expected that lowering the CRP would reduce cardiovascular risk and prospective studies have shown that treatment with methotrexate (although not other DMARDs) can reduce mortality, in particular cardiovascular mortality.[13] Drugs that inhibit both TNF α and reduce the CRP are likely to be even more effective at reducing cardiovascular risk, although this has not yet been proven.

Patients with rheumatoid arthritis also have higher plasma homocysteine levels than controls. Homocysteine is an independent risk factor for cardiovascular disease, possibly by causing direct endothelial damage. Whether reducing plasma homocysteine levels by dietary supplementation with vitamin B6 or folic acid can reduce the risk of cardiovascular disease is unclear, but avoiding hyperhomocysteinaemia seems logical. Methotrexate increases plasma homocysteine levels, but this effect is reversed with folic acid supplements that are usually co-prescribed with methotrexate to mitigate some of the adverse effects.

Angiotensin II promotes endothelial dysfunction and vascular smooth muscle proliferation and can indirectly increase pro-inflammatory cytokines, effects that are reversed by ACE inhibitors. Although plasma levels of renin and ACE are not elevated in rheumatoid arthritis, synovial levels of both substances are, and may contribute to local joint damage. ACE inhibitors and angiotensin receptor blockers have therefore been proposed as potential disease-modifying agents in RA, but although they seem effective in mouse models, clinical data are lacking.

Patients with lupus are at an even higher risk of cardiovascular disease: women aged 35–44 with lupus have a 50-fold increased risk of myocardial infarction compared to controls (although the absolute risk in this age group

[12] Vaudo *et al.* Rheum Dis (2004) 63: 31–35.

[13] Choi *et al.* Lancet (2002) 359: 1173–1177.

is of course still small).[14] The link between systemic inflammation and endothelial dysfunction is the subject of much ongoing research.

Cachexia in rheumatoid

Measures of muscle strength (such as grip strength) are inversely related to life expectancy in both elderly patients (irrespective of chronic disease) and in those with RA.[15] A change of mindset (on the part of both doctors and patients) is required: exercise and exercise hard!

Although the majority of patients with rheumatoid arthritis are not underweight, most have a relative excess of body fat and lack muscle mass. This paradox is known as 'cachectic obesity' and is associated with insulin resistance and the development of type 2 diabetes. Inflammatory cytokines, particularly TNF α and interleukin-1 beta, may also contribute to decreased insulin sensitivity and increased protein catabolism. Reduced lean body mass is related to the number of swollen joints and the levels of circulating TNF α. Treatment of the acute phase process with DMARDs may improve insulin sensitivity, although this alone is unlikely to improve muscle mass. Although it seems illogical, perhaps even sadistic, to suggest that patients with inflamed joints should exercise, progressive resistance training in the gymnasium can improve both lean body mass and physical function in patients even with moderately bad rheumatoid arthritis, with no worsening of symptoms.[16] The challenge of persuading elderly people who have previously been told to rest painful joints to even buy a pair of trainers, let alone exercise, is real.

NSAIDs, cardiovascular disease and gastrointestinal complications

Following the withdrawal of rofecoxib in September 2004, there has been a confusing and sometimes contradictory rash of studies showing an increased cardiovascular risk with both selective and non-selective COX inhibitors. Many patients with inflammatory arthritis have had their NSAID changed or stopped, and both patients and professionals remain muddled. Patients with inflammatory arthritis often use NSAIDs continuously for many years

---

[14] Manzi et al. Am J Epidemiol (1997) 145: 408–415.

[15] Pincus et al. J Rheumatol (1992) 19: 1051–1057.

[16] Marcora et al. J Rheumatol (2005) 32: 1031–1039.

and a balance has to be struck between individual benefits and the risks of both gastrointestinal and cardiovascular adverse effects.

NSAIDs act by inhibiting cyclo-oxygenase (COX), of which there are two main forms. COX-2 is thought to play a major role in inflammation whereas the gastrointestinal adverse effects associated with NSAIDs are thought to be mediated mainly by the inhibition of COX-1.

Selective COX-2 inhibitors (such as celecoxib and etoricoxib) inhibit prostacyclin (PGI_2) but not thromboxane A_2 (TXA_2). The imbalance between PGI_2 and TXA_2 inhibition may be the basis of increased atherogenesis with selective COX-2 inhibitors. 'Non-selective' NSAIDs have varying degrees of COX-2/COX-1 selectivity. Diclofenac is COX-2 'preferential', whereas ibuprofen and naproxen have more effects against COX-1. Non-selective NSAIDs also reversibly inhibit TXA_2, although this does not reliably inhibit platelet aggregation except in the case of aspirin (where inhibition is irreversible).

The issue of an increase in cardiovascular events with selective COX-2 inhibitors was first raised following the VIGOR study of rofecoxib in 2000.[17] The increase in myocardial infarction rates in those taking rofecoxib was largely ignored because of methodological criticisms of the study. It took another 4 years for rofecoxib to be withdrawn as a result of another study that showed a doubling of cardiovascular events in patients who had used rofecoxib for 18 months or more.[18] Increased rates of cardiovascular events have also been found for other COX-2 selective agents celecoxib and valdecoxib. These complications were initially considered to be a 'class effect' of COX-2 selective agents but several studies have also now shown an increase in cardiovascular events with non-selective NSAIDs. Most of the data relate to diclofenac, naproxen and ibuprofen.

COX-1 must be inhibited by at least 95% before an anti-platelet effect is evident. This does not apply to most non-selective NSAIDs. An exception may be naproxen, which in high doses does inhibit TXA_2, seems to have an anti-platelet effect and may be cardioprotective. By contrast, the ADAPT study using low-dose naproxen showed a higher risk of cardiovascular events with naproxen than placebo over 3 years (possibly because of inadequate COX-1 inhibition).

[17] Bombardier et al. NEJM (2000) 343: 1520–1528.

[18] Bresalier et al. NEJM (2005) 352: 1092–1102.

A further complicating factor in patients with inflammatory arthritis is that many take aspirin for concurrent cardiovascular disease. Furthermore, ibuprofen may antagonize the anti-platelet and therefore cardioprotective effects of aspirin.[19]

The rate of hospitalization for gastrointestinal complications of NSAIDs is around 0.5–1% of patients per year. Indeed, for patients taking chronic NSAIDs (for whatever reason), a 'number needed to kill' (through bleeding or ulcer perforation) of between 870 and 2500 has been calculated.[20] Although the rate of troublesome gastrointestinal side effects has declined, the reasons for this are not necessarily attributable to the use of COX-2 inhibitors, but probably also to the more judicious use of NSAIDs and gastroprotective drugs. Although several trials, notably those sponsored by pharmaceutical companies, have shown an advantage of COX-2 selective over non-selective NSAIDs in terms of adverse gastrointestinal complications, the advantage has not been shown over conventional NSAIDs plus gastroprotection. [16,21] Furthermore, favourable reports of a gastroprotective effect of celecoxib in the CLASS study, were not substantiated in subsequent analysis. Although this study was widely reported as showing a benefit of celecoxib over ibuprofen and diclofenac, celecoxib had no benefit on the major outcome measures, gastrointestinal ulcer complications (bleeding, perforation and obstruction), and any extant benefit only applied to those patients not taking concurrent aspirin.

In summary, the gastroprotective advantage of selective COX-2 inhibitors over non-selective NSAIDs plus gastroprotection is debatable. These drugs probably double the risk of cardiovascular events. The risk of cardiovascular disease with traditional NSAIDs may also be increased, but the situation remains confusing. Naproxen may be the safest NSAID in terms of cardiovascular risk and naproxen plus a proton pump inhibitor is an attractive recipe (where a NSAID is essential). In the real world, patient preference and individual benefits over risks are critical. The NICE guidelines on the prescription of COX-2 inhibitors now need to be balanced against cardiovascular risk, making NICE still less enthusiastic about their use.[22]

---

[19] Catella-Lawson et al. NEJM (2001) 345: 1809–1817.

[20] Tramer et al. Pain (2000) 85: 169–182.

[21] Silverstein et al. JAMA (2000) 284: 1247–1255.

[22] TA027 (July 2001) (www.nice.org.uk)

OSTEOPOROSIS

Although the subject of osteoporosis is not particularly glamorous, the compelling facts are that it affects an increasing number of people and costs the NHS about £5 million a day. Half of all women and one-fifth of men will have a fracture after the age of 50 years.[23] Only about half of those who fracture a hip regain their previous level of independence, about a fifth need institutional care: the 2-year survival in men may be as low as 37%.[24]

Most patients with uncomplicated osteoporosis can be managed in primary care. Some require specialist referral, not least because of the expense of some drugs, particularly recombinant human parathyroid hormone (teriparatide) and confusion about the interpretation of bone mineral density (BMD) scores (see table below). Such scores are a statistical representation of the bone density related to normal young adults (the T-score). The risk of osteoporotic fracture increases with decreasing scores, although fracture risk also depends on bone strength which relates to bone geometry and trabecular microstructure. Predicting fracture risk for an individual by BMD alone is therefore unreliable. The inherent errors in measuring BMD mean that DXA scans should not be performed more often than at 2-yearly intervals. Standard DXA scores were developed for white adult women. Results in children, men and other ethnic groups are therefore unreliable. This also applies to patients with severe osteoarthritis, as bone sclerosis produces spuriously high scores.

WHO definition of osteoporosis

- Normal: T-score of −1 or above
- Osteopenia: T-score between −1 and −2.5
- Osteoporosis: T-score of less than −2.5
- Established osteoporosis: T-score of less than −2.5 with one or more documented low trauma or fragility fractures

Markers of bone turnover provide a more timely estimate of changes in bone composition and structure than DXA, and in future they may be used to predict fracture risk. Probably the most useful at present (although not universally available) is the serum amino-terminal propeptide of type 1 procollagen (P1NP).

[23] www.nos.org.uk

[24] Pande *et al.* Ann Rheum Dis 2006; 65: 87–92.

P1NP reflects osteoblast activity, and levels decline in patients taking bisphos-phonates. It can therefore also be used to monitor compliance.

Drug companies promoting therapies for osteoporosis are usually keen to provide information that their product increases BMD. Although this is important, fracture reduction is the critical issue. Although spine fractures are painful and debilitating, they cause less morbidity and mortality than hip frac-tures. Reduction in the rates of hip fracture should therefore be the main outcome of treatment for osteoporosis. Some pharmaceutical companies are perhaps intentionally vague on this point: a reduction in spine fractures does not necessarily equate with a reduction in hip fracture, since the two areas have a different bony micro-architecture. Nasal calcitonin and the selective oestro-gen receptor modulator, raloxifene both increase BMD and reduce spinal frac-tures, but have no effect on the rates of hip fracture. Hormone replacement therapy is no longer suitable for treatment of osteoporosis because other agents are more effective and because of the increased risk of breast cancer. The standard weekly bisphosphonates alendronate and risedronate, increase BMD and reduce vertebral and non-vertebral fractures. Unfortunately long-term compliance may be as low as 40%. The newer bisphosphonates, such as monthly ibandronate and yearly zolendronate, are likely to improve compliance, and results for hip fracture prevention are pending.

Supplementary calcium and vitamin D are usually given with other treat-ments for osteoporosis, and have a small but significant effect, particularly since about 50% of patients with osteoporosis are vitamin D deficient. Severe vitamin D deficiency must be excluded or treated before osteoporotic patients are treated with bisphosphonates or other drugs.

Recombinant parathyroid hormone (teriparatide) is the most effective treat-ment for osteoporosis. It stimulates new bone formation by acting on osteo-clasts, increases bone density by up to 10% per year and dramatically reduces the risk of vertebral and non-vertebral fractures. When bisphosphonates follow a course of teriparatide, the gains in bone mass may be maintained. PTH is unfortunately very expensive and therefore limited to those with the most severe osteoporosis who either continue to have fractures in spite of bisphosphonates or are intolerant of them. It may also have unpleasant effects such as dizziness, GI disturbance, muscle cramps and injection site reactions, making it intolerable in some cases.

Strontium inhibits bone resorption and stimulates increased calcium uptake into bones. It reduces the rates of both vertebral and non-vertebral fractures. Its effects cannot be monitored by bone densitometry since it is taken up into bones, and is denser than calcium. This increases the apparent BMD, and makes monitoring by DXA complicated.

GOUT

I confidently affirm that the greater part of those who are supposed to have died of gout, have died of the medicine rather than the disease...

Thomas Sydenham (1624–1689)[25]

Gout results from the deposition of urate crystals in joints or soft tissues. Humans and Dalmatian dogs are amongst the few mammals lacking in uricase, the enzyme that converts uric acid to a soluble (and excretable) compound. Gout is a common affliction with a prevalence of 1.4% amongst patients registered in general practice.[26] Men have higher uric acid levels than women and there is an impressive male preponderance for clinical disease (up to 9-fold). The incidence of gout over a 5-year period is strongly correlated with random plasma uric acid levels but that said, gout can occur in those with normal levels, and many people with quite profound hyperuricaemia manage to evade clinical disease.[27]

Uric acid is formed from purine compounds by the enzyme xanthine oxidase. About 30% of purine is of dietary origin, with the remainder arising from the degradation of endogenous purines (in DNA) and *de novo* purine synthesis. Hyperuricaemia (> 0.42 mmol/l) may therefore result from the under-excretion or over-production of urate. Excretion of urate is predominantly renal and is reduced by alcohol, hypertension, renal failure and a number of drugs (including diuretics, low-dose aspirin, ciclosporin and several anti-tuberculosis drugs). Over-production may be due to dietary excess, myeloproliferative disease or one of a number of rare hereditary enzyme defects.

A typical male patient with acute gout is middle aged, with one or more of obesity, hypertension, hyperlipidaemia, ischaemic heart disease and insulin resistance. A typical female patient is postmenopausal, on diuretic therapy with gouty tophi over the distal interphalangeal joints. Acute attacks typically involve a single lower limb joint which becomes red, hot, swollen, intensely painful, often with periarticular swelling and erythema (gouty cellulitis), followed by exfoliation as the acute attack regresses within 7–10 days. *Podagra* (gout affecting the hallux) is the first presentation in up to 70% but gout is

---

[25] McDonald, *The Oxford Dictionary of Medical Quotations*. Oxford University Press, Oxford, 2004.

[26] Mikuls *et al.* Ann Rheum Dis (2005) 64: 267–272.

[27] Campion *et al.* Am J Med (1987) 82: 421–426.

often polyarticular and any joint can be affected. In addition to arthritis, gout may manifest as chronic tophi (said to affect up to 70% of sufferers 20 years after the initial presentation in pre-treatment days), renal tract stones and rarely, renal failure through interstitial nephritis.[28]

The gold standard for the diagnosis of an acute attack of gout is the visualization of crystals on microscopy of synovial fluid. Other clues, aside from a characteristic history and examination, include raised inflammatory markers (which can be dramatic). Many general physicians greatly value plasma uric acid levels for diagnosis, although others feel the test is not tremendously useful as hyperuricaemia and gout do not necessarily go hand in hand: indeed, uric acid levels may fall at the time of an acute attack (as the uric acid is sequestered) and are said to be within the normal range in about 40% of patients. However, a uric acid level below 0.33 mmol/l is generally regarded as inconsistent with a diagnosis of acute gout. The crucial differential diagnosis not to miss is that of septic arthritis. Another common problem is that of pyrophosphate arthropathy (pseudogout) in elderly patients with osteoarthritis. If the diagnosis is not clinically straightforward, the joint should be aspirated: if this is not a task suited to the admitting physician, then an expert should be summoned.

Acute gout is self-limiting but the symptoms tend to be sufficiently disabling to demand treatment. This generally involves a non-steroidal: the precise form not being important. In those for whom non-steroidals are contra-indicated, colchicine is an option. It is thought to act by inhibiting leucocyte micro-tubules, preventing the migration of inflammatory cells to the gouty hotspot. Diarrhoea is a reliable and predictable side effect and often determines the dose: it is not a symptom welcomed by middle-aged overweight men, immobile through gout. For acute attacks, although the British National Formulary (BNF) advises doses of 1 mg followed by 500 mg every 2–3 h until either symptom relief or diarrhoea or vomiting occur, most patients are unable to tolerate more than 500 mg once or twice daily. The dose to accompany allopurinol or uricosuric agents, for prophylaxis, is 500 mg 2 or 3 times a day. Although renal failure can often trigger the avoidance of non-steroidals, it can also pose problems for colchicine users as it increases the chances of side effects such as myopathy or neuropathy with long-term use (which is therefore rarely indicated). However, colchicine does not lead to fluid retention making it a reasonable choice for those with heart failure.

----

28 Yu *et al.* Am J Med Sci (1967) 254: 893–907.

The other option for the acute treatment of gout is steroids, which can bring about dramatic relief within hours. A short course (perhaps 15 mg a day for 10 days) is reasonable for patients with multiple other co-morbidities and is an underused strategy. Another alternative (when gout is localized) is the intra-articular injection of steroids, although this can be awkward for smaller joints.

There are a number of agents that can help prevent further attacks of acute gout. There is a general consensus for treating those with more than one attack in a year, more than two attacks ever, the presence of tophi, or urate stones within the renal tract. The pharmacological workhorse for the prevention of gout is the xanthine oxidase inhibitor allopurinol. Sulfinpyrazone and probenecid increase the excretion of uric acid but are rarely used. Hyperuricaemia *per se* does not warrant treatment unless severe. In order to avoid precipitating a resurgence of gout, it is sensible to wait a few weeks after an acute attack before starting allopurinol (some wait far longer) and to consider the use of a prophylactic (non-steroidal, steroid or colchicine) when starting the drug. Allopurinol treatment can be titrated to reduce uric acid levels to within the normal range but many pharmacologists question the meaning of levels and doubt the value of such monitoring. If a patient is taking allopurinol when hit by an attack of acute gout, it should be continued, with acute therapy added in. A rash is not infrequent with allopurinol (around 2%) and a rarer side effect is a serious hypersensitivity syndrome characterized by exfoliative dermatitis, eosinophilia, hepatitis and interstitial nephritis. Some patients end up on long-term low-dose steroids as an alternative to allopurinol.

Aside from drug therapy, a number of lifestyle modifications are to be encouraged, not least because of the co-morbidities found in patients with gout. Weight loss is certainly associated with a fall in uric acid levels and a reduction in clinical gout.[29] However, a number of traditional views on gout have been challenged in recent times. Curiously, gout seems to be associated with high purine intake derived from meat and seafood, but not from vegetables.[30] Although patients are often advised to avoid red wine, a recent study suggested moderate consumption was without detriment.[31] Heavy beer intake continues to be discouraged.

---

[29] Dessein *et al.* Ann Rheum Dis (2000) 59: 539–543.

[30] Choi *et al.* NEJM (2004) 350: 1093–1103.

[31] Choi *et al.* Lancet (2004) 363: 1277–1281.

Chapter 18

Catherine Sargent, Aamir Aslam and Richard Steele

IMMUNOLOGY

ALLERGY

Allergy is an enormously common problem in the developed world, with approximately 20% of the population suffering from some sort of allergic disease. The spectrum of clinical manifestations is wide and allergic disease may be seen by the general physician in a number of different guises.

Hygiene hypothesis

Vaccination, antibiotics and improved hygiene have greatly reduced the mortality and morbidity associated with childhood infections. However, it is postulated that this reduction in infection is itself responsible for the marked rise in allergic disease. There is direct evidence that treating bacterial and helminthic infections increases skin test reactivity to common allergens. Furthermore, epidemiological data show that early childhood TB, hepatitis A and helminthic infections reduce the risk of allergy, as does being nurtured in an environment that increases the likelihood of encountering infections (such as having siblings, attending day-care or living on a farm). It appears that childhood infections generate regulatory T-cells that prevent allergic disease, possibly through inhibitory cytokines such as IL-10 and TGFβ. Indeed, individuals with the IPEX syndrome (who are deficient in regulatory T-cells) characteristically develop elevated IgE concentrations and allergic disease. The hygiene hypothesis is still controversial, as there are some conflicting data. For example, there is a high prevalence of asthma in some developing countries, particularly in urban slums.

Anaphylaxis

The three most common causes of anaphylaxis are drugs (most commonly penicillins and non-steroidal anti-inflammatory drugs), foods (most commonly peanuts, true nuts, seafoods, milk and eggs) and insect stings. At the moment of presentation, the patient requires immediate intramuscular adrenaline into the lateral aspect of the thigh and any procrastination increases the chance of death. In addition, resuscitative measures should be instituted including the securing of the airway and intravenous fluids. If possible the patient should be kept flat: one recent study suggested that death from anaphylaxis was associated with sitting the patient up.[1]

Antihistamines and hydrocortisone should usually be administered at the same time, to prevent a subsequent recrudescence of symptoms. However, these medications do not save lives and are no substitute for adrenaline. The precipitant may be clear from the history of the reaction. A useful adjunct to the history in the diagnosis of anaphylaxis (especially where other diagnoses are being considered) is a blood test for mast-cell tryptase: this should be taken between 30 min and 6 h of the reaction. If the serum tryptase is raised, it should be repeated after 24 h to document a return to normal levels. A persistently raised serum tryptase suggests an underlying mastocytosis.

If the causative agent is a drug, this should be prominently recorded in the notes and explained to the patient. A MedicAlert emblem should be worn. All patients who have had anaphylaxis should ideally be referred to a specialist clinic where they will be taken through an action plan outlining the signs and symptoms of anaphylaxis and also how and when to use an adrenaline pen.[2]

Reactions to insect venoms can be severe. Contrary to popular belief, it is the honey bee that is the most dangerous creature in Australasia, killing more people through fatal reactions than any of the venomous snakes and spiders. Any adult who has suffered a systemic reaction to an insect bite and who has a positive IgE (or skin test) to the relevant venom should be offered venom immunotherapy. This is usually continued for 3–5 years and should be initiated by a physician who has experience in this form of therapy. In children, there is evidence to suggest that those with cutaneous symptoms only do not require immunotherapy as their likelihood of more serious reactions to subsequent stings is low.

Urticaria and angioedema

These conditions represent a spectrum of the same disease. Urticaria is an intensely itchy raised erythematous rash which is due to swelling of the skin layers. Lesions usually resolve spontaneously leaving no scarring. It is

---

[1] Pumphrey, J Allergy Clin Immunol (2003) 112: 451–452.

[2] www.allergy.org.au/anaphylaxis/index.htm

extremely common, affecting about a fifth of the population at some point. Angioedema is due to swelling of deeper tissues so that patients tend to present with more diffuse symptoms, typically of the face, periorbital region, mouth and throat. It is usually not particularly itchy.

Diagnosis is based on clinical examination although a skin biopsy can be useful when there is suspicion of a vasculitis. When assessing a patient with this syndrome, it is useful to ask the following three questions:

- Is the presentation one of urticaria (with or without angioedema) or lone angioedema?

- If urticaria, is it acute (less than 6 weeks) or chronic?

- If chronic, is there some physical precipitant (for example, heat, cold, water or pressure) and is there any evidence of vasculitis (lesions lasting more than 24 h, painful lesions or lesions leaving bruising or scarring)?

If lone angioedema, then it is important to ask about ACE inhibitors and (less commonly) angiotensin II receptor blockers, as these medications are the most common causes and should be stopped. Hereditary angioedema should also be considered. This is rare. It is an autosomal dominant condition, so a family history may be available. There is also an acquired form of this condition. Patients may present to surgical teams with abdominal pain due to angioedema of the gut. The condition is due to a deficiency (or abnormality) of C1 esterase inhibitor such that there is failure of inactivation of the complement and kinin cascades. It is often precipitated by trauma or infections. Quantitative and functional assays can be performed to establish the diagnosis. The C4 level is a useful screen, as it is usually reduced, even between attacks. Patients who have a confirmed diagnosis will have a supply of the inhibitor to use when they have attacks. In addition, medications can be used to prevent attacks, including danazol and tranexamic acid. Prior to surgical procedures, an immunologist may wish to consider prophylaxis.

In those with acute urticaria, it is important to take a forensically detailed history in order to rule out a specific precipitant. Common culprits are similar to anaphylaxis and include infections, foods, drugs and venoms. By its very definition, acute urticaria is self-limiting and requires only symptomatic therapy with antihistamines. When debilitating, it may prompt a short course of oral corticosteroids.

In chronic urticaria/angioedema, it is important to differentiate the physical from the idiopathic form. In most cases, the physical urticarias (whether cholinergic or cold-, pressure- or exercise-induced) can be deduced from the history and physical examination. Confirmation with an appropriate test (for example, an ice cube for cold-induced urticaria) can be helpful. Dermographism (the induction of hives after firmly scratching the skin) is also a useful sign as it does suggest a physical component. In a significant proportion of patients with chronic urticaria/angioedema, the cause is not certain. It has been shown that many of these patients have antibodies directed against a portion (epsilon-R1) of the Fc receptor and also (in a minority) to IgE. It is likely that these patients have autoimmunity rather than allergy as the basis of their problem.

Urticarial vasculitis is a rare problem. The lesions are generalized wheals or erythematous plaques, occasionally with central clearing, which last for more than 24 h in a fixed location. Petechiae may be noted within the lesions and they may resolve with bruising or post-inflammatory hyperpigmentation. They can be associated with systemic symptoms such as fever, arthralgia and lymphadenopathy. Complement, urinalysis and ANA studies are indicated as such lesions may represent an early manifestation of SLE. Confirmation is with a deep (punch) biopsy, looking for the histological features of a leukocytoclastic vasculitis. Treatment may require immunosuppressives.

The extent of investigation for the urticarias is usually determined by how frequently the episodes occur and if they are resistant to treatment with simple antihistamines. When patients suffer from continuous and irritating attacks, they can be referred to an immunologist who may consider other therapies including elimination diets, doxepin and various forms of immunomodulation. It is important to tell the patient that in most cases, chronic urticaria will resolve with time (1–2 years), and that in the interim, therapy is directed at minimizing the impact of the condition on their lives.

Drug allergy

Drug allergy is a large topic and is well beyond the scope of this chapter. It is important to distinguish drug allergy (immunologic) from other adverse effects of drugs (non-immunologic). Drugs can cause many types of immunologic reactions including IgE-mediated reactions (type I), antibody-mediated cytotoxic (type II), immune complex-mediated (type III) and cell-mediated (type IV). Although previously classified through the Gell and Coombes system it is clear that for some immunologic reactions to drugs, the underlying mechanisms are not well understood and may involve other important immune mechanisms (for example, cytokine release, direct mast cell activation, granulomatous reactions and drug-induced autoimmunity).

When assessing a patient with possible drug allergy, the history is the most important tool. Attention needs to be paid to what drugs were taken, and the time course, in relation to the reactions that occurred. Other important factors include the patient's age, genetic background and medical conditions. The usefulness of diagnostic tests depends upon the drug in question and the immunological mechanism involved. The issue of testing remains problematic, particularly as new drugs come onto the market continually as older drugs become obsolete: the playing field is not static.

Management is always a balance between a number of factors including:

- the therapeutic importance of the drug;
- the severity of the reaction;
- the availability of alternative medications; and
- the preferences of the patient.

Management includes a combination of treatment of the acute reaction and avoidance/minimization of further exposure. Where the causative agent is not certain, graded challenges may be indicated. The decision to do this should however be judged against the severity of the reaction. For example, in patients who suffered a life threatening reaction such as Stevens-Johnson syndrome and toxic epidermal necrolysis, graded challenges with the implicated drug would be inappropriate. When continuation of the drug outweighs the risk of further reactions and no good alternative exists, then other management strategies can be considered. These include treating through where the reaction is mild and, for more severe reactions, desensitization. Examples where desensitization has been used include beta lactams, sulphur-based antibiotics (such as co-trimoxazole), allopurinol and aspirin. Where life threatening reactions have occurred then the patient should also be offered an MedicAlert emblem in order to reduce the risk of inadvertent exposure in the future. Also, the information should be reported to the appropriate adverse drug reaction surveillance authority and where available, added to an electronic alert system.

Where the responsible drug is not clear and where further testing may be helpful (for example, skin testing or graded oral challenge), referral to an immunologist for assessment is appropriate – likewise where desensitization may be of clinical benefit.

Allergen immunotherapy

The current mainstays of treating allergic disease are avoidance and drugs. Allergen avoidance can be simple but in the common allergic diseases such as allergic rhinitis, it is impossible. Some allergic disease can be cured by immunotherapy – which involves the administration of allergen in increasing doses. Indeed allergen immunotherapy is the only treatment that successfully utilizes the induction of clinical tolerance. Immunotherapy is available for aeroallergy (allergic rhinitis, ocular allergy and asthma) and venom allergy.

As the treatment involves injecting allergic patients with allergen, there is a risk of precipitating anaphylaxis and patients have to be treated where there is ready access to resuscitation equipment and drugs. Allergen-specific immunotherapy was first used in London before the First World War and in more recent times, it was taken up with enthusiasm in mainland Europe and America. During the 1980s, injecting pollen extract into hayfever sufferers became fashionable in GP surgeries in the UK: like other fashions, the vogue for this treatment was short lived. In 1986, the Committee on Safety of Medicines reported 26 deaths over three decades and the use of this treatment in primary care (in the absence of such resuscitation equipment) was promptly abandoned.[3] Its mechanism has yet to be fully elucidated but it is thought that immunotherapy generates IL-10-secreting regulatory T-cells and IgG antibodies that block the binding of allergen to IgE-coated mast cells and basophils.

As a consequence of the iatrogenic risk of anaphylaxis, alternative treatments have been researched. One approach that has been used in bee venom and cat allergy is only to use allergen-derived T-cell epitopes, which will lack the IgE epitopes responsible for anaphylaxis. Another is to manipulate the allergen such that it promotes a T-helper 1 (Th1) subset response, rather than the allergic Th2 response: an example of this is the conjugation of Amb a 1 (a ragweed allergen) to an immunostimulatory sequence of DNA. More recently sublingual immunotherapy has been used extensively in Europe, particularly for allergic rhinitis. It appears to be safe and effective. However, to date there are limited data on safety and efficacy when compared to conventional immunotherapy by subcutaneous injection. In addition, the reagents are substantially more expensive.[4]

Anti-IgE therapy

The generation of allergen-specific IgE molecules is critical in the pathogenesis of allergic disease. Thus, the recent development of omalizumab – a humanized anti-IgE antibody – is a rational step. Omalizumab binds free IgE which is then removed by the reticulo-endothelial system via FcG receptors. The IgE receptor is prevented from entering a catabolic pathway if it binds IgE, thus reduction in serum IgE levels also reduces the number of IgE receptors on mast cells and basophils.[5] Trials have demonstrated reductions in the frequency of symptoms, hospital visits and in the use of inhaled corticosteroids in asthmatics receiving omalizumab – the benefit being greatest in severe asthmatics.[6]

[3] Committee on Safety of Medicines, BMJ (1986) 293: 948.

[4] Wilson et al. Cochrane Database Syst Rev (2003, updated 2006) CD002893.

[5] MacGlashan et al. J Immunol (1997) 158: 1438–1445.

[6] Holgate et al. Clin Exp Allergy (2005) 35: 408–416.

Syndromes of drug allergy

Syndrome	Mechanisms	Examples	Potentially useful tests
Anaphylaxis, urticaria and angioedema (IgE mediated)	IgE (type I)	Penicillin Insulin	Skin testing Specific IgE testing Serum tryptase
Anaphylaxis, urticaria and angioedema (non-IgE mediated)	Various	Radiocontrast Aspirin NSAIDs	Complement Serum tryptase
Drug-induced cytopenias	Drug-induced cytotoxicity (type II)	Penicillin-induced haemolytic anaemia Quinine-induced thrombocytopenia Heparin-induced thrombocytopenia and thrombosis	Coomb's testing (direct and indirect with drug in question) Platelet antibody testing
Serum sickness	Immune complexes (type III)	Penicillin	Complement studies
Contact dermatitis	Delayed hypersensitivity (type IV)	Topical antibiotics	Patch testing
Drug-induced bullous pemphigoid	Unknown (possibly drug-induced cytotoxicity or cell-mediated immunity, CD8+)	Diuretics Antibiotics	Direct (skin biopsy) and indirect (serum) immunofluorescence
Asthma Rhinitis	Unknown (possibly through cyclo-oxygenase pathways)	Aspirin-induced asthma	Nil (challenge testing only)
Stevens-Johnson Syndrome Toxic Epidermal necrolysis	Unknown (possibly Fas mediated)	Carbamazepine Sulphonamides Penicillin Nevirapine	Nil
Drug-induced vasculitis	Unknown	Minocycline	ANCA ANA, Anti-dsDNA
Drug-induced lupus	Unknown	Hydralazine Isoniazid Phenytoin	ANA Anti-dsDNA

There is a similar picture in allergic rhinitis with improvements in symptoms in birch, ragweed, house-dust mite, cat and dog-induced rhinitis. Anti-IgE treatment has also been used in peanut allergy where it increases the amount of peanut flour that peanut-allergic patients can tolerate before they develop symptoms. As the severity of anaphylactic reactions in peanut allergic patients cannot be reliably predicted and since avoiding peanuts is difficult, treatment with anti-IgE should prevent anaphylaxis if peanuts are mistakenly ingested.[7] The place of omalizumab in the treatment of allergic disease is uncertain and is dictated by its huge cost (around £10,000 per year), which restricts its use to severe asthmatics and prohibits its use for all but the most severe allergic responses. Long-term safety data are also not yet available.

IMMUNODEFICIENCY

There are numerous very rare conditions that give rise to congenital immunodeficiency. The advance in molecular biology has in more recent times revealed a vast number of specific defects. The study of primary immunodeficiency ('experiments of nature') has also increased our understanding of the immune system in general. Their diagnosis and treatment is the province of the specialist immunologist. Such people are susceptible to recurrent and opportunistic infections but may also present with failure to thrive in childhood, or with end-organ damage (such as bronchiectasis).

Alongside these congenital defects are a multitude of secondary or acquired defects. They may be iatrogenic due to immunosuppressive regimes (including the use of cytotoxic drugs, radiation, steroids or monoclonal therapies) or physiological (as in diabetes and pregnancy). Patients with autoimmune disease, including SLE and rheumatoid, and haematological malignancy, may also be immunocompromised. Splenectomy following trauma, or functional asplenia as occurs in sickle cell disease, may also result in a propensity to acquire serious infections that would normally pose little threat.

Results of investigations that may alert the physician to immunocompromise are the absolute numbers of neutrophils and lymphocytes and the quantity of immunoglobulins in the serum. Many cytotoxic drugs reliably induce neutropenia after a specific number of days (cyclophosphamide produces a nadir at day 10). These patients are at increased risk of developing bacterial infections and if they present with fevers, they should undergo a thorough screen in an attempt to locate the source, before early administration of broad-spectrum antibiotics.

....

[7] Leung *et al.* NEJM (2003) 348: 986–993.

Lymphopenia is commonly seen in cases of acute infection but as the patient recovers, so does the number of lymphocytes. A persistent lymphopenia should be investigated, the most common causes being underlying HIV or malignancy.

Though not commonly picked up by general physicians, there are a number of patients who have recurrent bacterial infections in childhood. A proportion of these may have hypogammaglobulinaemia. They should be referred to an immunologist who may consider treatment with intravenous immunoglobulin (IVIG) every few weeks. Treated patients suffer fewer bacterial infections and have a better overall prognosis. Immunoglobulins are well tolerated and patients can often be taught how to perform infusions at home. Subcutaneous administration, using an infusion pump, is another home option.

Depending upon the severity of the underlying immunological defect and its manifestations, other treatments can also be useful in these patients including prophylactic antibiotics and sinus rinses. For severe combined immunodeficiency (SCID), bone marrow transplantation and more recently gene therapy is the treatment of choice. The earlier in life this condition is found, the better the prognosis, therefore a high degree of suspicion for this condition should be exercised by those clinicians who work with children.

INTRAVENOUS IMMUNOGLOBULIN (IVIG)

IVIG is extracted from the pooled plasma of thousands of donors and has been used as an immunomodulatory agent in a wide range of diseases. IVIG is relatively well tolerated and free from the cytopenias, hepatic and pulmonary toxicities that often complicate conventional treatment. Its cost is the main barrier to its use. Randomized controlled trials have established the efficacy of IVIG in a number of diseases (see table), although there are other diseases where 'evidence' remains anecdotal and there is precious little data to suggest benefit.

Diseases in which IVIG has proven efficacy

System	Disease
Neurological	Guillain-Barré syndrome
	Chronic inflammatory demyelinating polyneuropathy
	Myaesthenia gravis (acute crisis only)
	Eaton–Lambert syndrome
	Stiff person syndrome
	Multi-focal motor neuropathy
Haematological	Idiopathic thrombocytopenic purpura
Rheumatological	Kawasaki disease
	Dermatomyositis

Although IVIG has a favourable side effect profile when compared with conventional immunosuppressives, its use is not without risk. Common side effects include headache, backache and flu-like symptoms, which can be treated with simple analgesics. IVIG raises plasma viscosity and if given to patients with underlying arterial disease, may precipitate a vascular event. As it is a blood product, there is a risk of transmitting infectious diseases: a number of cases of hepatitis C transmission through IVIG were reported in the mid-1990s in the UK. Additional precautions have since been added to the manufacturing process but concerns about prion and other diseases apply as much here as with other blood products, especially when used in younger patients with more benign conditions.

As IVIG contains antibodies from many donors, it contains a large variety of antibody specificities that are capable of binding to a large number of antigens. These antibody–antigen interactions may play a role in abrogating immune-mediated disease (for example, in toxic epidermal necrolysis, where fas-ligand-mediated apoptosis can be blocked by antibodies contained in IVIG). Many antibody functions are mediated through the interaction of the Fc portion of the molecule and Fc receptors found on macrophages in the reticulo-endothelial system. Autoimmune cytopenias are caused by the removal of autoantibody-coated cells by macrophages via the antibody and Fc receptor interaction. Antibodies in IVIG compete with host autoantibodies for binding with these receptors, thereby reducing the removal of antibody-coated cells from the bloodstream. The neonatal Fc receptor (named due to its role in the trans-placental transfer of IgG, although it exists in adults too) is important in the homeostasis of IgG. IgG is non-specifically pinocytosed by endothelial cells before being 'trafficked' to acidic endosomes where it eventually undergoes lysosomal degradation. However, if IgG binds to the neonatal Fc receptor (which is found on endothelial surfaces) it is prevented from entering this pathway and is returned to the circulation. IgG antibodies in IVIG may competitively displace pathogenic antibodies from the neonatal Fc receptor, thereby increasing their breakdown.

THE IMMUNOLOGY LABORATORY AND THE GENERAL PHYSICIAN

The modern immunology laboratory offers a bewildering array of tests, some of which may help in the diagnosis and management of patients! However, the tests are all too often requested inappropriately causing difficulty in their subsequent interpretation.

Anti-nuclear antibodies

Anti-nuclear antibodies should only be requested in adults if a specific autoimmune disease is suspected such as SLE, Sjogren's syndrome, sclero-derma, dermatomyositis and autoimmune liver disease (that is to say in a population with a high pre-test probability of having a disease). As ANA lacks specificity for the diagnosis of autoimmune diseases, 'screening' general medical patients will yield many false-positive results. Therefore, testing patients who present with lethargy, non-specific aches and pains, headaches and other poorly defined symptoms should generally be discour-aged. However, ANA is sensitive and SLE is highly unlikely in the absence of a positive ANA. Recent studies have shown that autoantibodies may be pres-ent up to years before the onset of an autoimmune disease. Although this is interesting, for most antibodies, the predictive value of a positive test in the absence of other signs and symptoms of an autoimmune disease is not known, therefore the presence of autoantibodies in these patients tends to cause unnecessary anxiety and unwanted investigations. There are poten-tially thousands of antigens that can give rise to the immunofluoresence seen in a positive ANA test, yet we measure antibodies specific to only the few of these that are associated with particular diseases: double stranded DNA, Smith, RNP, Ro (SS-A) and La (SS-B) with lupus; Ro and La with Sjogren's and Jo-1 for dermato/polymyositis.

Testing in coeliac disease

Anti-endomysial antibodies (EMAs) are so specific for coeliac disease (CD) that their detection should prompt endoscopy and duodenal biopsy to confirm the diagnosis. Gliadin antibodies, are less sensitive and specific than EMA, and their use for the investigation of CD is declining. Reticulin antibodies are just as sensitive but much less specific for CD than EMA and should not be ordered. A recent addition to the immunological toolkit is an ELISA for IgA/IgG to tissue transglutaminase (TTG) – the specificity is said to be similar to EMA and the sensitivity is potentially higher. In many labo-ratories, anti-TTG antibody testing is replacing EMA as the test of choice to screen for CD. Most experts also suggest that a total IgA be asked for when testing for CD. This is because many of the tests are IgA-based therefore it is more likely that a false-negative test can occur in those deficient in IgA. In addition, the prevalence of CD is said to be higher in patients with IgA deficiency, therefore the threshold to perform upper GI endoscopy and duodenal biopsy should be lower. It is also important to realize that all CD blood testing (and the biopsy) tends to normalize on a gluten-free diet, therefore in general all those tested should remain on a gluten containing diet until the diagnosis is confirmed.

The area of testing and treatment in CD continues to change rapidly. For example, commercial testing kits have become available for gliadin peptides. These peptides are based on the B cell epitopes found on de-amidated gliadin in CD. Preliminary data suggests that these tests are just as sensitive and specific as TTG for the diagnosis of CD. In addition, there are specific HLA-DQ subtypes associated with CD and some laboratories will offer this testing, especially in cases where the diagnosis is not clear.

Anti-neutrophil cytoplasmic antibodies (ANCAs)

Anti-neutrophil cytoplasmic antibodies (ANCAs) are well established as markers of the Wegener's/microscopic polyangiitis spectrum of small vessel vasculitides. They are detected by immunofluoresence of neutrophils and give characteristic perinuclear (p-ANCA) and cytoplasmic (c-ANCA) patterns: the important antigens responsible for these patterns are myeloperoxidase and proteinase 3, respectively. However, given the rarity of the small vessel vasculitides, detecting ANCA in an unselected population most likely represents a false-positive result. It is therefore critical to limit their use to clinical scenarios where small vessel vasculitis is a plausible diagnosis. Suggested clinical situations where ANCA would be tested are shown below. The diagnosis of small vessel vasculitis is histological, so a biopsy should always be sought to confirm a diagnosis.

Clinical situations in which ANCA has utility
Glomerulonephritis (especially rapidly progressive)
Pulmonary haemorrhage (especially pulmonary renal syndrome)
Cutaneous vasculitis with systemic features (myalgia, arthralgia, arthritis)
Multiple lung nodules
Chronic destructive disease of the airways
Longstanding sinusitis or otitis
Sub-glottic tracheal stenosis
Mononeuritis multiplex or other peripheral neuropathy
Retro-orbital mass

Immunoglobulins

Serum immunoglobulin concentrations are frequently requested and usually IgA, IgM and IgG will be measured. Where marked deficiencies are found in acutely unwell patients, they are most commonly secondary to lymphoproliferative disease or myeloma.

Serum immunoglobulin concentrations should be requested when considering a diagnosis of multiple myeloma, lymphoproliferative disease or primary immunodeficiency, which are associated with a marked depression in one or more subtype of serum immunoglobulin. Immunoelectrophoresis should also be requested in these circumstances in order to detect serum paraproteins. However, it is important to note that 10% of myeloma cases secrete light chains only that require urine immunoelectrophoresis for their detection. Some are unhelpfully non-secretory! A common finding on serum electrophoresis, is the presence of a relatively small monoclonal band without any immunoparesis. This condition is sometimes termed monoclonal gammopathy of undetermined significance (MGUS) and is discussed further in Chapter Fourteen. Recently, serum-free light chain analysis has become helpful in the diagnosis of non-secretory myeloma and for prognostication in MGUS.

T-cell subsets

Flow cytometry can be used to quantify the number of CD4/CD8 cells in peripheral blood. It should only be requested routinely to monitor the progress of patients with HIV or to investigate primary immunodeficiency. If a new diagnosis of HIV is suspected, a very few doctors may think that a CD4 count is a crafty way to avoid a tricky conversation with the patient: all but the sleepiest of laboratories will be wise to this unacceptable (and expensive) practice!

Cryoglobulins

Cryoglobulinaemia is a relatively rare disorder in everyday practice but may appear in a list of differentials more frequently when a member of the team is due to take their membership examinations. Cryoglobulins are abnormal immunoglobulins that form complexes (with each other and complement) and precipitate out of the serum at low temperatures. Cryoglobulins can manifest in a variety of ways, causing skin lesions, Raynaud's, arthralgia, nephritis and neurological conditions such as stroke and mononeuritis multiplex.

Over and above these presenting features, cryoglobulinaemia tends to be associated with other diseases. Amongst them are connective tissue disorders (such as rheumatoid disease and SLE), chronic viral infections (such as hepatitis C and infectious mononucleosis) and malignancies, notably those of the B cell lineage and multiple myeloma.

Testing for cryoglobulins is a tricky business as false negatives result if the serum is allowed to cool below body temperature between phlebotomist and immunology laboratory. In general, a flask warmed to the appropriate temperature is a better idea than walking down hospital corridors holding test tubes underarm or elsewhere!

Chapter 19

Ashley Cooper and Barbara Leppard

DERMATOLOGY

Dermatology is one of those smaller medical specialties that is sometimes seen as arcane and subjective by other colleagues. However, it is also one where a proper diagnosis can transform a patient's life and end weeks or months of misery. On hasty ward rounds, mantras such as 'if it's wet, dry it' or 'if it's dry, wet it' can often be heard but when a rash fails to respond to simple treatments, most patients and their admitting teams are thoroughly grateful when a specialist arrives. Likewise, there is often a flurry of interest in dermatology from medics around the time of postgraduate exams or whenever an unusual mole is spotted on their person. For every skill level, there is a multitude of dermatology texts, filled to the rafters with beautiful colour pictures; however, these only give a two-dimensional view.[1]

Few dermatological conditions are 'catching' but there is often marked reluctance to actually feel the skin during a clinical examination. It is extremely helpful, if not essential, to touch the rash or lesion to clinch the diagnosis in many skin diseases. Here, we attempt to present some of the important life-threatening dermatological conditions that are encountered in general medicine and also to discuss the common causes of itching.

Red for danger

Dermatology has few emergencies but when they occur they are often catastrophic. With more and more patients ending up taking multiple medications, drug eruptions are becoming increasingly common. The three discrete entities seen are erythema multiforme (EM), Stevens–Johnson syndrome (SJS)

----

[1] Ashton *et al. Differential Diagnosis in Dermatology. Radcliffe Medical Press,* 2005.

and toxic epidermal necrolysis (TEN). A study from Boston suggested that the overall incidence of hospitalization for EM, SJS or TEN (due to all causes) was 4.2 per million person-years. The incidence of the three conditions, when associated with drug use, was 7.0, 1.8 and 9.0 per million person-years, respectively, for those under 20 years of age, 20–64 years of age, and 65 years and older.[2] In an average UK district general hospital, one can expect to see between two and four serious drug eruptions per year.

The most feared of the three diseases is TEN. The first description of 'an eruption resembling scalding of the skin' was provided by Alan Lyell in 1956, and it is known in many earlier texts as Lyell's Disease.[3] However, it is probable that Lyell's original patient had staphylococcal scalded skin syndrome (SSSS) rather than TEN. SSSS is clinically similar to TEN but is due to a staphylococcal infection and mainly occurs in infants and young children.

Most cases of TEN and SJS are drug-induced, usually by a medication initiated 7–14 days previously. However, if a patient has had the drug before, development can be more rapid.[4] The highest-risk medications used on a short-term basis are trimethoprim-sulfamethoxazole (Septrin), nitrofurantoin and other sulphonamide antibiotics, chlormezanone, aminopenicillins, quinolones, and cephalosporins. Among longer-term medications, the worst offenders are carbamazepine, phenobarbitone, phenytoin, sodium valproate, oxicam nonsteroidal anti-inflammatory drugs, allopurinol and corticosteroids.

Epidemiological studies have shown that TEN and SJS occur more commonly in patients infected with HIV and those with acute graft-versus-host disease than in the general population. There is also a reportedly higher incidence of TEN among those suffering from systemic lupus erythematosus, leukemia, lymphoma, ulcerative colitis and Crohn's disease. Clearly, this may be on account of the types of drugs used in these conditions; however, there are articles in the literature suggesting that individuals presenting with these diseases do indeed have more severe eruptions with a worse prognosis than might otherwise be expected.

The clinical hallmark of TEN is the rapid development of extensive dusky erythema (erythroderma), with sheets of skin becoming detached due to epidermal necrosis, either spontaneously or on minimal pressure. With loss of

2 Chan *et al.* Arch Dermatol (1990) 126: 1103–1104.

3 Lyell, Br J Dermatol (1956) 68: 355–361.

4 Roujeau *et al.* NEJM (1995) 333:1600–1607.

the epidermal covering of the skin, there is loss of body fluid and electrolytes and the risk of secondary infection (similar to that occurring in extensive burns). There is a considerable mortality with this condition (between 30 and 75%, depending on which series one reads). The risk of death depends on what percentage of skin covering is lost, which is mainly determined by how quickly the diagnosis is made and when treatment is started.

The diagnosis can be confirmed by biopsying the erythematous skin or a piece of skin that has sheared off. Urgent frozen sections will distinguish between TEN and SSSS. In TEN, the detached skin is made up of the full thickness of the epidermis but the cells will be dying or dead. In SSSS, the detached skin is just keratin. Apoptosis of keratinocytes involves an interaction between a cell-surface 'death receptor', known as Fas, and its receptor ligand, to form a Fas-ligand pairing (FasL). High concentrations of soluble FasL have been detected in the serum of patients with TEN.[5] Keratinocyte cell death can be blocked *in vitro* by a FasL-blocking antibody and by antibodies present in pooled human immunoglobulin. Several open-label human studies have suggested that intravenous immunoglobulin (IVIG) can be very useful in TEN, halting progression of skin necrosis within 24–48 h and reducing mortality.[6] Time is of importance when it comes to management, as nothing can reverse apoptosis once it has occurred. Treatment should be started with an infusion of IVIG as soon as the diagnosis is suspected and continued for 3 days. The only fly in the ointment is a recent study showing that levels of FasL-blocking antibody differ between preparations of IVIG – some appear to have virtually none – which may explain why other studies have not reported such good results.[7] Also, it is worth remembering that IVIG can induce a hyperviscous circulation and is not without its risks. These patients should be managed in intensive care by a multi-specialist team composed of a dermatologist, anaesthetist, respiratory physician and microbiologist (and perhaps even others).

Stevens-Johnson syndrome can also be a dermatological emergency. This is erythema multiforme with extensive involvement of the mucous membranes. The skin lesions are round target-like papules and plaques made up of rings of different colours. The main pathology is in the mouth with extensive erosions making eating and drinking difficult. The eyes, urethra and vagina may also be involved. The skin lesions are sometimes extensive, and it is not always possible

---

5   Viard *et al.* Science (1998) 282: 490–493.

6   Prins *et al.* Arch Dermatol (2003) 139: 26–32.

7   Bachot *et al.* Arch Dermatol (2003) 139: 33–36.

to distinguish it from TEN. The pathology is very similar with necrosis of the lower half of the epidermis. Most patients with SJS are not too unwell; the mortality rate is far lower than that for TEN (probably around 5%). As with TEN, medications are the most important provoking factor, although the herpes viruses and mycoplasma infection may also be responsible in some cases.

'Ordinary' erythema multiforme (EM) is a far more innocuous process lasting about 10–14 days. It is characterized by discrete 'target' lesions, with or without central blisters, occasionally coalescing but mainly found in a symmetric acral distribution. Oral involvement with superficial erosions is relatively common. Most cases are thought to be due to an abnormal immunological cross-reaction to the herpes simplex virus (a history of cold sores is a useful diagnostic clue), although other viral and bacterial infections and various drugs can also precipitate EM. Although the condition has low morbidity and no mortality, viral EM is often recurrent, which can be a real nuisance for patients. Long-term, low-dose prophylaxis with aciclovir can prevent episodes, if caused by herpes simplex.

There is often a desire on the part of the generalist to instigate large doses of oral prednisolone for any alarming skin rash. Experience has shown that this is definitely detrimental in TEN, probably of no benefit in SJS and useless in EM. So, apart from IVIG in TEN and limited use of aciclovir in recurrent SJS or EM, the management of the three conditions involves stopping all suspect medications, screening for atypical organisms and supportive skin care.[8] In TEN, nursing care is paramount, as simply turning a patient in bed can cause extensive skin tearing. Airflow mattresses are employed; as are copious quantities of topical 50% white soft paraffin and 50% liquid paraffin, single-layer tubigauze bandaging and nonadherent dressings (such as Mepetal) for eroded areas. There has been some debate as to the role of potent topical steroids, perhaps mainly as vasoconstricting agents, but these are mostly not used. Cool fanning of the skin, meticulous fluid balance with CVP monitoring and hawk-like observation for the development of sepsis is essential. The skin itself rarely becomes infected; sepsis usually originates from the chest or urinary tract. Unfortunately, inflammatory markers such as ESR and CRP are often elevated due to the condition, and pyrexia can be misleading. The neutrophil count can be a helpful indicator of antibiotic requirement (assuming that steroids have not been given in error). Prophylactic antibiotics are not indicated in TEN, as the general feeling is that since there has clearly

8 Ghislain et al. Dermatol Online J (2002) 8: 5.

been an abnormal response to the drug that initiated the epidermal necrolysis, it is best not to tempt a second episode with another potential precipitant. Clearly, for less impressive eruptions, greasy emollients are still very important to make the patient comfortable. Painful oral ulceration can be relieved with Difflam or tetracycline mouthwashes. The whole process usually runs a course of 10–14 days.

Survivors of significant epidermal disorders may experience numerous long-term sequelae, including ocular conjunctival cicatrization (scar formation for those who would rather be spared a trip to the dictionary) and other potentially disabling lesions that may cause blindness. The skin may heal, leaving varying patterns of hyper- and hypo-pigmentation. Fingernails and toenails may be shed and often regrow abnormally, sometimes with 'Beau's lines' (transverse lines) across the nail plate. Erosions in the mucous membranes of the genitourinary system may stick together, leading to phimosis or vaginal synechiae.

Skin sepsis

Necrotizing fasciitis (streptococcal gangrene) is a very serious condition in which infection with *Streptococcus pyogenes* (a group A β-haemolytic streptococcus) causes an acute fulminant illness that may kill the patient before one can even think of the diagnosis.[9,10] Here, the infection is in the subcutaneous fat and the deep fascia. In this site, the streptococcus produces a toxin that causes thrombosis within the blood vessels in the skin and sometimes disseminated intravascular coagulation. The skin lesions initially look like either cellulitis or erysipelas with the cardinal features of *rubor, calor* and *tumor*. Within 24–48 h, the skin begins to turn dusky red or purple and then obviously necrotic areas appear. Anti-DNAase B levels are very high and can confirm the diagnosis if it is considered.[11] However, surgical debridement of all necrotic tissue may be life saving and should be carried out as soon as possible – one should not wait patiently for the immunology lab to open on Monday morning! Benzyl penicillin is not adequate because it will be unable to access the affected areas, owing to the thrombosed vessels. In some patients, necrotizing fasciitis is less fulminant, and slow necrosis of the skin occurs over weeks or months. These patients often spend long periods in hospital until the

9 Hawkey *et al.* BMJ (1980) 281: 1058.
10 Cruickshank *et al.* BMJ (1981) 282: 1944–1945.
11 Leppard *et al.* Br J Dermatol (1983) 109: 37–44.

black eschar has lifted off. High levels of anti-DNAase B will support the diagnosis and trigger early surgery, which is likely to be curative.

Superficial skin infections with *S. pyogenes* are less common but perhaps more serious than those due to *Staphylococcus aureus*. Cocci will not penetrate intact skin, and the infection that occurs depends on the depth of inoculation of the organism. Erysipelas is one such streptococcal infection of the upper half of the dermis. It is an acute illness with the patient complaining of fever, rigors and general malaise, more than the rash. There is a very well-defined area of red swollen skin, often with blisters in the centre. There is usually no lymphangitis or lymphadenopathy and often no obvious portal of entry for the organism. Streptococcal antibodies (ASOT, anti-DNAase B and anti-hyaluronidase – AHT) are sometimes normal. Penicillin is the treatment of choice and results in the temperature returning to normal within 24 h and rapid healing of the skin. Treatment needs to be given for 5–7 days.[12]

Cellulitis is typically an infection of the lower half of the dermis caused by gram-positive cocci – streptococci or staphylococci. There is usually an obvious skin lesion that has allowed entry of the organism, such as a leg ulcer, eczema or athlete's foot. The patient complains of a red, hot swollen area of skin rather than general malaise, although there is often a fever. The rash is less well defined than in erysipelas, and there are typically no blisters. Lymphangitis and lymphadenopathy are nearly always present. When caused by streptococci, the ASOT is usually high and the AHT can be used to distinguish between infections due to group A, C and G streptococci. Culturing the blood is of course a rather more traditional way in which to single out the culprit organism. Treatment is surprisingly controversial: in hospital, many choose intravenous benzyl penicillin in addition to flucloxacillin, although some authorities advocate high-dose intravenous flucloxacillin alone or a cephalosporin. There does not appear to have been a randomised controlled trial comparing these approaches. In those known or suspected to be colonised with methicillin-resistant *Staphylococcus aureus* (MRSA), treatment of cellulitis should be tailored accordingly, usually with the addition of intravenous vancomycin. Cellulitis it is often slow to settle, taking up to 25 days (mean 12 days) to resolve fully.[8] It is vitally important to also treat the disease that has allowed entry to the bugs, or else recurrent infections may occur, predisposing to chronic lymphoedema.

Viruses can also cause serious skin problems, most notably herpes simplex virus type I (HSV-1), which can produce the 'Kaposi Varicelliform eruption',

---

12 Leppard *et al.* Br J Dermatol (1985) 112: 559–567.

often referred to as eczema herpeticum. This predominantly impacts on atopic individuals, or the immunocompromised, and can affect any age group. Before the development of aciclovir, mortality was over 50%, but this has now decreased to less than 10% if intravenous antiviral treatment is started promptly. Patients are usually very unwell with fever and malaise, often with a preceding history of cold sores on a background of poorly controlled eczema. Clinically, the most common diagnostic sign is the presence of umbilicated vesicles or sometimes multiple circular 'punched-out' erosions around the periphery of an extremely angry patch of eczema. Depending on local laboratory preferences, viral swabs, Tzanck smears or PCR of vesicle exudate are vital to diagnose the condition.

Angioedema and urticaria

Another cause for great concern in the emergency department is the patient with swollen lips and/or tongue (angioedema), which is a localised form of urticaria (discussed below). In the majority of cases, this seems to be precipitated by foods or medications (typically ACE inhibitors – when the angioedema is unaccompanied by hives, and is caused by the inhibition of enzymatic degradation of tissue bradykinin).[13] The patient may be clear as to the trigger, since the reaction develops very quickly after exposure to the offending agent.

If the respiratory tract is involved, the first priority must be to secure the airway and establish an intravenous line. Intramuscular adrenaline will reduce the oedema and should be given. Diphenhydramine is helpful, and hydrocortisone may reduce the possibility of relapse. Patients with severe angioedema should be admitted for at least 24 h of observation, particularly where laryngeal oedema has occurred. Patients with angioedema should be advised to wear a Medic Alert emblem.

Hereditary angioedema (HAE) is a rare genetic condition inherited as an autosomal dominant trait. The incidence of HAE is estimated at 1:10,000 to 1:150,000, with most authors quoting a range of 1:10,000 to 1:50,000. The gene encoding C1-INH maps to chromosome 11q12-q13.1. There are two classically described forms. Type I, which accounts for the vast majority, is characterized by low plasma levels of C1-esterase inhibitor. Type II exhibits normal or elevated levels of C1-esterase inhibitor but the protein is a dysfunctional mutant. In both forms, reduced functional levels of C1-esterase

---

13 Kaplan *et al.* J Am Acad Dermatol (2005) 53: 373–388.

inhibitor cause auto-activation of the first component of the complement cascade (C1) with consumption of C4 and C2 – which may be low when measured. A third type of hereditary angioedema has been defined by several groups. Occurring exclusively in women, it is unhelpfully not associated with detectable abnormalities of the complement system![14] Angioedema caused by a C1-esterase inhibitor deficiency can also be acquired in several clinical settings, including lymphoma and autoimmune connective tissue disease. It can also occur because of specific anti-C1 esterase autoantibodies in some patients.

The end result is spontaneous non-itchy swelling of soft tissues, most often orofacial but sometimes genital and even gastrointestinal. These attacks often occur entirely randomly, but some patients relate them to stress or trauma. Danazol or stanozolol may be used prophylactically to prevent attacks if they are occurring frequently (more than once a month), although these are not without side effects. There are various protocols and recommendations, but usually danazol 200 mg/day is started and adjusted according to response. Another option is tranexamic acid in females. Antihistamines and cortico-steroids are not helpful.

Acute attacks of HAE are best treated with commercially available C1-esterase inhibitor replacement peptide (C1INHRP), or if not severe and in the prodromal phase, some patients already on danazol can simply increase the dose and might be able to abort an attack. Most patients should be offered home-use C1INHRP. The role of fresh-frozen plasma is controversial and, theoretically, might worsen attacks, but it is often used without good evidence if nothing else is available.[15]

Urticaria (hives) is one of those dermatological conditions that looks impressive and may frighten the patient, but the rash has usually long gone by the time they arrive in the hospital. In acute urticaria, the cardinal feature in the history is that the individual lesions come and go within a few hours and always in less than 24 h. If the lesions appear to be lasting longer than this, then the diagnosis might be urticarial vasculitis and a biopsy needs to be under-taken to confirm it. In classical urticaria, a biopsy is not normally necessary as the history and clinical picture are so distinctive. The pathophysiology revolves around 'unstable' mast cells, which dump histamine and other inflammatory cytokines at the slightest provocation.[16] Histamine causes extravasation

[14] Bork *et al.* Lancet (2000) 356: 213–217.

[15] Bowen *et al.* J Allergy Clin Immunol (2003) 114: 629–637.

[16] Kaplan, J Allergy Clin Immunol (2004) 114: 465–474.

of fluid, vasodilatation and a considerable amount of itching. In most patients with urticaria, no obvious cause can be found. However, it can be due to a Type 1 allergic reaction to foodstuffs (e.g. nuts, shellfish, strawberries), drugs (e.g. penicillin) or bee stings. It may be due to direct degranulation of mast cells without any allergic reaction being involved; aspirin, n-acetylcysteine and the opioids are common causes here. Characteristically, patients get episodes of urticaria whenever they take aspirin for a cold or pain.

Antihistamines and not systemic steroids are the treatment of choice. The newer-generation antihistamines, such as cetirizine and levocetirizine, are highly specific for histamine H1 receptors and seem safe for long-term use. Standard hay-fever-type doses are often inadequate, and patients with chronic idiopathic urticaria may end up on combinations of different antihistamines, at 2 or 3 times the normal dosage. Contrary to what one might expect, there may also be a role for the addition of an H2 blocker in the small number of patients who fail to completely respond to adequate doses of H1 blockers. H2 blockers have also been reported to have some benefit in patients with pressure urticaria or dermographism.[17] It is said that about two-thirds of those affected by acute urticaria will be free of symptoms by 2 weeks, and the remainder by 3 months. However, in dermatology clinics, one is often faced with those few that enter the chronic pattern and end up having treatment for many years.

Blisters

There are two main categories of blistering, autoimmune and toxic. Probably the most frequent condition causing generalised blistering, encountered in the hospital setting, is bullous pemphigoid. This has a predilection for older people and presents with a very itchy, nonspecific rash (a bit like eczema and a bit like urticaria, but not quite right for either) before the characteristic tense, fluid-filled (and sometimes haemorrhagic) blisters materialise and give the game away. The pathophysiology involves the development of auto-antibodies to two proteins (BP180 and BP230), which are part of the hemidesmosome that anchors the basal layer of keratinocytes to the basement membrane.[18] Hence, the roof of the blister is made up of the full thickness of the epidermis, so blisters can reach a good size — up to several centimetres in diameter. The diagnosis can be confirmed by immunofluorescence of serum, blister fluid or urine (in some centres) or via a skin biopsy of perilesional skin

---

[17] Cook *et al.* Acta Derm Venereol (1983) 63: 260–262.

[18] Fairley *et al.* J Invest Dermatol (2005) 125: 467–472.

that will show IgG along the basement membrane. Treatment is with prednisolone (initially 30–40 mg/day) but this is often needed for several years,
so appropriate bone protection is indicated. Because of this, many dermatologists will substitute a second-line agent such as azathioprine at the earliest
opportunity. The development of the thiopurine methyl-transferase assay that
can detect those individuals with genetically low levels of the azathioprine-
metabolizing enzyme potentially makes treatment safer.[19] However, idiosyncratic
reactions still occur and regular blood monitoring, principally to detect
drug-induced agranulocytosis, is necessary. In many patients, the disease
seems to burn itself out over 5 years or so but some elderly patients require
treatment for life.

Pemphigus vulgaris is the other autoimmune blistering condition of which
most doctors have heard. It is very rare indeed. Here, the circulating autoantibody is directed against an anchoring protein present higher up in the
epidermis (desmoglein 3, plus or minus desmoglein 1). Blisters occur within
the epidermis, so the blister roof is very fragile. Blisters, when present, are
therefore small. Clinically, the patient rarely has visible blisters, but instead has
larger erosions and weepy areas. It is much nastier and harder to treat than
bullous pemphigoid. Therapy relies upon very large doses of corticosteroids
(60–120 mg/day) plus a steroid-sparing agent such as azathioprine,
mycophenylate mofetil, ciclosporin or other modalities such as intravenous
immunoglobulin and extracorporeal plasma- and photophoresis. A light at the
end of the tunnel for sufferers comes in the form of the monoclonal antibody,
rituximab, which selectively targets and destroys B-cells, the site of most
antibody production.[20] It definitely helps but it is extremely expensive and
does not affect plasma cells, which can also be responsible for producing the
pathogenic autoantibody.

Itching

Itching (pruritis) is defined as an unpleasant cutaneous sensation leading to
the desire to scratch. It serves as a physiological self-protective mechanism
to help defend the skin against harmful external agents, including
parasites. When a patient presents with itching, the first thing to sort out is
whether they also have a rash. If no rash is present, the cause may be iron
deficiency anaemia, uraemia, cholestatic jaundice, hypo- or hyperthyroidism,

[19] Snow, Arch Dermatol (1995) 131: 193–197.

[20] Salopek, J Am Acad Dermatol (2002) 47: 785–788.

lymphoma or carcinoma, and these should all be considered. In the elderly, itching may be due to frequent bathing (especially when they are admitted to the hospital), causing drying out of the skin.

If a rash is present, then hopefully the diagnosis can be made and treatment instituted. Many common skin diseases induce itching, especially eczema, urticaria, scabies and lichen planus. Itching is an important symptom because it needs to be alleviated. If patients have uncontrollable itching at night, think of scabies or dermatitis herpetiformis. The latter is much rarer but should be thought of in a young adult with an itchy rash.[21] Characteristically, it is made up of grouped blisters on the elbows, knees, sacrum and scalp. It may be that no blisters are seen because the patient has scratched them all away. To confirm the diagnosis, antigliadin and antiendomysial antibodies should be sought in the serum and a skin biopsy of perilesional skin taken for immunofluorescence. This will show IgA in the upper dermis. Dapsone will stop the itching within a few hours, but these patients should be treated with a gluten-free diet as well, since they also have a gluten enteropathy.

Scabies is much more common than dermatitis herpetiformis. It causes an itchy rash over the whole body except the face and scalp, and there will usually be other family members or close contacts who are itching too. It is an infestation with a newly fertilised female *Sarcoptes scabiei* mite, which is passed from one person to another, usually while they are asleep. Prolonged contact is needed, as the mites propagate very slowly. The itching starts 4–6 weeks after infestation, and the accompanying rash is often rather nonspecific. One can be sure of the diagnosis by finding burrows along the sides of the fingers or on the ventral aspect of the wrist. These are S-shaped tracks where the fertilised female has burrowed into the stratum corneum to lay her eggs. Treatment is with 5% permethrin cream, applied to the whole body except the face and scalp (including all the nooks and crannies) and left in place for 24 h. All close contacts must be treated at the same time, whether or not they are itching or have a rash (as the rash also takes 4–6 weeks to appear). 24 h after treatment, clothes and bedsheets should be changed, washed and ironed but there is no need to go to any elaborate lengths to fumigate the house. A single treatment will usually cure but many dermatologists recommend two treatments, each a week apart.

Crusted scabies (Norwegian scabies) is an infestation with the same creature that causes ordinary scabies but in which there is a different host response.

---

21 Karpati, Dermatol Sci (2004) 34: 83–90.

In patients who are immunosuppressed or who have had a stroke or some other kind of sensory loss, the scabies mites multiply uncontrollably, and there are thousands or millions of mites in the skin (rather than the 10 or so which is the average in ordinary scabies). This situation is highly contagious, not just to close contacts but to virtually anybody who walks by. The patient has thick hyperkeratotic scale on the palms, soles, flexures and under the nails. Eventually, a widespread scaly rash appears, which is often mistaken for eczema. Scratching results in huge numbers of mites being shed into the environment — onto the furniture, soft furnishings, bedding, floor, walls and, of course, onto someone else's skin if they are in the vicinity: are you itching yet?

Crusted scabies causes large outbreaks in nursing and residential homes and in hospitals, among staff, patients and relatives alike. The diagnosis usually comes to light when most of the staff start to itch. The treatment of such outbreaks is much more complex than simply applying 5% permethrin cream to the patient and any close relatives. The nursing home or ward needs to be closed, the patient with crusted scabies treated and put into a clean room. All other inmates of a home, ward (or indeed prison), together with all members of staff and their close relatives, must be treated. All bedding and soft furnishings must be laundered; the walls and floors need to be cleaned with an acaricide. It is important to explain to everyone (other than the patient with crusted scabies) that they have the ordinary kind of scabies that is only infectious to close contacts. Oral ivermectin is an alternative to topical permethrin and is much easier to administer.[22] It is, however, much slower to work than topical permethrin, taking 4–8 weeks for the itching to stop.[23] Another disadvantage is that it is only available on a named-patient basis.

If one suspects crusted scabies, scrape off some of the scale and examine under a microscope – it will be stacked full of eggs, larvae, nymphs and adult mites!

[22] Meinking, NEJM (1995) 333: 26–30.

[23] Leppard, Br J Derm (2000) 143: 520–523.

Chapter 20

Deborah Harrington and Christopher Redman

OBSTETRIC MEDICINE

Obstetric medicine is a unique and fascinating branch of medicine. There are two patients, mother and baby, the population is young and resilient, there are conditions that occur only in pregnancy and the immediate time course of events is short, at most 9 months. However, medical care for pregnancy may need to begin before conception (for example, with type 1 diabetes) and new diagnoses made in pregnancy may indicate a lifelong health issue (for example, chronic hypertension).

The pregnant woman is different. Oxygen consumption and ventilation are increased (such that breathlessness is common); plasma volume is expanded; cardiac output is increased by about 40%; the blood pressure falls early in pregnancy and rises to non-pregnant levels towards delivery and the clotting system is more prothrombotic. An increase in glomerular filtration rate of 50% is accompanied by a significant fall in plasma osmolality. Metabolic changes are profound and include an increase in insulin resistance and hyperlipidaemia creating an apparently pro-atherogenic profile.

Normal laboratory indices are also different, rendering some tests, such as ESR, unhelpful during pregnancy. Plasma creatinine falls: even values close to 90 mmol/l are likely to be abnormal except possibly very near term. Episodic glycosuria is common and a poor indicator of hyperglycaemia. Physiological adjustments of pregnancy begin early in the first trimester – for example, the increase in cardiac output, the fall in blood pressure and enhanced renal function.

The demands of pregnancy can reveal latent pathology. Pre-existing borderline insulin resistance may be revealed as type 2 diabetes or become manifest as gestational diabetes. The large increase in cardiac output may reveal intrinsic cardiac problems that were previously clinically unapparent, such as severe mitral stenosis.

Laboratory indices in pregnancy	Change in pregnancy
Full blood count	
Haemoglobin concentration	↓
Haematocrit	↓
Red cell count	↓
Leucocytes	↑
Platelets	↔
ESR	↑
Coagulation factors	
Factors VIII, IX and X	↑
Fibrinogen	↑
Protein S	↓
D-dimer	↑
Biochemistry	
Creatinine	↓
Urea	↓
Total protein	↓
Bilirubin	↔
Albumin	↓
Alkaline phosphatase	↑

Some medical illnesses are specific to pregnancy (for example, pre-eclampsia), or more severe because of pregnancy (for example, thromboembolism). The health of the foetus and how it might be affected by maternal drug use, or special investigations such as imaging are a source of much anxiety. Diagnoses that are considered first by physicians who predominantly look after older individuals (including men) may not be appropriate in pregnant women because of their rarity, for example, coronary thrombosis. Lastly, the time course of pregnancy is short but the implications of severe illness have a particular resonance for the long-term health of the family concerned (for example, if a mother dies or is permanently disabled).

The impact of pregnancy on pre-existing medical conditions varies according to the disorder and from individual to individual. Some improve dramatically (such as rheumatoid arthritis), some remain unchanged (such as hypothyroidism) and some inevitably worsen (as occurs with type 1 diabetes). For many, the changes are unpredictable: SLE and migraine amongst others.

Pregnancy-specific medical conditions
Hyperemesis gravidarum
Gestational diabetes
Pre-eclampsia
Cholestasis of pregnancy
Skin disorders of pregnancy (e.g. pemphigoid gestationalis)
Peripartum cardiomyopathy
Puerperal psychosis
Postpartum depression
Postpartum thyroiditis

This chapter focuses on some important and common problems in pregnancy, including hypertension, thromboembolism, epilepsy and diabetes together with diagnostic imaging and prescribing. There are numerous important conditions that present in pregnancy which keep maternal medicine specialists thinking, and busy. Their number is too great to cover here and the interested reader is directed to a more comprehensive review.[1]

MEDICATING THE MOTHER OR FOETUS?

Almost all drugs cross the placenta and have the potential to affect the foetus. They may be teratogenic during organogenesis in the first trimester (for example, thalidomide), foetotoxic by the direct pharmacological actions of the drug in the second or third trimesters (for example, COX-2 inhibitors) or both (for example, warfarin). Furthermore, *in utero* exposure may cause delayed problems such as those following on from the early pregnancy use of diethylstilboestrol. Hence, drug use in pregnancy is a difficult issue. Over-caution may deny vital or life-saving medication to the mother. In contrast, injudicious therapy may cause undesirable or unnecessary foetal problems. Epidemiological studies of drug exposure in pregnancy may be superficially reassuring, but they are frequently too small to exclude modest foetal risks. There are fewer than 20 drugs or groups of drugs that are definitely known

---

[1] De Swiet (Ed), *Medical Disorders in Obstetric Practice*. Blackwell Publishing, Oxford, 2002.

to predispose to birth defects. However, more than 90% of pregnancies exposed to known teratogens during the first trimester will be normal.

Drugs should be prescribed only if they are essential in pregnancy, at the lowest dose and after adequate counselling. Pre-natal screening is essential so that termination can be offered for obvious and debilitating foetal abnormalities. Drugs that are known teratogens, are foetotoxic, that may cause delayed problems in adulthood or that are contraindicated during breast feeding are shown in the table below.

Those women on long-term medication should ideally be offered pre-pregnancy counselling in order to optimize their drug regimens. All women should be advised to take pre-conceptual folic acid supplements to reduce the risk of neural tube defects.

Prescribing in pregnancy

Drugs that should not be used at any stage of pregnancy
Antifungal drugs
fluconazole, griseofulvin, ketoconazole
Cytotoxic drugs
methotrexate, busulfan, cyclophosphamide, chlorambucil
Retinoids
acitretin, isotretinoin, etretinate
Sex hormones
danazol, diethylstilboestrol
Others
thalidomide, lithium, penicillamine, misoprostol
Drugs that are relatively contraindicated
Oral anticoagulants
warfarin
Anticonvulsants
sodium valproate, phenytoin, carbamazepine, phenobarbitone, lamotrigine
Cardiovascular drugs
high-dose beta blockers
ACE inhibitors
Drugs that may or do adversely affect the foetus without teratogenesis
Antibiotics
aminoglycosides, quinolones, chloramphenicol
Anti-inflammatory drugs
NSAIDs, COX-1 inhibitors

Antipsychotic drugs
  phenothiazines

Hypoglycaemic and hypolipidaemic agents
  sulphonylureas, statins, fibrates

Opioid analgesia
  morphine, methadone, pethidine

Drugs that cause long-term effects on the child after exposure in utero

Diethylstilboestrol

Tetracyclines

Valproate

Drugs that are contraindicated during breast feeding

Amiodarone and iodides

Antibiotics
  chloramphenicol, tetracycline, ciprofloxacin

Cytotoxic drugs
  methotrexate, cyclophosphamide, doxorubicin

Dapsone

Antidepressants
  doxepin, fluoxetine, citalopram

Ergotamine

Gold salts

Immunosuppressive drugs
  azathioprine, hydroxychloroquine, high-dose prednisolone

Lithium

Sex hormones
  oestrogens, androgens

Phenindione

Retinoids
  acitretin, isotretinoin, etretinate

UNDER PRESSURE

Hypertension in pregnancy may be longstanding, pregnancy-induced (including pre-eclampsia) or, extremely rarely, a new coincidental presentation. Chronic, longstanding hypertension is evident by raised blood pressure levels in early pregnancy, and predisposes to placental abruption or pre-eclampsia. Antihypertensive drugs may be continued if necessary. None is definitely teratogenic but ACE inhibitors are contraindicated (fetotoxic after the first trimester). Diuretics are avoided because they deplete plasma volume and may adversely affect placental perfusion. β-blockers (especially in high doses) slow foetal growth.

Pregnancy-induced hypertension (PIH, > 140/90 mmHg) occurs only in the second half of pregnancy and regresses after delivery. It may be a harbinger of pre-eclampsia or an expression of latent chronic hypertension. The earlier it presents, the more likely it is to evolve into pre-eclampsia, which comprises both PIH and pregnancy-induced proteinuria (> 0.3 g/24 h).

Pre-eclampsia affects about 3% of pregnancies. The foetus may be involved directly, owing to placental insufficiency, or indirectly through iatrogenic preterm delivery. The onset and course of pre-eclampsia are unpredictable and much of modern antenatal care, which in the UK occurs in the community, is geared to its detection. But pre-eclampsia can also present for the first time during labour or after delivery, which is usually in hospital. Recent NICE guidelines recommend a reduced number of scheduled antenatal visits for healthy women at low risk, which presupposes accurate risk prediction.[2] The most substantial risk factors are a previous history (RR 7) or the presence of antiphospholipid antibodies (RR 10), the latter being rare. Pre-existing diabetes, morbid obesity, nulliparity, multiple pregnancy, a family history of pre-eclampsia and advanced maternal age also significantly increase the risk.[3]

The definition of pre-eclampsia hides its protean and variable nature, as it can affect the maternal liver, clotting system, lungs or brain. There may be neither hypertension nor proteinuria in 10% of eclamptic women (unheralded eclampsia) although these signs appear afterwards.[4]

Complications of pre-eclampsia

Eclampsia
HELLP syndrome
Placental abruption
Pulmonary oedema
Acute renal failure
Acute liver failure
Cerebrovascular haemorrhage
Maternal death
Intrauterine growth restriction
Preterm delivery

[2] CG006 (2003) (www.nice.org.uk)

[3] Duckitt et al. BMJ (2000) 330: 565–571.

[4] Douglas et al. BMJ (1994) 309: 1395–1400.

The HELLP (haemolysis, elevated liver enzymes and low platelets) syndrome can present in the community or in hospital emergency departments as sudden and extremely severe abdominal pain, which mimics a surgical abdominal catastrophe. The pain arises from the liver. The typical features of pre-eclampsia may not be evident at first but become so within hours. HELLP syndrome is a possible diagnosis in all pregnant women presenting in the second half of pregnancy with an acute abdomen.

Timely delivery is the cornerstone of management. Severe pre-eclamptic hypertension should be treated to reduce the risk of cerebral haemorrhage, which accounts for half of the attributable maternal deaths.[5] The choice of antihypertensive agent for acute control includes hydralazine, labetalol and oral nifedipine.

In a large meta-analysis, prophylaxis with low-dose aspirin was shown to bring about a 19% reduction in pre-eclampsia in women thought to be at risk of developing it.[6] High hopes that anti-oxidant vitamins (C and E) may confer similar benefits have not been realized.

Long-term epilepsy is the commonest cause of seizures in pregnancy. Eclampsia is rarer and occurs in one in 2000 pregnancies in the UK. It is associated with a 2% maternal mortality and may occur antepartum, intrapartum or postpartum. Magnesium sulphate is the drug of choice to prevent further fits.[7] Its prophylactic use is only effective if the immediate risk of eclampsia is high, which is currently impossible to judge with accuracy, and magnesium sulphate should probably be reserved for women with the HELLP syndrome or related crises, or those who have already had one eclamptic seizure.[8]

Women who develop pre-eclampsia are at increased risk of cardiovascular disease in later life.[9] In addition, foetal growth restriction (which is commonly due to pre-eclampsia) has been shown to be a risk factor for premature arterial disease or type 2 diabetes in the later life of the child (the so-called 'foetal origin of adult disease' hypothesis).[10]

5 Confidential Enquiry into Maternal and Child Health. *Why mothers die 2000–2002*. RCOG Press (2004).

6 Knight *et al.* Cochrane Database Syst Rev (2000) 2: CD000492.

7 CLASP, Lancet (1995) 345: 1455–1463.

8 Duley *et al.* Lancet (2002) 359: 1877–1890.

9 Sattar *et al.* BMJ (2002) 325: 157–160.

10 Barker *et al.* Lancet (1993) 341: 938–941.

THE SILENT KILLER

Pulmonary thromboembolism is the commonest direct cause of maternal death in the UK. [5] The risk per day is greatest in the puerperium and most events occur following discharge from hospital after delivery. However first trimester events contribute substantially to the overall problem.

There is a 10-fold increase in the risk of VTE in pregnancy. The risk is enhanced by venous stasis in the lower limbs, in part owing to the bulk of the uterus. After caesarean section, it is about 1–2% and higher still after emergency surgery during labour.

Risk factors for VTE in pregnancy

Previous VTE

Thrombophilia

Antiphospholipid syndrome

Obesity (BMI > 30 kg/m^2)

High parity

Maternal age $\geq$ 35 years

Ovarian hyperstimulation syndrome

Pre-eclampsia

Sickle cell disease

Inflammatory disorders

Nephrotic syndrome

Excessive blood loss

Immobility

Long haul travel

Confirming venous thromboembolism

Anticoagulants should not be given to pregnant women for VTE without a clear diagnosis except as a brief interim measure – otherwise a woman is marked for life: she may be denied oral contraception, exposed to added measures during pregnancy not to mention the general concerns of air travel and post-operative risks.

The clinical diagnosis of acute VTE is unreliable. The vast majority of DVTs are left-sided. Ileo-femoral thromboses are more likely to embolise and are associated with greater post-phlebitic complications. It is possible for a woman with a DVT to present with abdominal pain caused by extension of the clot into the pelvic veins. When accompanied by a mild pyrexia and leucocytosis, it is easy to misdiagnose as urinary tract infection or appendicitis. Although diagnostic confirmation is important, initial treatment should not be unduly delayed where there is a high level of clinical suspicion. Circulating D-dimer is normally elevated in late pregnancy. Pending establishment of a pregnancy-specific normal range, it cannot be used with confidence to aid diagnosis. However, a normal result by non-pregnancy criteria (although found infrequently) does reduce the odds of a positive diagnosis.

Doppler ultrasound is the initial diagnostic investigation for suspected DVT. If ultrasound is negative and there is a low level of clinical suspicion, anticoagulant treatment can be withheld. If ultrasound is negative but a high level of clinical suspicion persists, the patient should undergo venography of the femoral and more distal veins. With adequate shielding of the uterus, the direct radiation to the foetus is negligible (see table overleaf).

The diagnosis of a major pulmonary embolus is usually obvious. However, a major pulmonary embolus is often preceded by smaller emboli. It is too easy to attribute these to another cause but efforts should be made to exclude clot. The chest X-ray may be normal but is an essential part of the investigation to rule out other chest pathology. The radiation to the foetus from one chest X-ray is equivalent to that received in a single long-haul flight. As in the general medical population, the electrocardiogram may be normal and the 'S1, Q3, T3' pattern can be caused by pregnancy alone. Blood gas measurement helps because normoxaemia excludes a substantial acute problem by criteria that are unchanged for pregnancy.

The diagnosis of pulmonary embolism must be confirmed. The usual way to do this would be with a lung scan, although there is an argument for the use of bilateral Doppler ultrasound leg studies (which if positive, provide an indication for treatment). The lung scan of choice is a perfusion (Q) scan where the chest X-ray is normal, with the addition of a ventilation (V) scan where it is not. The isotopes used in these scans have very short half lives and the radiation to the foetus is minimal (less than 400 µGy) and well below the maximum recommended exposure in pregnancy (50,000 µGy). [11] Computed tomographic pulmonary angiography (CTPA) may be used in pregnancy, and in some hospitals is becoming the standard diagnostic investigation for pulmonary thromboembolism. There is significant radiation to the maternal breast but the radiation dose to the foetus is up to 1000 µGy, well within safety limits. Magnetic resonance imaging (MRI) is safe in pregnancy but there is limited experience of its use in this context.

----

[11] Toglia *et al.* NEJM (1996) 335: 108–114.

The use of radiation for diagnostic imaging understandably raises anxiety for both the pregnant woman and her doctors. Although safer alternative imaging techniques such as ultrasound and MRI have dramatically reduced the use of diagnostic radiography, there are situations in which the conventional tests are necessary and unavoidable. In these cases, the benefits have to be weighed against the risks. Women can be reassured that there is no evidence of increased incidence of congenital malformation, genetic disease or intrauterine death at the dose levels associated with diagnostic radiography. Certainly, the lives of pregnant women and their babies must not be put at risk by denying them appropriate investigations on the misguided basis that pregnancy is a contraindication to such tests.

Estimated radiation to the foetus from imaging studies

Procedure	Foetal radiation; dose (μGy)
Chest X-ray	< 10
Abdominal plain film	2000–3000
Limited venography	< 500
CT chest	300
CT abdomen	25,000
Perfusion lung scan (technetium-99m)	60–120
Ventilation lung scan	10–190
CT pulmonary angiogram	60–1000
Pulmonary angiography (brachial route)	< 500
Pulmonary angiography (femoral route)	2200–3700

Maximum recommended exposure in pregnancy = 50,000 μGy

Treatment of thromboembolism

If there is a high level of clinical suspicion, treatment should be started before diagnostic confirmation. The majority of cases of venous thromboembolism are treated initially with low molecular weight heparin (LMWH). Both unfractionated and low molecular weight heparin are strongly polar and do not cross the placenta.

Doses are based on weight but higher doses, similar to those used for unstable angina, are required in pregnancy. Thus, LMWH is given twice daily in this context. This dose adjustment occurs on account of the increased glomerular filtration rate in pregnancy. In life-threatening pulmonary embolus, the use of both thrombolysis and embolectomy has been reported.

Following the acute phase, women with antenatal VTE can be managed with subcutaneous LMWH as pregnancy continues, as it is easier to use, more predictable in its actions and associated with a lower risk of heparin-induced thrombocytopenia and osteoporosis than unfractionated heparin.[12,13] Treatment should be continued for at least 6 months (or 3 months for below knee episodes) and if the VTE occurred early in pregnancy, prophylactic doses should be continued for the remainder of pregnancy and well into the puerperium but stopped briefly to facilitate delivery.

Prophylaxis and pregnancy

Women with a history of multiple thromboses may be on long-term warfarin, which is teratogenic, particularly between 6 and 12 week's gestation, and foetotoxic in the second two trimesters. It is safe to use after delivery and is compatible with breastfeeding. It is recommended that such women should receive LMWH as soon as pregnancy is established and resume warfarin after delivery. However this presents special difficulties in women with metal cardiac valve prostheses, where warfarin is the safest for the mother but not for the foetus. Doses below 5 mg/day are safer for the foetus than higher doses. At the moment there is no agreement as to what is the best therapeutic strategy. It is a specialized area of obstetric medicine and should be managed as such.

Complications of warfarin in pregnancy
Teratogenesis (first trimester)
Miscarriage
Stillbirth
Foetal haemorrhage
Maternal haemorrhage

Should a woman without antiphospholipid syndrome who has had only one previous VTE be treated with heparin prophylaxis? This is controversial and there are few objective data for guidance. Where the previous episode was associated with a temporary risk factor, antepartum prophylaxis with heparin is not justified.[14] However, thromboprophylaxis with LMWH should be given

---

[12] Sanson *et al.* Thromb Haemostat (1999) 81: 668–672.

[13] Leperq *et al.* BJOG (2001) 108: 1134–1140.

[14] Brill-Edwards *et al.* NEJM (2000) 343: 439–444.

for 6 weeks post delivery and consideration should also be given to (empirical) antenatal low-dose aspirin. An increasing number of women are presenting in pregnancy with known thrombophilia, but no personal history of VTE, identified by family screening. They should be stratified according to the level of risk associated with their thrombophilia. Antenatal thromboprophylaxis is usually not necessary.

It is important that where epidural analgesia (or spinal anaesthesia) is proposed for pain relief in labour, consideration is given to managing the use of anticoagulants, to avoid the potentially devastating consequences of an epidural haematoma.

DIABETES

Pre-pregnancy counselling for women with diabetes is often neglected. If there is good blood glucose control and a lower HbA1c level at conception, the risks of congenital abnormalities in the foetus and pre-eclampsia are reduced, and pregnancy outcome is improved. Pre-pregnancy counselling also enables the assessment of complications such as hypertension, retinopathy and nephropathy in order to give an accurate estimation of the risk of developing pregnancy complications such as pre-eclampsia. Women with type 2 diabetes should be converted to insulin either before or in early pregnancy. Oral hypoglycaemic drugs are usually avoided as they cross the placenta and theoretically may cause foetal hypoglycaemia. Metformin may be safe but further evidence is required.

Principles of diabetes management in pregnancy

Pre-pregnancy

- optimize diabetic control
- assess and manage diabetic complications (hypertension, renal impairment, retinopathy)
- give folic acid pre-natally and in the first trimester

During pregnancy

- multidisciplinary clinics
- frequent home blood glucose monitoring
- aim for near-normal maternal glycaemia
- strict adherence to low sugar, high-fibre diet
- periodic detailed ophthalmic examination
- relatives and partners instructed how to give glucagon
- convert women with type 2 diabetes to insulin

Diabetic nephropathy may deteriorate in pregnancy with worsening renal function and increasing proteinuria. These changes may be irreversible if there is severe renal impairment pre-pregnancy. Retinopathy may develop or progress during pregnancy, and the risk is higher with type 1 than type 2 diabetes.

The main objective of management is to achieve maternal normoglycaemia with target capillary glucose concentrations of < 5.0–5.5 mmol/l fasting, < 7.0–7.5 mmol/l postprandial, and an HbA1c below 6. Women with poorly controlled diabetes have an increased risk of congenital abnormalities or miscarriage (with the level of risk directly related to the degree of glycaemic control around the time of conception); stillbirths, foetal macrosomia or neonatal hypoglycaemia are also important complications. The risk is minimized if HbA1c levels are normalized. Tighter control means more hypoglycaemic attacks and there is often a loss of awareness of hypoglycaemia in pregnancy. Most maternal deaths caused by diabetes are due to hypoglycaemia.

Pregnant women with diabetes should be managed in joint obstetric diabetic clinics by obstetricians and physicians supported by specialist midwives and dieticians with expertise in the care of such women.

EPILEPSY

As for diabetes, the management of women with epilepsy should begin pre-conceptually. Anticonvulsant treatment should be optimized with the lowest dose of the most effective treatment. Polytherapy should be avoided if possible.

All anti-epileptic drugs (AEDs) cross the placenta and are potentially teratogenic. The major congenital malformations are neural tube defects (particularly associated with carbamazepine and sodium valproate), congenital heart defects (particularly with phenobarbitone, sodium valproate and phenytoin), and orofacial clefts (particularly with carbamezipine, phenytoin and phenobarbitone). Prospective registers such as the UK Epilepsy and Pregnancy Register show that sodium valproate has the highest risk of congenital malformation that increases from the background of 2–3% to about 5–9% with monotherapy and 10–15% or more for polytherapy. Lamotrigine and sodium valproate in particular, show a dose-dependent effect. Although animal studies are reassuring, there are few human data on the use of newer anticonvulsants drugs (gabapentin, levetiracetam, tiagabine) in pregnancy.

All epileptic women on treatment should take folic acid 5 mg daily before conception as AEDs interfere with folate metabolism. This should be continued throughout pregnancy as there is also a risk of folate-deficiency anaemia. Women taking valproate may wish to be changed (under careful supervision) to a different AED pre-conception. If valproate is continued, the use of divided doses or slow-release preparations lowers peak levels and reduces the risk of malformations. Vitamin K (10 mg orally) should be prescribed in the last month of pregnancy for women on hepatic enzyme-inducing drugs as a means of protecting the infant against haemorrhagic disease of the newborn.

Seizure frequency increases in about 25% of pregnancies. This is most likely in those with poorly controlled epilepsy and is often attributable to reduced plasma concentrations of anticonvulsant drugs owing to an increased plasma volume and enhanced renal and hepatic drug clearance. If seizures occur during pregnancy, drug levels should be monitored regularly so that doses can be adjusted to optimize concentrations of the free drug. Such monitoring is not required in pregnant women who remain seizure free.

The main risk of seizures to the foetus is hypoxia. The foetus is relatively resistant to short episodes of hypoxia but status epilepticus is dangerous for both the mother and the foetus and must be treated vigorously.

MEDICAL CONTRAINDICATIONS TO PREGNANCY – RELATIVE AND ABSOLUTE

There are only a small number of absolute medical contraindications to pregnancy. Women with pulmonary hypertension are at risk during pregnancy, whether it is 'primary' or due to Eisenmengers's syndrome, lung disease (such as cystic fibrosis) or connective tissue disease (such as scleroderma). The maternal mortality rate is 30–50% and such women should be actively advised against pregnancy and if they do become pregnant, offered a termination. Other contraindications to pregnancy include previous cardiomyopathy of pregnancy with residual ventricular dysfunction, severe left heart obstruction from critical mitral or aortic stenosis, severe impairment of left ventricular function, and a dilated aortic root of over 4.5 cm. A dilated aortic root, as may be seen in Marfan's syndrome, can potentially be tackled surgically in advance of conception. Non-cardiac contraindications include severe renal impairment, respiratory disease complicated by cor pulmonale, severe impairment of hepatic function, severe diabetic retinopathy and advanced AIDS.

Even in the twenty-first century, women in the UK continue to die unnecessarily during and shortly after pregnancy. For those with chronic, complex illnesses, specialist attention from one of the rare breed of obstetric physicians is important. For the others, where illness presents acutely, general physicians remain the first port of call: it is vital that their presentations are not lightly dismissed as 'normal for pregnancy' and that necessary investigation is not deferred on the misplaced but well-intentioned desire to 'protect the baby'.

Chapter 21

Michael Browning and Christopher Bass

LIAISON PSYCHIATRY

One of the great pleasures of psychiatry is that with very few exceptions, there are no diagnostic investigations. Psychiatric diagnosis continues to rest on clinical judgements based on information garnered from the patient and other interested parties. A consequence of this is that when things go well, it is easy to believe that it is due to one's own clinical acumen. Of course, the down side is that there are fewer objective tests to bring one down to earth when one's diagnoses are becoming a little fanciful. This disadvantage was eloquently demonstrated in Rosenhan's famous paper from 1973.[1] In this study, 8 stooges presented to 12 different hospitals describing simple auditory hallucinations with no other symptoms. All were admitted, most with a diagnosis of schizophrenia and given a variety of drugs despite displaying no abnormal symptoms following admission. Thus one of the great worries about psychiatry is that with very few exceptions, there are no diagnostic investigations.

Defying the physician

In truth however, some psychiatrists are jealous of their medical colleagues and would love to have some super-duper scanning test (hopefully producing three-dimensional, multi-coloured pictures of the brain) that would tell us definitively whether our patient is schizophrenic, depressed or manic. So far, the promise of biological psychiatry has only delivered diagnostically useful tests for neuro-syphillis, anorexia (simply calculating the BMI of the patient) and dementia (essentially a neurological illness hijacked by psychiatry). But perhaps we should not be jealous as it seems that diagnosis in medical clinics may not be quite so straightforward. A recent study of neurology out-patients

---

[1] Rosenhan, Science (1973) 179: 250–258.

suggested that about one-third of new patients presented with symptoms that the neurologist could not explain by demonstrable pathology (a finding that reflects rates in other specialties).[2] So a fair proportion of medical out-patients will present with problems that the physician cannot attribute to a physical pathology, despite employing all of the diagnostic measures at their disposal.

The real difficulty with the group of patients who present with medically unexplained symptoms (MUS) is that they do not play fair. They break all the rules that we learned in medical school (and had reinforced by *ER* and *Dr Kildare*). The rules tell us that our patients will turn up at clinic with a list of symptoms that we can reconstruct using our arcane medical knowledge in order to produce masterful conclusions such as 'It is perfectly clear to me, Mr Smith, that you have Halovordan–Spatz disease'. Unfortunately, patients with MUS refuse to give us symptoms which we can easily understand, our medical knowledge returns an error message and we are left with generally less than masterful conclusions along the lines of 'hmm ... yes ... well I'm afraid, Mr Smith, that I'm not really sure what's going on'. To make matters worse, these patients are obviously disabled by their symptoms and are thus just the sort of people who we, as doctors, should be helping. So is there anything that one can do to help this large group of patients? Time to put away the medical model and dust off that bio-psycho-social model that may have been mentioned at medical school.

A common reaction when dealing with patients with MUS is anxiety – what have I missed? Indeed, an oft quoted paper by Slater in the 1960s suggested that patients diagnosed with functional weakness actually turned out to have missed organic pathology when they were followed up 10 years later.[3] However, the study has been repeated since (the topic has even been subjected to a systematic review) and because of advances in medical practice and diagnostic techniques it is actually very unusual for patients with functional symptoms to turn out to have an organic illness.[4,5] Thus the consensus opinion is that once patients have had the initial investigations that have reasonably excluded organic pathology, leading to a diagnosis of MUS, the investigations should not be repeated unless the symptoms change. As a medic though, one is probably a fairly obsessional character, preferring to have something to worry about. It has been suggested that colluding with the concerns of patients with MUS by repeatedly investigating

2 Carson *et al.* J Neurol Neurosurg Psychiatry (2000) 68: 207–210.

3 Slater *et al.* J Psychosom Res (1965) 9: 9–13.

4 Crimlisk *et al.* BMJ (1998) 316: 582–586.

5 Stone *et al.* BMJ (2005) 331: 989–991.

them can actually make matters worse, so perhaps one should worry about the risks of over-investigating rather than that of missing a diagnosis? [6,7]

Another common reaction to patients with MUS is to feel rather despondent and hopeless – their symptoms are difficult to understand and it may seem unlikely that they can be improved. The whole experience in psychiatric parlance is not very 'ego syntonic'. This can understandably lead to a dismissive attitude towards the patient, in its worst form an 'it's all in your mind' statement. Patients often find this sort of approach insulting; it can suggest to them that their illness and suffering are not real or that you are questioning their veracity. In general, if one does opt for this approach in patients with MUS, it is worthwhile holding an up-to-date subscription to a medical defence organization, as it is likely that their services will be called upon in the not too distant future!

So how should one approach these patients? In our experience the most useful strategy is a thorough assessment of the patient during which one *listens* to him or her. Trying to rush this part of the process is often a false economy. It may well be that the medical clinic is not the most appropriate place for the patient to be treated but if things are handled well at this early stage, the patient may feel better and be less likely to shop around for a more sympathetic opinion. Indeed, there is a proven association between strength of physician–patient interaction (measured by factors such as the physician recording a psychosocial history and discussing the treatment with the patient) and the number of return visits for irritable bowel syndrome (IBS) – the stronger the physician–patient interaction, the fewer the number of return visits.[8] During the assessment it is often useful early on to make a list of all the symptoms (it can be a long list) that the patient reports. Even more importantly, try and the get a feel for what the patient believes about his or her illness and what their main concerns are. Once one has reached the conclusion that there is no evidence of organic illness, the patient should be informed. If one's belief is that they are suffering from IBS, fibromyalgia or one of the other myriad of functional syndromes, then the diagnosis ought to be communicated confidently. Importantly, the patient should be reassured that although the aetiology of their problem is not understood, no evidence of any disease or organ damage has been uncovered and that they do not have a life threatening condition. Salmon and colleagues

6 Page *et al.* J Roy Soc Med (2003) 96: 223–227.

7 Bass *et al.* BMJ (2002) 325: 588–591.

8 Owens *et al.* Ann Intern Med (1995) 122: 107–112.

suggested in a qualitative study that the real 'gold star' explanation of a diagnosis of MUS is one which:[9]

- suggests a tangible, usually physical, causal mechanism (e.g. spasm of the muscles in the gut wall);
- is exculpatory, attributing symptoms to a cause for which the patient cannot be blamed (e.g. current work stress);
- involves the patient in self-management of the condition (allowing them to take responsibility for getting better, without feeling guilty for being ill).

If it is felt that the patient has a co-existing psychiatric illness (commonly depression or anxiety) or that they would benefit from seeing a psychiatrist, the subject should be approached gently. Patients with MUS are often exquisitely sensitive to the 'it's all in your mind' brush-off, so the referral needs to be framed as a positive intervention in the diagnosis and treatment of the symptoms that the patient is suffering from. An approach that we have found useful is:

- You have a problem that is likely to be caused by both physical and psychological factors.
- It is as important to address the psychological as the physical causes.
- Would you like me to organize a referral to a psychologist/psychiatrist who has a special interest in these problems?
- This person works in the general hospital and has had a lot of experience dealing with these problems.

If one does not have a friendly local psychiatrist with an interest in liaison psychiatry then the first step will be persuading the hospital managers to purchase one; the recent joint report from the Royal Colleges of Physicians and Psychiatrists may provide useful leverage in this undertaking.[10]

Of course, patients with MUS are not solely encountered in the out-patient clinic; they are frequently admitted as emergencies. If a functional diagnosis is suspected during an emergency admission, the first and most important investigation is a phone call to the GP. This simple step seems to be becoming a progressively less standard aspect of practice: this is a pity, as the longer term perspective gained through the general practitioner's relationship with a patient often yields the most useful information – has the patient had previous functional symptoms and have they experienced any important life events or setbacks?

[9] Salmon et al. BMJ (1999) 318: 372–376.

[10] The Psychological Care of Medical Patients: A Practical Guide. Report of a joint working party of the Royal College of Physicians and the Royal College of Psychiatrists, 2nd Ed, 2003.

There is a sub-group of patients with MUS who will continue to re-present to services regardless of the skill of the practitioner, often accruing the psychiatric diagnosis of somatization disorder. The best management strategy for these patients is probably to use the long-term relationship with the patient's GP (or occasionally with a liaison psychiatrist). The doctor involved should see the patient on a regular basis, regardless of symptomatology. This allows the patient to communicate their feelings about their symptoms and other psychosocial problems and allows the involved medic to act as a gatekeeper to secondary services. If a primary care doctor can fulfil this role then so much the better. For patients at the less extreme end of the spectrum, there is increasing evidence for the efficacy of both cognitive behavioural therapy and graded exercise in many of the functional syndromes.

Fighting fit

There has been a torrent of recent publications addressing the prevalence of non-epileptic attack disorder (NEAD) in specific populations (generally tertiary neurology centre patients) and an increasing acknowledgement of the lack of services in place for these patients.

Again the first hurdle with this patient group is diagnosis. NEAD is commonly encountered in A&E. One study of consecutive patients transferred to a neurological intensive care unit (ICU) with a diagnosis of status epilepticus found that 23% of patients had status *non-epilepticus* (a similar proportion of patients had medication-induced coma).[11] Other epidemiological studies suggest that approximately 20% of patients considered to have epilepsy actually had NEAD; to complicate matters approximately the same proportion (20%) of patients with epilepsy also seem to have concomitant non-epileptic attacks.

How does one tell the difference between epilepsy and NEAD? As psychiatrists we prefer our NEAD patients to have already been subject to the mysterious arts of our neurology colleagues, ideally having had video EEG telemetry demonstrating non-epileptic attacks. There are, however a number of factors which suggest a positive diagnosis of NEAD. First, the semeiology of the attacks tends to differ from epilepsy; NEAD attacks tend to last longer than epileptic seizures with NEAD sufferers being more likely to retain consciousness throughout an attack or having a waxing and waning level of responsiveness. If standing next to a patient in the midst of a non-epileptic attack, one is apparently more likely to be hit, while conversely if one holds the arm of the patient above his or her head

---

[11] Walker *et al.* QJM (1996) 89: 913–920.

and then lets go, the arm of the patient with the non-epileptic attack will tend to miss the patient's head on descent, while that of the epileptic patient will not. There is also the suggestion that the clonic movements of epileptic seizures tend to be in phase while those of NEAD are more likely to be out of phase.

The second class of positive predictors of a NEAD diagnosis includes both psychological and social elements. Patients with NEAD are more likely than those with epilepsy to have a family or personal history of psychiatric disorder, to have attempted suicide or to be currently experiencing affective symptoms. There is also evidence for high rates (around 80%) of previous sexual or physical abuse in NEAD patients.

Despite this long list of associations a definitive diagnosis of NEAD often remains difficult, the ideal service for assessing these patients probably being a neurology centre with good links to local liaison (or neuro-) psychiatrists. Regrettably few such links exist.

Another slightly thorny issue with NEAD patients is what one does to treat them once a diagnosis has been made. There is very little published material on the treatment of this disorder except a preliminary trial of Cognitive Behavioural Therapy (CBT) that showed some promise. Some generally accepted (although not evidence-based) pointers include reduction, and if possible, cessation of anti-epileptic drugs in those with pure NEAD, taking as broad a history as possible (including social and psychological information which may be relevant to the onset or maintenance of the attacks) as well as offering a non-judgemental explanation of the diagnosis which explicitly differentiates the condition from epilepsy. Providing factsheets can be helpful, especially in busier clinics.[12] A full psychiatric assessment and treatment of any concurrent psychiatric disorder is often helpful, especially as it has been suggested that a subset of NEAD patients represents an atypical presentation of panic disorder. It is, however, only in the minority of patients that a straightforward association between attacks and mental state can be found, with the majority of patients presenting with a complex array of predisposing and maintaining factors.

Panic and depression – sniffing them out

Panic disorder is a common anxiety disorder for which there are a number of effective treatments. Often the trick with panic is thinking of it in the first place. The panic attacks that are characteristic of the disorder generally include a number of somatic sensations coupled with catastrophic interpretations of these sensations along the lines of 'I'm going to die' or 'I'm having a heart attack'.

---

[12] Stone *et al.* J Neurol Neurosurg Psychiatry (2005) 76(Supplement 1): i13–i21.

It is therefore not surprising that if one really wants to find somebody with panic disorder, the A&E department or the cardiology clinic is a good place to start looking.

There are no generally agreed screening tools for panic in medical patients, although there are two very useful basic questions:[13]

- 'In the past 6 months have you ever had a spell or an attack when all of a sudden you felt frightened, anxious or very uneasy'?

- 'In the past 6 months have you ever had a spell or an attack when for no reason your heart suddenly began to race, you felt faint, or you couldn't catch your breath'?

A positive response to one of these questions should prompt further enquiry. It is recommended that panic should be considered in those patients with ongoing symptoms and negative investigations (e.g. chest pain with normal angiogram) but none of the more complex questionnaires used in research in this area has yet made the leap to standard clinical practice (the recent NICE guidelines on anxiety and panic provide a useful review of the available questionnaires).[14] For the closet psychiatrist, the real clincher in making a diagnosis is what the patient was thinking when they had the physical symptoms. It is often difficult to pin down but a diagnosis of panic disorder is strongly supported if catastrophic thoughts, associated with the physical sensations of panic, can be demonstrated.

Once the diagnosis has been made, the primary treatment for panic disorder is CBT, with pharmacotherapy (generally SSRI anti-depressants) coming in a poor second. If, however, one is able to find a local service that can provide CBT within a clinically meaningful timeframe, the authors would likely fall to the ground in shock.

Depression is a rather different fish – its treatments are generally more protracted than those for panic and they are often less effective. It is similar to panic though in that its detection remains poor in many settings. Population-based studies suggest that only a minority of people with depression reach the point of diagnosis and treatment. Many depressed individuals never contact the health services and those that do often present with somatic rather than psychological symptoms. Much recent work, particularly focusing on primary care, has examined ways of increasing the detection rate for this large cohort

---

[13] Stein *et al.* J Psychosom Med (1999) 61: 359–364.

[14] CG022 (December 2004) (www.nice.org.uk)

of depressed patients. An enormous number of screening tools have been evaluated, but perhaps the most user-friendly is simply asking the following two questions:

- 'During the last month, have you often been bothered by feeling down, depressed or hopeless'?
- 'During the last month, have you often been bothered by having little interest or pleasure in doing things'?

Eliciting these core symptoms of depression has been found to offer a reasonable sensitivity and specificity as well as obviously being simple to administer. If one receives an affirmative answer to either of these questions, it is worth pursuing further – treating depression will not only improve the quality of life of the patient but it will also reduce the burden of symptoms and functional limitations.

Capacity

Assessment of capacity is a common reason to consult with psychiatrists, and if Scotland's experience is a reasonable marker, it is likely that the coming implementation of the Mental Capacity Act will lead to a focusing of attention on the capacity of patients to agree to or refuse treatment.[15] In 2007, the Act will essentially transfer the current legal position on capacity issues, which has largely arisen through Case Law, to Statute Law. The guiding principles behind capacity law will not change, namely that there is a presumption of capacity; that everything should be done to improve an individual's capacity before it is decided that it is not present; that making an unwise decision does not mean that an individual lacks capacity to make that decision; that any act done for an individual who lacks capacity must be done in their best interests and finally that the least restrictive (to the individual's rights or freedom of action) option must be chosen.

Before assessing a patient's capacity (or lack of it), the Act states that there must be 'an impairment of, or disturbance in, the functioning of the person's mind or brain'; if not, then by definition the person has capacity. The actual assessment of capacity to make a decision remains largely unchanged in that an individual should be able to understand the information pertinent to the decision, retain that information, use the information in coming to a decision and finally communicate that decision. Importantly, capacity assessments are made for *a particular decision at a particular time*, so one could assess the capacity of a patient

---

15 www.opsi.gov.uk/acts/acts2005/20050009.htm

to refuse a particular treatment today but could not, in theory, find that a patient is generally incapable of making decisions from this point in time on.

The Act goes a little further than this with some changes to the current arrangement. Perhaps most notable is the introduction of a statutory service of 'independent mental capacity advocates'. There will be a requirement of 'responsible bodies' (acute or primary care trusts in the health arena) to arrange for these advocates to be involved in significant decisions made about incapacitated patients who have no one else (generally family or friends) to help them. Significant decisions include administering or withholding treatment (some treatments will apparently be specified) and moving a patient (this will include transferring a patient to a different hospital for a period greater than 28 days). So before enacting significant decisions about the care or placement of incapacitated patients without any (interested) family or friends, the NHS Trust will have to arrange for a person, independent of itself, to review the decision.

So what proportion of patients lacks capacity to agree to the treatment we are providing? More than one would think if Raymont and colleagues are to be believed.[16] They found that of 302 consecutive acute medical admissions, 24% were severely cognitively impaired or unconscious (and therefore were felt to lack capacity about treatment decisions), and a further 31% of those remaining patients who were willing to be interviewed were found to lack capacity (giving a total of 40% of all admissions). Of the latter group of patients, only 24% were identified by the medical team responsible as lacking capacity to agree to their treatment. The Act should not change the management of the great majority of these patients, although as such a high proportion of medical inpatients have impaired capacity, even a change only affecting a small proportion of the incapacitated is likely to be felt by most busy acute medical teams.

Low-weight anorexia

Low-weight anorectics are often admitted under general medical teams or gastroenterologists for the management and treatment of extreme low weight. This can occur either informally or formally, with a recent clarification that re-feeding can be considered as treatment under the Mental Health Act. Re-feeding a very low-weight patient is a hazardous undertaking medically with a number of potential complications: one would probably prefer to be told about these by a gastroenterologist rather than a psychiatrist.[17] However, the most

---

16 Raymont, Lancet (2004) 364: 1421–1427.

17 www.iop.kcl.ac.uk/IoP/Departments/PsychMed/EDU/downloads/pdf/RiskAssessment.pdf

difficult aspect of managing a low-weight anorectic patient is often centred on ensuring that the prescribed nutrition is actually ingested, that the patient does not purge either by vomiting or through the use of laxatives and that other compensating behaviours (such as exercise) do not undo all the benefit of the ingested nutrition.

The expectant reader awaiting a pithy and practical description of just how this can be achieved on a medical ward will, we are afraid, be disappointed. There are no particularly easy methods of ensuring that the patient is absorbing sufficient calories to survive – the only apparently effective strategy that the authors are aware of (although there are no published data supporting it) is the use of experienced, vigilant staff who can monitor the patient's behaviour particularly in the early stages of treatment so that long trips to the toilet and hiding of food are minimized, while working with the patient in as collaborative a manner as possible. This is, of course, enormously easy to write while being enormously difficult to achieve, particularly on a general medical ward where it may be difficult to even have a patient weighed on an intermittent basis. Similar problems may be encountered on general psychiatry wards, where some anorectic patients can languish for months without significant gains in weight. Patients do seem to do better on specialist units where the system is designed specifically with the purpose of supporting anorectic patients in the struggle to gain weight and the staff is understandably more experienced in detecting and dealing with attempts to sabotage treatment. These units tend to employ group-based techniques similar to certain therapeutic communities, where for instance all the patients will eat together and stay at the table until everyone has finished. Unfortunately, it can often be a struggle to find a placement for patients in specialist centres and there is a sub-group of patients who lose weight even in environments as protected as these, occasionally resulting in transfer to the general hospital. The only other advice we can offer on the management of these challenging patients is to invite the local eating disorders consultant round to one's house for dinner, as early specialist input is often key to preventing the deaths of these patients on medical wards.

Index

Abram's needle biopsy 292
ACCENT trial 261
ACE inhibitors 21, 121, 126, 145
N-acetylcysteine 61, 140
achalasia 245
acromegaly 83
activated charcoal 58
acute confusional state 365–7
acute coronary syndrome 2
acute disseminated encephalomyelitis 167
acute fatty liver of pregnancy 223
acute liver failure 220–2
  aetiology 222
acute renal failure 134–6
  diagnosis and management 136–8
  dialysis in 140–1
  intervention in 138–9
  vs chronic renal disease 141–2
acute terminal haemorrhage 356
Addisonian crisis 73
adrenal disease 76–83
  adrenal incidentaloma 83
  adrenal insufficiency 76–9
  Cushing's disease 81–3
  phaeochromocytoma 79–81
AIDS 193–7
alcohol 64
alcoholic hepatitis 219
alcohol-related liver disease 231–2
aldosterone 116
allergen immunotherapy 391–2
allergy 387
ALLHAT trial 103, 121
alpha glucosidase inhibitors 99
Alport's syndrome 129
Alzheimer's disease 182
aminophylline 278
5-aminosalicylic acid 260–1
amiodarone 28–30, 75–6
anaemia 250–2
analgesic ladder 349–50
anaphylaxis 387–8
ANCA 133, 398
angina 1
angioedema 388–90, 407–9
angioplasty 3–6
angiotensin receptor blockers 21, 121–2
anorexia 435–6
anticoagulation 30–2
antidotes 59
antihypertensives 120–1, 121–2

anti-IgE therapy 392–4
anti-neutrophil cytoplasmic antibody
  see ANCA
anti-nuclear antibodies 374, 397
antithyroid drugs 69–70
aortic dissection 16–17
aortic regurgitation 40
aortic stenosis 39
aortic syndromes 16–17
aplastic anaemia 330
apoplexy 86–7
arrhythmogenic right ventricular
  dysplasia 33
arterial dissection 155–6
artificial heart valves 37
ascites 225–7
ASCOT trial 122
asthma 276–9
ASTRAL trial 119
atrial fibrillation 28–30
  risk of embolic stroke 32
autoimmune hepatitis 219, 234–5
AV nodal reentrant tachycardia 34
azathioprine 134, 148, 261

barium swallow 244
Barrett's oesophagus 271–2
basilizimab 148
Behçet's disease 170
Bell's palsy 183
benign paroxysmal positional
  vertigo 161
berry aneurysm 152
bevacizimab 250, 311, 319
biliary disorders 233–4
biliary duct dilatation 218
biological psychiatry 427–31
blisters 409–10
bone pain 350
bovine spongiform encephalopathy 200
brain natriuretic peptide 20, 26
breast cancer 312–16
breathlessness 352–3
Brugada syndrome 32
Budd-Chiari syndrome 220, 223–4
bulbar function 172–3
bullous pemphigoid 409
cachexia 379
CADASIL 169
calcium channel blockers 122
capacity 434–5

capillary refill time 45
CAPRIE trial 11, 188
CAPTIM study 5
captopril 21–2, 125
carbimazole 70
carcinoma of unknown origin 324–5
cardiac arrhythmias 28–37
  anticoagulation 30–2
  atrial fibrillation 28–30
  pacing 34–5
  sudden cardiac death 36–7
  syncope 32–4
cardiac failure 3, 17–27
  acute left ventricular failure 17–19
  chronic cardiac failure 19–22
  diagnosis 26–7
  diastolic failure 24–5
  resynchronization 27–8
  symptoms 24–5
cardiac enzymes 2
cardiogenic shock 48
cardiology 1–40
  aortic dissections and aortic
      syndromes 16–17
  cardiac failure 17–28
  ischaemic heart disease 1–16
  rhythm disturbance 28–37
  valvular heart disease 37–40
CARDS trial 102
carotid sinus hypersensitivity 364
CAST trial 187
cellulitis 406
central venous pressure 46
cetuximab 311
CHARM trial 22
cholangiocarcinoma 219
cholecystitis 219
chronic kidney disease 142–6
  classification 143
chronic liver failure 234–5
  causes of 230
  screening 229–30
chronic lymphocytic leukaemia 341–2
chronic obstructive pulmonary
      disease 279–83
chronic viral hepatitis 232–3
ciclosporin 148, 262
circulation, assessment of 44–7
clonidine 129
clopidogrel 11–12
Clostridium difficile 254
  diarrhoea 207–8
cluster headache 159
coarctation of aorta 119
Cockcroft Gault equation 143
coeliac disease 265–6, 397–8
  untreated 266
cognitive impairment 362

colitis 254–5
colloids 46
colorectal cancer 249, 318–20
  screening 270–1
coma 180–2
COMMIT trial 11
community acquired pneumonia 297–8
COMPANION-HF trial 27–8
Congo-Crimean haemorrhagic
      fever 204–6
Conn's syndrome 119
continuous positive airways
      pressure 50, 282
COOPERATE trial 144
coronary artery bypass grafting 13–14
coronary spasm 1
corticobasal degeneration 180
crescentic nephritis 133
Creutzfeldt-Jakob disease, new
      variant 200–1
Crohn's disease 259–60
cryoglobulins 399–400
CURE trial 11
Cushing response 164
Cushing's syndrome 81–3, 119
cystic fibrosis 299–301

D-dimer test 285
death rattle 355
decompensated shock 48–9
delirium 180–2, 365–7
dementia 180–2
dengue fever 204
depression 356–7, 432–4
dermatology 401–12
  angioedema and urticaria 407–9
  blisters 409–10
  drug eruptions 401–5
  itching 410–12
  skin sepsis 405–7
desferrioxamine 59
diabetes mellitus, in pregnancy 424–6
diabetes mellitus type 1 103–5
  insulin therapy 106–7
  surgery in 106
  ulcers 108–9
diabetes mellitus type 2 93, 95–103
  diet 96
  initial management 96–8
  insulin therapy 100–1
  managed care 102
  escalating therapy 98–100
diabetic ketoacidosis 103–4
diabetic nephropathy 126–8
diarrhoea
  acute 252–5
  chronic 255–7
  Clostridium difficile 207–8

diet
  diabetes mellitus 96
  see also nutrition
Dieulafoy lesion 242
diffuse parenchymal lung disease 306
dipyridamole 188
disease-modifying anti-rheumatic
    drugs 373, 375–6
disseminated intravascular
    coagulation 335–6
diverticulosis 249
diving 201–2
dizziness 160–3
L-dopa 178–9
dopamine 139–40
dopexamine 139
drotrecogin alfa 215
drug allergy 390–1
drug eruptions 401–5
drug resistance 210
dyspepsia 246–7
dysphagia 243–5

Ebola virus 204–6
ECST trial 192
Ehlers-Danlos syndrome 152
ejection fraction 24–5
electrocardiogram 32–4
end diastolic volume 24
endocrinology 67–89
  adrenal disease 76–83
    adrenal incidentaloma 83
    adrenal insufficiency 76–9
    Cushing's disease 81–3
    phaeochromocytoma 79–81
  hyperparathyroidism 87–9
  pituitary disease 83–4
    apoplexy 86–7
    hyperprolactinaemia 84–5
    hyponatraemia 86–7
  thyroid dysfunction 67–76
    antithyroid drugs 69–70
    hypothyroidism 72–3
    myxoedema coma 73–4
    overactive thyroid 68–9
    radioiodine 70–1
    subclinical thyroid disease 74–5
    surgery 71
    thyroid storms 72
endoscopic retrograde
    cholangiopancreatography 218
endoscopy 242
end stage renal disease 118
  drugs in 150
Entamoeba histolytica 254
epilepsy 176–8
  and pregnancy 425–6
Epworth Sleepiness Scale 304

erlotinib 318
erythema multiforme 401, 404
erythropoietin 343

faecal occult blood testing 271
falls 361–3
fentanyl 350
flaccid paresis 173–4
flecainide 30
fluid replacement 46
  in palliative care 355–6
flying 302–3
fomepizole 59
funny turns 176–8
furosemide 138

gallstones 219
gastric antral vascular ectasia 242–3
gastric lavage 57–8
gastroenterology 239–72
  acute diarrhoea 252–5
  anaemia 250–2
  Barrett's oesophagus 271–2
  bleeding 239–43
  chronic constipation 257–9
  chronic diarrhoea 255–7
  coeliac disease 265–6
  colorectal cancer 270–1
  dyspepsia 246–7
  dysphagia 243–5
  inflammatory bowel disease 259–64
  irritable bowel disease 264–5
  nutrition 267–9
  rectal bleeding 248–50
  screening 269–70
gastrointestinal bleeding 239–43
gastro-oesophageal reflux
    disease 246, 283–4
gefitinib 318
gemcitabine 321
geriatric medicine 359–71
  acute confusional state 365–7
  ageing population 359
  assistive technology 369–70
  carotid sinus hypersensitivity 364
  falls 361–3
  geriatricians 359–61
  geriatric syndromes 361
  orthostatic hypotension 363–4
  patient wishes 367–8
  prescribing 368–9
  prolonging life 370–1
  syncope/collapse 363
  vasovagal syncope 364–5
Gilbert's syndrome 217, 219
glitazones 96
glomerular filtration rate 126, 229
glomerulus 115–16

glucagon-like peptide 1 99
goitre 69
Goodpasture's syndrome 132
gout 384–6
GRACIA-1 trial 6
Graves' disease 68, 69
Guillain-Barré syndrome 165, 173, 253
GUSTO thrombolytic trial 4
gut decontamination 57–8

HAART therapy 194
  metabolic complications 196
haematemesis 242
haematology 329–45
  chronic lymphocytic leukaemia 341–2
  disseminated intravascular
      coagulation 335–6
  haemorrhage 336–7
  heparin-induced thrombocytopenia
      and thrombosis 331–3
  immune thrombocytopenic purpura 333–5
  multiple myeloma 339–41
  myelodysplasias 344–5
  myeloproliferative disorders 342
  pancytopenia 329–31
  paraproteinaemia 339–41
  polycythaemia 342–3
  thrombocytopenia 331
  thrombocytosis 343–4
  thrombophilia 337–9
haematuria 129–30
haemochromatosis 235–6
haemodialysis 58, 148–9
haemofiltration 141
  see also renal replacement therapy
haemorrhage 336–7
  acute terminal 356
haemorrhoids 248
Hashimoto's thyroiditis 73
headache, acute 151–63
  arterial dissection and venous sinus
      thrombosis 155–6
  dizziness 160–3
  imaging studies 160
  intracranial haemorrhage 156–7
  migraine 158–9
  raised intracranial pressure 157–8
  subarachnoid haemorrhage 151–5
Health Protection Agency 193
Helicobacter pylori 246, 247
HELLP syndrome 223
Henoch-Schönlein purpura 133
heparin-induced thrombocytopenia and
      thrombosis 331–3
hepatology 217–37
  abnormal liver function tests 236
  acute liver failure 220–2
  alcohol-related liver disease 231–2

hepatology (Continued)
  ascites 225–7
  biliary disorders 233–4
  Budd-Chiari syndrome 223–4
  chronic liver failure 229–30, 234–5
  chronic viral hepatitis 232–3
  hepatorenal syndrome 228–9
  jaundice 217–19
  liver lesions 237
  malignant infiltration 234
  paracetamol 222
  pregnancy-related liver disease 223
  spontaneous bacterial peritonitis 227
  variceal haemorrhage 228
  Wilson's disease 234
hepatoma 219
hepatorenal syndrome 228–9
herpes zoster 184
high-dependency medicine 41–53
  circulation assessment 44–7
  continuous positive airway pressure 50
  decompensated shock 48–9
  mixed venous oxygen saturation 47
  non-invasive ventilation 50–1
  pump failure 43–4
  recognition of sick patients 42–3
  renal failure 51–2
  respiratory inadequacy 49–50
  sepsis 52
  treatment limitation 52–3
  vasoactive drugs 47–8
HIV 193–7
HOPE trial 123
Horner's syndrome 155
hospital-acquired infections 206
hydralazine 129
hydrocephalus 164–5
hygiene hypothesis 387
hyperaldosteronism 119
hypercalcaemia 327, 352
hyperemesis gravidarum 223
hyperkalaemia 145
hyperosmolar non-ketotic
      hyperglycaemia 103
hyperparathyroidism 87–9, 119
hyperprolactinaemia 84–5
hypertension 116–25
  coarctation of aorta 119
  definition of 117
  endocrine abnormalities 119
  malignant 124–5
  NICE guidelines 122–3
  in pregnancy 128
  renovascular disease 118–19
  salt intake 121
  secondary 117–18
  target blood pressure 123–4
  target organ damage 119–20

hypertension *(Continued)*
  treatment 120–1, 121–2
  white coat 117
hypertensive crisis 125
hypoglycaemia 105–6, 161
hyponatraemia 86–7
hypothyroidism 72–3
hypovolaemia 45, 136

immune thrombocytopenic purpura 333–5
immunodeficiency 394–5
immunoglobulins 399
  intravenous 395–6
immunology 387–400
  allergen immunotherapy 391–2
  allergy 387
  anaphylaxis 387–8
  anti-IgE therapy 392–4
  anti-neutrophil cytoplasmic antibodies 398
  anti-nuclear antibodies 397
  coeliac disease 397–8
  cryoglobulins 399–400
  drug allergy 390–1
  hygiene hypothesis 387
  immunodeficiency 394–5
  immunoglobulins 399
  intravenous immunoglobulin 395–6
  T-cell subsets 399
  urticaria and angioedema 388–90
immunology laboratory 396
immunosuppression 148
impaired glucose tolerance 94
infections of CNS 182–4
infectious diseases 193–215
  Clostridium difficile diarrhoea 207–8
  dengue 204
  drug resistance 210
  extended-spectrum beta-lactamases 213
  HIV and AIDS 193–7
  hospital-acquired 206
  influenza 197–8
  intravascular cannulae 206–7
  malaria 202–4
  MRSA 210–11
  prion diseases 200–1
  SARS 199–200
  sepsis and septic shock 214–15
  travel-related 201–2
  urinary catheter-associated
    infection 208–10
  vancomycin-intermediate
    S. aureus 211–12
  vancomycin-resistant enterococci 212–13
  vancomycin-resistant
    S. aureus 211–12
  viral haemorrhagic fevers 204–6
  West Nile virus 198–9
infective gastroenteritis 253

inflammatory bowel disease 259–64
inflammatory CNS disease 166–71
infliximab 261
influenza 197–8
insulin therapy 100–1, 106–7
International Subarachnoid Aneurysm
    Trial 154
intracranial haemorrhage 156–7
intravascular cannulae 206–7
ipecacuanha 58
irritable bowel disease 256, 264–5
ischaemic heart disease 1–16
  investigations 8–10
  sexual function 15–16
  surgery 15
  treatment 306
IST trial 187
itching 410–12

jaundice 217–19

Kaposi varicelliform eruption 306–7
kidney 115–16
kidney disease 125–34
  diabetic kidney 126–8
  haematuria 129–30
  nephrotic syndrome 131–2
  in pregnancy 128–9
  proteinuria 130–1
  rapidly progressive 132–4
  see also renal failure; renal impairment
    syndromes
kidney transplantation 147–8

labetolol 129
labyrinthitis 162
lactic acidosis 45
Lambert-Eaton myasthenic syndrome 175
lamotrigine 176
Lassa fever 204–6
Lhermitte's phenomenon 167
liaison psychiatry 427–36
  biological psychiatry 427–31
  capacity 434–5
  low-weight anorexia 435–6
  non-epileptic attack disorder 431–2
  panic and depression 432–4
lipid disorders 89–92
lithium 75–6
liver *see* hepatology
liver function tests, abnormal 236
liver lesions 237
Liverpool Care Pathway for the Dying 353
low molecular weight heparin 286
lumbar puncture 156
lung cancer 294–5, 316–18
  screening for 296–7
Lyell's disease 402

MADIT-2 trial 37
magnesium 278
magnetic resonance
   cholangiopancreatography 218, 257
malabsorption 267–8
malaria 202–4537
malignant bowel obstruction 352
malignant hypertension 124–5
malignant infiltration 234
mannitol 139–40
Marburg fever 204–6
MATCH trial 188
medical emergency team 43
medically unexplained symptoms 428–9
meglitinides 99
Menière's disease 162
Mental Capacity Act 2007 357, 434–5
6-mercaptopurine 261
MERLIN trial 7
mesothelioma 292, 293–4
metabolic syndrome 113–14
metastatic cancer 219
metformin 96, 97
methyldopa 129
metronidazole 261
microalbuminuria 123, 126
migraine 158–9
mitral regurgitation 38
mixed venous oxygen saturation 47
morphine 350
MRSA 210–11
multiple endocrine neoplasia type 2 81
multiple myeloma 339–41
  mortality 341
multiple sclerosis 166–71
multisystem atrophy 180
myasthenia gravis 173, 174
mycophenolate 148
myelodysplasias 344–5
myeloproliferative disorders 342
myocardial infarction national audit
   project (MINAP) 14
myocarditis 3
myoglobinuria 129
myxoedema coma 73–4

naloxone 59
NASCET trial 192
National Acute Spinal Cord Injury Studies 165
nausea and vomiting 351–2
necrotizing fasciitis 109, 405
nephrotic syndrome 131–2
neurology 151–84
  acute headache 151–63
  infection 182–4
  inflammatory CNS disease 166–71
  neurosurgery 163–6
  progressive weakness 171–82

neuromuscular respiratory failure 172
neuropathic pain 350–1
neurosurgery 163–6
  raised intracranial pressure 163–4
  shunts 164–5
  spinal cord compression 165–6
neutropenia 325–7
NICE guidelines
  cardiology 20, 21
  diabetic nephropathy 127
  dyspepsia 246
  hypertension 122–3
  obesity 111–12
  stroke 188
nifedipine 129
nonalcoholic fatty liver disease 235
nonalcoholic steatohepatitis 219
non-epileptic attack disorder 431–2
non-invasive ventilation 50–1, 279, 281–2
non-small cell lung cancer 316–18
non-steroidal anti-inflammatory drugs
   see NSAIDs
NSAIDs 373
  complications of 379–81
nutrition 267–9
  dying patients 355–6
nutritional deficiencies 267–8

obesity 93–4, 109–14
  metabolic syndrome 113–14
  pharmacotherapy 111–12
  surgery for 112
obstetric medicine 413–26
  diabetes mellitus 424–5
  drug use in pregnancy 415–16
  epilepsy 425–6
  hypertension 416–19
  medical contraindications to
   pregnancy 426
  venous thromboembolism 420–4
odynophagia 245
oedema 136
oliguria 44
oncology 309–28
  breast cancer 312–16
  carcinoma of unknown origin 324–5
  colorectal cancer 318–20
  emergencies 325–7
  hypercalcaemia 327
  lung cancer 316–18
  ovarian cancer 320–1
  prostate cancer 321–4
  spinal cord compression 328
  superior vena cava obstruction 327–8
ophthalmoparesis 174
opioids 64–5
optic neuritis 168
oral glucose tolerance test 94

organophosphorous agents 65
orlistat 97, 112
orthostatic hypotension 363–4
oseltamivir 198
Osler-Weber-Rendu syndrome 249
osteoporosis 382–3
ovarian cancer 320–1
oxprenolol 129
oxyhaemoglobin 153

pacing 34–5
paclitaxel 320
pain control 349–50
palliative care medicine 347–57
  acute terminal haemorrhage 356
  bone pain 350
  breathlessness 352–3
  depression 356–7
  hypercalcaemia 352
  malignant bowel obstruction 352
  nausea and vomiting 351–2
  neuropathic pain 350–1
  nutrition and fluids 355–6
  pain control 349–50
  prescribing 354–5
  spinal cord compression 351
  superior vena caval obstruction 353
  symptom management 348–9
  terminal phase 353–4
pancreatic cancer 219
pancreatitis 219
pancytopenia 329–31
panic disorder 432–4
paracetamol 61–2, 222
  overdose 221
paraproteinaemia 339–41
paresis
  flaccid 173–4
  with retained reflexes 174–82
Parkinsonian syndromes 178–80
pemphigus vulgaris 410
peptic ulcer 247
peritoneal dialysis 149–50
phaeochromocytoma 79–81
phlebotomy 26–7
pioglitazone 98
pituitary disease 83–4
  apoplexy 86–7
  hyperprolactinaemia 84–5
  hyponatraemia 86–7
platelet clumping 331
pleural effusion 290–2
  Light's criteria 291
Pneumocystis carinii 307
pneumonia 292–3
  community acquired 297–8
pneumothorax 281, 286–90
  iatrogenic 289

poisoning 55–66
  active elimination 58
  alcohol 64
  definition of poison 55–6
  general principles 59
  gut decontamination 57–8
  opioids 64–5
  organophosphorous agents 65
  paracetamol 61–2
  psychiatric input 66
  risks of 56–7
  role of laboratory 60–1
  salicylates 62
  selective serotonin reuptake inhibitors 62–3
  toxicokinetics 57
  toxidromes 59
  tricyclic antidepressants 63–4
polycystic kidney disease 129
polycythaemia 342–3
polypharmacy 368
postherpetic neuralgia 184
prazosin 129
prednisolone 148
pre-eclampsia 128–9, 223, 418
pregnancy
  kidney disease in 128–9
  laboratory indices in 414
  liver disease in 223
  medical contraindications to 426
  respiratory disease in 303–4
  see also obstetric medicine
pregnancy-specific medical conditions 414–15
prescribing
  in geriatric medicine 368–9
  palliative care medicine 354–5
  in pregnancy 415–18
primary biliary cirrhosis 219, 233
primary sclerosing cholangitis 234
prion diseases 182–3, 200–1
progressive supranuclear palsy 180
progressive weakness 171–82
  bulbar function 172–3
  flaccid paresis 173–4
  neuromuscular respiratory failure 172
  paresis with retained reflexes 174–82
prolonging life 370–1
  see also palliative care medicine
propofenone 30
prostaglandins 116
prostate cancer 321–4
proteinuria 130–1
  diabetic nephropathy 127
  orthostatic 130
  in pregnancy 128
pruritus 410–12
pulmonary embolism 284–6
  in pregnancy 420
pulmonary fibrosis 306–7

pulmonary nodules 295–6
pump failure 43–4

quality-adjusted life years 312

radioiodine 70–1
raised intracranial pressure 157–8
rapidly progressive glomerulonephritis 132–4
REACT trial 7
rectal bleeding 248–50
Reiter's syndrome 253
renal bone disease 145
renal failure 51–2
    acute 134–6, 138–9, 140–2
    dopamine in 139–40
    end stage 118, 150
renal impairment syndromes 134–50
    acute renal failure 134–6, 138–9, 140–2
    chronic kidney disease 142–6
    diagnosis and management 136–8
    renal replacement therapy 146–50
renal replacement therapy 146–50
    acute renal failure 140–1
    choice 147–8
    haemodialysis 58, 148–9
    peritoneal dialysis 149–50
    rates of 147
renin 116
renovascular disease 118–19
respiratory inadequacy 49–50
respiratory medicine 273–307
    asthma 276–9
    chronic obstructive pulmonary
        disease 279–83
    community acquired pneumonia 297–8
    cystic fibrosis 299–301
    diving 201–2
    flying 302–3
    lung cancer 294–5, 296–7
    mesothelioma 293–4
    pleural effusion 290–2
    pneumonia 292–3
    pneumothorax 286–90
    pregnancy 303–4
    pulmonary embolism 284–6
    pulmonary fibrosis 306–7
    pulmonary nodules 295–6
    sleep apnoea 304–6
    smoking 273–6
    wheeze 283–4
resynchronization 27–8
rheumatoid arthritis 373–81
    cachexia in 379
    cardiovascular risk 377–9
    diagnosis 373–4
    differential diagnosis 373–4
    immunological basis 376–7
    NSAIDs 373, 379–81

rheumatoid arthritis (Continued)
    outcome prediction 375
    treatment 375–6
rheumatology 373–86
    gout 384–6
    osteoporosis 382–3
    rheumatoid arthritis 373–81
rimonabant 112
rituximab 134
Rockall scoring system 240–1
rosiglitazone 98

saccular aneurysm 152
salicylates 62
salt intake 121
salt restriction 226
SARS 199–200
scabies 411–12
screening 269–70
    colorectal cancer 270–1
    lung cancer 296–7
seizures 176–8
selective serotonin reuptake inhibitors 62–3
sentinel headache 152
sepsis 52, 214–15
    skin 405–7
septic shock 214–1581
severe combined immunodeficiency 395
shunts 164–5
sibutramine 112
sirolimus 148
SITS-MOST 189
Sjögren's syndrome 170
skin sepsis 405–7
sleep apnoea 304–6
SLUDGE syndrome 175
small cell lung cancer 316
smoking 273–6
smoking cessation 274–6
sodium nitroprusside 125
SPARTAC trial 195
spinal cord compression 165–6, 328, 351
Spongiform Encephalopathy Advisory
    Committee (SEAC) 200
spontaneous bacterial peritonitis 227
sputum 283
statins 91
status epilepticus 176–8
ST elevation myocardial infarction see STEMI
stem-cell therapy 6
STEMI 2, 3
    treatment 3–6
steroids 278–9
Stevens-Johnstone syndrome 401, 403–4
Streptococcus pyogenes 405
stroke medicine 185–92
    aetiology of stroke 191–2
    definition of stroke 185–6

stroke medicine *(Continued)*
  physiology 186–7
  stroke units 190–1
  thrombolysis 188–90
  transient ischaemic attacks 190
  treatment 187–8
subarachnoid haemorrhage 151–5
  grading 152–3
sudden cardiac death 36–7
sulphonylureas 97
superior vena cava obstruction 327–8, 353
syncope 32–4
  elderly patients 363
  vasovagal 364–5
syndrome of inappropriate antidiuretic
    hormone 87
syndrome X 1
syringe drivers 348–9

tachycardia 44
tacrolimus 148
target blood pressure 123–4
T-cell subsets 399
Terson's syndrome 152
thrombocytopenia 331
thrombocytosis 343–4
thrombolysis 2, 3–6, 188–90
  risks of 4
thrombolytic chaser 7
thrombophilia 337–9
thunderclap headache 152
thyroid dysfunction 67–76
  amiodarone and lithium 75–6
  antithyroid drugs 69–70
  hypothyroidism 72–3
  myxoedema coma 73–4
  overactive thyroid 68–9
  radioiodine 70–1
  subclinical thyroid disease 74–5
  surgery 71
  thyroid storms 72
total parenteral nutrition 269
TOXBASE 55
toxic epidermal necrolysis 402
toxicokinetics 57
toxidromes 59
transient ischaemic attacks 190
transjugular intrahepatic portosystemic
    shunt 228
trastuzumab (Herceptin) 311, 313–14
travel-related infections 201–2
tricyclic antidepressants 63–4

trigeminal autonomic cephalgia 159
troponin 2
tumour necrosis factor-α 376

Uhthoff's phenomenon 167
UK National Poisons Information
    Service 55–6
ulcerative colitis 263
ulcers, diabetic 108–9
ultrafiltration 141
urinary casts 137
urinary catheter-associated
    infection 208–10
urticaria 388–90, 407–9

Val-HEFT trial 21
VALIANT trial 21
valsartan 21
valvular heart disease 37–40
  aortic regurgitation 40
  aortic stenosis 39
  mitral regurgitation 38
valvuloplasty 38
vancomycin-intermediate
    S. aureus 211–12
vancomycin-resistant enterococci 212–13
vancomycin-resistant *S. aureus* 211–12
variceal haemorrhage 228
vasoactive drugs 47–8
vasovagal syncope 364–5
venous sinus thrombosis 155–6
venous thromboembolism 420–4
  diagnosis 420–2
  prophylaxis 423–4
  treatment 422–3
viral haemorrhagic fevers 204–6
viral hepatitis 219
  chronic 232–3
vomiting *see* nausea and vomiting
von Hippel Lindau disease 81

Warfarin versus Aspirin for Secondary
    Stroke Prevention trial 155
Wernicke's encephalopathy 181
West Nile virus 198–9
wheeze 283–4
  see also asthma
white coat hypertension 117
Wilson's disease 220, 234
Woolf-Parkinson-White syndrome 32, 33

xanthochromia 153